Hay Fever & Allergies

Discovering the Real Culprits
and
Natural Solutions for Reversing
Allergic Rhinitis

By Casey Adams, Ph.D.

Hay Fever and Allergies: Discovering the Real Culprits and Natural Solutions for
    Reversing Allergic Rhinitis
Copyright © 2011 Casey Adams
LOGICAL BOOKS
Wilmington, Delaware
http://www.logicalbooks.org
All rights reserved.
Printed in USA
Front Cover image © Alina Isakovich
Back Cover image © Christian Wagner

Publishers Cataloging in Publication Data
Adams, Casey
Hay Fever and Allergies: Discovering the Real Culprits
    and Natural Solutions for Reversing Allergic Rhinitis
First Edition
1. Medicine. 2. Health.
Bibliography and References; Index

Library of Congress Control Number: 2011932532

ISBN-13 paperback: 978-1-936251-21-6
ISBN-13 ebook: 978-1-936251-22-3

Table of Contents

Introduction

With each passing spring, more people find themselves faced with uncontrollable fits of sneezing, blocked nose and watery eyes. What used to be the most beautiful time of year, with colorful flowers and an unfolding of life has become, for many, the most dreaded time of year.

For many, these seasonal bouts are increasingly becoming year-round scenarios: Not only are the seasons becoming more variable; sensitivities to one allergen are crossing over to other allergens.

Why are allergies and hay fever increasing so dramatically? And what causes them?

There are currently two strategies at work in conventional medicine in response to hay fever and allergies. The first is the removal of the symptoms. As a result, finding better antihistamines and decongestants, together with anti-inflammatory medications consumes most of the focus of research regarding hay fever and allergies.

In addition to prescribing these medications, most health professionals and medical writers have focused their recommendations upon how to avoid allergen exposure. This calls for various strategies to purify our air, close our windows, turn on our air conditioning, and in general, attempt to remove ourselves as far away as possible from nature.

Do these strategies provide any long-term opportunities to permanently eliminate allergies and/or hay fever? Nada.

As most of us realize, removing the symptoms will not eliminate the issue. It will only produce a permanent dependency upon the medication as the symptoms return. In addition, medication typically comes with a variety of side effects—the most notable among many antihistamines is daytime drowsiness and lethargy.

And as far as trying to eliminate exposure to pollens, molds, dust, insect endotoxins and other allergens, this has proven close to impossible. Unless we live in a bubble, we will have to be exposed to pollen as we attempt to breathe. And unless we are wearing a hazmat suit replete with oxygen tanks and gas mask, we will be exposed to all the other allergens that nature produces constantly.

This last point is where this text picks up. While in this text we do discuss allergen exposure and its place in reversing allergies, we leave behind the entire discussion of the possible medications that may or may not relieve allergy symptoms.

This is because this text goes further. Way further. Here the condition of allergies and hay fever is the subject of a mission. That mission is to solve the mysteries of the real underlying causes of hay fever and allergic rhinitis—and provide the solutions to reverse those causes.

We say 'mystery' because modern medicine has yet to—even with its billion-dollar research budgets and expensive medical treatment centers—solved the mysteries surrounding hay fever and allergic rhinitis.

What are those mysteries? As we'll discuss in more detail, the first is that hay fever has arrived among human society only about 200 years ago. Before this, there is virtually no record of humans having hay fever or allergic rhinitis.

No allergies? Certainly humans had allergies, yes? Maybe, but the historical record is virtually bare. Especially when it comes to pollens, molds, dust mites and so on. Allergies by and far are a modern development. Humans have suffered from a multitude of infections and diseases related to infection, along with other ailments related to nature's challenges to our physiology. But our immune systems historically have not been hypersensitive to pollens, molds and insect endotoxins.

Animals also rarely if ever suffer from allergies. The few animals that appear to suffer from allergies are those who have—curiously—become domesticated by humans or have otherwise come to rely upon humans for their feeding. Thus we find that cats, horses, dogs and to some degree pigs and other farmed animals, have—to a far less degree than humans—developed allergies. The rest of the animal kingdom—like humanity before the industrial age—has been practically immune to allergies.

This presents a mystery that modern medical researchers and physicians have pondered over the past century-plus. There have been many theories, including, of course, its namesake, "hay fever." While some thought that hay or alfalfa itself was the cause for what is now called allergic rhinitis, others thought it was caused by sunshine, rain and even the shape of the nose—as many of the aristocratic that had allergies so happened to also have larger-than-normal noses.

Like any sleuth detective mystery, this text sets out to discover and unveil the real culprits of allergic rhinitis. The text explores the many suspects, the history of the disease, and the various symptoms and means used to diagnose the condition.

Then the text digs deeper. The precise physiology of the condition is laid out clearly for the reader. Armed with these tools, the reader is then plunged into the depths of the research—most led by accomplished university and medical school professors and scientists. The plethora of research exposes the very underlying conditions that lie at the foundation of not only what causes allergies, but also why our modern society is now bound in the grips of this epidemic.

The text does not stop there. It then takes the reader through numerous strategies that rebuild those deficiencies, to help us arrive at that place where our bodies can once again tolerate nature's wealth of springtime fresh air, sunshine, colorful flowers and fields of grasses.

As we embrace these conclusions, we find, like the teapot in the image below, that the solution was right in front of our eyes (and noses) the whole time.

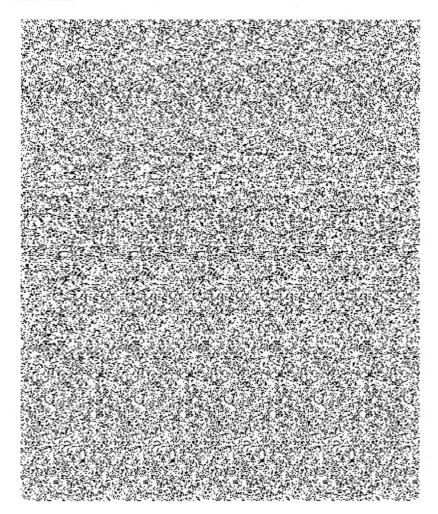

Stereogram: Can you see the teacup?

Chapter One

First Clues

A Modern Ailment?

The term 'hay fever' appears to have originated around the 1820s, when the condition, found almost exclusively among the English elite, was hypothesized to be caused by the "effluvium from new hay." This namesake stuck, and since the condition often causes a redness of the face and eyes, the word 'fever' also stuck.

Among medical circles through the mid-twentieth century, the ailment was widely unrecognized, and even by many, unnamed.

Does this mean that allergies to pollen and other airborne ruminants is a recent ailment? Yes and no.

There is certainly evidence that some sensitivities have been around for centuries, though their widespread incidence is veritably impossible.

Among the elite aristocracy of the late Middle Ages, we find a few incidences of sensitivities here and there. Henry II, for example, apparently was sensitive to peaches, and Henry VIII's Anne Boleyn apparently suffered from cat sensitivities: *"Either that cat goes or I do,"* she is reported to have said. Both of these are still stretches in the face of today's disorder and magnitude. We might also note that peach allergies are indeed rare, even today.

The stonemasons of the ancient Greeks were also reported to have suffered nasal congestion to marble dust. Marble dust? This of course is reminiscent of any other type of occupational reaction to an environment full of dust, and may also be related to asthma, which was described by the Greek physician Celsus as "dysponea." Certainly this provides nothing resembling hay fever or otherwise allergic responses to plants, molds or insect endotoxins. Nearly everyone—even a healthy person—responds to a face full of dust with some sneezing and congestion. It is a practical physiological response—not typically an allergy.

Some have purported that the so-called War of the Roses—a series of battles fought amongst competitive elites vying for the English throne in the Fifteenth century—had something to do with rose allergies. This of course is a crock, as the reference to roses appeared four hundred years later when Sir Walter Scott applied the rose-like badges between the Lancaster and York houses in an attempt to juice up his novel.

Besides, roses are insect-pollinators—they rarely cause allergies. Their volatile essences, however, can cause some sensitivity in immunosuppressed people—as we'll discuss further later. But again, this is by no means an allergy.

Accordingly, we find Leonhardus Botallus of the Sixteenth century advising doctors to not use perfumes—another volatile oil source—advising that *"Sweet per-fumes temperately used are pleasing and likewise useful to doctors and to all men . . . but sometimes it happens that what is pleasing to many persons is injurious to one."* This may have in part been derived, at least in spirit, to the early Roman Naturalist Titus Lucretius Carus' attributed saying; *"What is one man's food is another man's poison."*

Certainly, from these few mentions of sensitivities, there is no doubt that some intolerances to certain compounds have existed over the centuries. This notion is supported by the reality that metallurgy and chemistry tinkering began in the Renaissance period.

Prior to this, we find—from the ancient medicine texts of the Egyptians, Chinese, Arabia, Greeks as well as Ayurveda—no mention of allergies, and particularly, hay fever.

Confirming this, one of the first historical inferences to seasonal allergies comes from the Flemish chemist, professor and physician John Baptist Van Helmont. He described an oddly seasonal case of asthma in the early seventeenth century, reporting that: *"He was asthmatic almost the whole summer; the entire winter he was free from this trouble."*

The only logical conclusion that can be made—confirmed by physicians and historians alike—is that the widespread occurrence of hay fever and airborne allergies is not found anywhere in the historical record before the Renaissance period. This condition has most certainly developed over the past two centuries or so. In other words, hay fever and allergies are phenomena of the modern industrial era.

One of the earliest collaborated records of multiple hay fever cases came at the turn of the nineteenth century by William Heberden. Heberden apparently described four persons who experienced a seasonal return of spring nasal symptoms.

Then in 1819, Doctor John Bostock of London submitted his first paper describing the condition to the Medical Society of London. Indeed, Dr. Bostock himself had suffered from this affliction from the age of eight years old. So he knew it well.

Dr. Bostock described the condition, which he named *"A Periodical Affection of the Eyes and Chest"* as follows:

> *"About the beginning or middle of June in every year the following symptoms make their appearance, with a greater or less degree of violence. A sensation of heat and fulness is experienced in the eyes, first along the edges of the lids, and especially in the inner angles, but after some time over all of the ball. At the commencement the external features of the eye are little affected, except that there is a*

6

slight degree of redness and a discharge of tears. This state gradually increases, until the sensation becomes converted into what may be characterized as a combination of the most acute itching and smarting, accompanied with a feeling of small points striking upon or darting into the ball, at the same time that the eyes become extremely inflamed and discharge very copiously a thick mucous fluid. This state of the eyes comes on in paroxysms, at uncertain intervals, from about the second week in June to about the middle of July. The eyes are seldom quite well for the whole of this period, but the violent paroxysms never occur more than two or three times daily, lasting an hour or two each time; but with respect to their frequency and duration there is the greatest uncertainty. Generally, but not always, their invasion may be distinctly traced to some exciting cause, of which the most certain is a close, moist heat, also a bright glare of light, dust, or other substances touching the eyes and any circumstance which increases the temperature. After the violent inflammation and discharge have continued for some time, the pain and redness gradually go off, but a degree of stiffness generally remains during the day.

"After this state of the eyes has subsided for a week or ten days, a general fulness is experienced in the head, and particularly about the fore part; to this succeeds irritation of the nose, producing sneezing, which occurs in fits of extreme violence, coming on at uncertain intervals. To the sneezings are added a further sensation of tightness of the chest, and a difficulty of breathing, with a general irritation of the fauces and trachea. There is no absolute pain in any part of the chest, but a feeling of want of room to receive the air necessary for respiration, a huskiness of the voice, and an incapacity of speaking aloud for any time without inconvenience. To these local symptoms, are at length added a degree of general indisposition, a great degree of languor, an incapacity for muscular exertion, loss of appetite, emaciation, restless nights, often attended with profuse perspirations, the extremities, however, being generally cold."

The record on this condition remained silent until Dr. Bostock published a second paper in 1828. During this period, Dr. Bostock had studied the condition in more detail. This nearly ten years of research found a grand total of 28 persons who also suffered from the malady. This of course is but a miniscule fraction of the millions among every industrial country now suffering from the condition.

Dr. Bostock had several hypotheses about the cause of the strange new ailment. This also agreed with the variable inquiries of other doctors, who investigated the few reports of the condition. After combing medical records throughout England and Greater Europe, Bostock noted that no other doctors had even reported the condition beyond a decade prior to his research.

Noting that most of the cases developed symptoms during hay harvest, the term "hay fever" was coined at some point between Bostock's two papers. Again, the hay culprit was only one of several possible causes proposed by Bostock and fellow doctors. Other theories included sunshine, neurosis, summer heat, benzoic acid and even ozone. Dr. Bostock's most firm position seems centered around the heat of the summer and sunshine itself. A logical choice, given the lack of sunshine through many winter months in Europe.

Despite these theories, from the beginning, it was unmistakable that most doctors observed the condition appeared almost exclusively among the elite—noblemen and those of the wealthier aristocracy.

The first solid hypothesis of pollen as the cause came from the English physician Dr. John Elliotson. In 1831, Dr. Elliotson conjectured that pollen causes hay fever:

> *"I believe certainly that it does not depend upon the hay and therefore ought not to be called hay fever, but upon the flower of the grass, and most probably on the pollen."*

Another nineteenth century physician, Dr. Charles Harrison Blackley of Manchester, England, provided the science for this hypothesis. Dr. Blackley was also a sufferer. Dr. Blackley conducted a number of tests between 1859 and 1871 to determine the precise causation elements for the condition. Dr. Blackley isolated and tested the possible culprits upon himself—including heat, light, various odors, benzoic acid, ozone and others—looking for reactions. None of these sparked the characteristic response. Eventually, he found that dust, collected from a country roadside, stimulated the symptoms.

As Dr. Blackley stared into his microscope, he found tiny grass pollens among the dust grains. These, he figured, could be the real cause for this newly emerging and rare ailment.

So Dr. Blackley then collected a variety of different grass pollens during the summer. He carefully stored them away until the winter, when the seasonal symptoms had passed. Upon exposing himself, he found the pollen produced immediate symptoms.

Dr. Blackley went on to conduct a variety of other experiments to establish the credibility of his hypothesis. He developed ingenious pollen traps. He flew kites with glued microscope slides to find the heights that pollen rose into the sky. He established a system of determining pollen counts—a term and general process still used today to determine pollen severity.

Dr. Blackley also documented that the condition was practically exclusive among the aristocratic classes. He also noted incredulously that pollen was curiously unknown among English farmers.

Dr. Blackley also noted in 1871 that Ireland was virtually devoid of the seasonal affliction.

The condition was still rare, and even questioned as real by a large majority of physicians around the world. We can thank Dr. Blackley for advancing the condition using a scientific approach.

Between Bostock's and Blackley's research, we find a scattering of reports by other physicians that also documented this odd malady among the aristocratic class. There is also reason to believe that the English Dukes and other aristocrats vacationed at the coast of Brighton to escape the countryside pollens.

The 'summer catarrh' was also described in the mid-nineteenth century by French and German doctors. This was soon followed by doctors in the United States. America's Dr. J.A. Swett described two types of hay fever, arising from alfalfa and other grasses, or from ragweed. These physicians were some of the first to document that the new condition was beginning to spread outside the aristocracy.

In other words, the disease was slowly moving from the wealthier classes of society to those of the rest of the population. In 1902, the Professor W. P. Dunbar published a paper noting that his conclusion, based on evidence, was that the new condition:

"is a disease caused by a poison derived from plants. These toxic substances are found in the dust of the blossoms of certain plants. They are present in the albumin of the pollen and are septic in nature."

What is Allergic Rhinitis?

While many still refer to this allergic condition as hay fever—as does this text—its proper medical name is allergic rhinitis. It is more precisely called seasonal allergic rhinitis when the condition occurs only during certain seasons of the year—usually connected with allergies to pollens or seasonal molds.

Strictly speaking, allergic rhinitis is a condition caused by an allergic response. It also describes the resulting symptoms that relate to inflammation among the nasal region. The root of rhinitis is the Greek word *rhino*, which means 'nose.'

Allergic rhinitis has thus been expanded outside the restriction of being caused by allergies to plant-borne allergens such as pollen proteins. Allergic rhinitis has been expanded to nasal inflammatory conditions related to allergies or sensitivities to molds, dust, soot, insect endotoxins, chemicals and other mostly airborne allergens—in addition to pollen proteins. Allergic rhinitis may also be triggered by other non-airborne allergens such as foods and skin applications.

There are a number of conditions that are related to allergic rhinitis, and are often (mistakenly) called allergic rhinitis. Some are also referred to as simply rhinitis. Vasomotor rhinitis, for example, is a condition that is typically attributed to hypersensitivity among the autonomic nerves among the nasal tissues.

Nonallergic rhinitis with eosinophilia, or NARES, is also often diagnosed as allergic rhinitis. This might be confusing, because allergic rhinitis can also be accompanied by an avalanche of eosinophils. We'll discuss eosinophils in greater detail later.

Rhinitis may also be caused by nasal polyps. Here orb-shaped growths will extend from the nasal tissues, where they can intrude upon the nasal cavities. They can block the nose and their inflammatory behavior will exert a thickening of the nasal mucous.

In fact, as we'll discuss more in detail later, NARES, vasomotor rhinitis and nasal polyps have a lot in common with allergic rhinitis when it comes to the underlying condition.

Another condition often related to allergic rhinitis is sinusitis—or rhinosinusitis. This is when both the sinuses and nasal tissues are inflamed. Rhinosinusitis and sinusitis are typically not related to allergic responses. Rather, they are typically inflammatory conditions related to a bacterial, viral or fungal infections of the sinuses and nasal region.

What the Heck is Pollen?

Most plants procreate from a distance. While most plants have both male and female parts—often right next to each other in the same plant—there are biochemical mechanisms in place that reject a plant's own pollen from germinating. This feat of nature keeps more variety among plants—and encourages the plant to reach out for other mates.

The male sex organs of a plant—the anthers—produce tiny pollen grains—typically less than 50 microns in size. These microscopic bits of pollen dust contain both procreative and non-procreative cells. The procreative cells have two nuclei, which will divide to form sperm cells within the pollen grains.

These tiny pollen grains are complex, typically spherical, and often beautiful structures that protect the sperm cells within. The pollen grains house structures that extend a tube out of the pollen grain to escort the sperm cells into the female organs—the stigma.

The stigma typically extends from the middle of the flower. As fortunate pollen grains make contact with the stigma, they go to work attaching themselves and inserting their contents into the stigma wall. The pollen grains produce special enzymes and proteins intended to attach and break down the surface of the stigma, allowing the insertion of the sperm cells.

This process might be compared to landing on the moon. The pollen grains are like lunar landing modules. As they are landing, they extend their landing gear (the pollen's enzymes and proteins) to penetrate and grab on to the moon's surface. Once landed, the module will extend a set of stairs (the pollen tube) down to the surface to escort the astronauts to the surface. Once extended, the astronauts will descend to the moon's surface by climbing down the stairs.

The analogy breaks down when we consider how deep the pollen tube can furrow into the stigma to deliver the sperm to the egg. As the pollen tube extends through the stigma, it will hopefully insert the sperm cells onto the egg. Depending upon the plant, the fertilized sperm cells will build into the endosperm of the seed. In the case of grains and other seeded plants, this is one of the more nutritious parts of the plant.

This also explains why pollens can be so insidious when they enter our nasal cavities. As they put their landing gear down on our nasal membranes, they instinctively want to complete the sexual act—with us!

Pollen can be transmitted through the air via the wind (anemophilous), via insects, or via the hair and feet of animals. Those plants that transmit their pollen via insects such as bees (entomophilous), or the hairs and feet of animals (zoophyilous) are not considered good candidates for allergies, simply because there are typically not enough of them floating around the air to populate the nose and stimulate allergic responses. This does not mean that these pollens—such as from many bee-managed flowers—cannot get into the nose or eyes to produce allergies. They can. But allergies from them are simply quite rare.

Furthermore, insect- and animal-carried pollen tends to be a bit sticky or otherwise more adhesive. This prevents them from typically reaching the nose. Pollens known to be transmitted via insects and animals include most of the edible fruits, most of the ornamental flowers, and many others. Insect- and animal-attached pollinators are more likely to meet with their sexual target, as insects and animals tend to go from flower to flower, harvesting among similar habitats.

Those more random pollinators that use the wind are typically profuse in the amount of pollen grains they produce. They will practically fill the air with their pollen, using their sheer numbers to insure landing on a plant of the same species. This 'conquest by sheer number' of pollen grains also insures that they will land in our noses as well. That is where the trouble can start: In some of us, but not others.

This does not mean that people cannot become allergic to insect- and animal-carried pollen. Ultra-sensitive people can certainly become sensitive to these pollens, especially if they have other allergies, and the underlying condition that predicates becoming allergic. Occupations that tend to handle these types of plants or their foods provide one of the greatest facilities to becoming sensitized to the proteins of these types of pollens.

We'll discuss at length why some people become allergic to these types of pollens, as well as why people become sensitized to pollen in general.

We'll also discuss in greater detail later that it is not the pollen grains that we can become allergic to. It is their proteins—and their protein fragments called epitopes. These pollen grains contain amino acid combinations particular to their species and DNA. The body's immune system becomes sensitized to these protein parts, eventually producing the allergic response. And once these protein parts are identified as foreigners by the body's immune system, those proteins—whether coming from the plant's foods or its pollens—can cause allergy symptoms among those who have become sensitized. We'll discuss the physiology of this shortly.

Who Gets Allergic Rhinitis?

Because allergic rhinitis embraces other allergies besides pollen protein sensitivities, the precise numbers can be a bit difficult to nail down.

According to the Centers for Disease Control's 2009 study, *Health Statistics for U.S. Children*, 7.2 million children were reported to have hay fever during the twelve-month period, totaling 9.8% of children. They also found that 8.2 million children, or 11%, reported respiratory allergies.

And according to the 2009 U.S. Centers for Disease Control *Health Statistics for U.S. Adults*, 17.7 million U.S. adults have hay fever. This is out of a adult population of 227.3 million, which means that about 7.8% of the U.S. adult population has hay fever. Men comprise 42% of this number, while women make up nearly 58%.

Most of this number is among adults between the ages of 18 and 64 years old. Among adults between the age of 18 years old and 44 years, 6.4% have hay fever, while nearly 10% of adults between the age of 45 and 64 years have hay fever. Among those between 65 and 74, 7.9% have hay fever, while 6.2% of those over 75 have hay fever. This means that adults in their middle ages (44-64) experience more hay fever than do adults of other ages.

As far as race, Caucasians have more hay fever by percentage (8%) than African-Americans (5.6%), Hispanic-Americans (5.6%), and Hawaiian/Pacific Islanders (6.3%). In terms of sex matched to race, Caucasian females lead the pack at 9.4%, while African-American males have the lowest rates, at 4.1% of their respective populations.

As far as education, the more educated the person, the higher incidence of hay fever. Of those with less than a high school diploma, 5.8% have hay fever. Of those with a high school diploma or GED, 7% have hay fever. Of those with some college, 8.3% have hay fever. Of those with a college degree or higher, 10% have hay fever.

Similar trends are seen amongst income. Generally, higher incomes have higher rates of hay fever. While 7% of those making $35k to $50k a year have hay fever, 9.2% of those making over $100k per year have hay fever. Meanwhile, among those making from $75k to $100k a year, 8% have hay fever.

These trends towards the more educated and those with higher incomes have remained consistent for most of the short history of hay fever. In fact, a century ago as discussed earlier, hay fever was almost exclusively a condition of the aristocratic class among the wealthier countries. Gradually over the years, hay fever has increasingly moved into populations with lower income and education levels.

Another interesting trend shows up with regard to marriage. Those who have never married or live with a partner have 6.6% and 5.9% incidence respectively, while 8.1% of those who are currently married have hay fever. Worse, 9.1% of those who are divorced or separated have hay fever, and nearly 10% of those who are widowed have hay fever.

With regard to where people with hay fever live, there is not a big difference between those living in big cities, small cities or rural areas. Those living in large metropolitan areas have a 7.5% hay fever incidence, while those living in smaller cities have an 8.3% hay fever incidence. Among those living in rural areas—where there are undoubtedly more pollens and molds—6.9% have hay fever.

Geographical region made little difference as well. However, hay fever rates among those living in the Midwest (6.8%) are noticeably lower than the rates of those living in the West, at 8.3%. Hay fever rates among those living in the Northwest match the rates of those living in the Northeast, at 7.7% of their respective populations.

It might be added that the West also hosts the most polluted region—Southern California—in the country.

As the CDC numbers are added up and combined with other resources, up to 50 million people in the U.S. have some sort of allergy. This includes being sensitive to any indoor and outdoor allergen, including those derived from pollen, foods, insects, mold, latex and other environmental sources. This number adds up to nearly 20% of the population.

We might want to mention that other research has confirmed that approximately 25% of people in England suffer from some sort of allergy (Walker and Wing 2010). Quite a change from the 28 cases found by Dr. Bostock over nearly ten years in the early 1800s.

Allergies are the fifth most prevalent chronic condition among all Americans, and the third most prevalent condition among children and adolescents (under 18). Allergies are more prevalent among children than adults, with 40% of children reporting activity-limiting allergy conditions.

Allergies are estimated to cost Americans $7 billion per year, of which $5.7 billion are required by medication and $300 million in health professional costs.

Hay fever is the fifth leading condition causing work absence. Almost four million workdays are lost to hay fever, costing an estimated $700 million in productivity loss.

Furthermore, multiple studies have shown that those who live in rural areas and have contact with farm animals—in combination with drinking raw cow's milk—have lower rates of hay fever (von Mutius and Vercelli 2010). We'll dig into the individual studies and their specifics later as we investigate these associations.

In Europe, hay fever tends to occur more in some areas than others. Seasonal plants may provide the link in some cases. In other cases, there appears to be other reasons. In some regions, being close to pollinating plants simply does not increase allergic rhinitis incidence. In others, there is no obvious connection. In many cases—especially among rural areas—higher exposure to pollen has no relationship to hay fever. This is especially true in rural farming areas of Europe.

Globally, one of the most consistent observations is that hay fever rates are higher among industrial countries than among third world and developing countries. And allergies are more prevalent among city-dwellers than rural-dwellers.

Hay fever and asthma rates in China, for example, have been far lower than Western countries. In research from the International Study of Asthma and Allergies in Childhood Steering Committee (ISAAC 1998), asthma and allergy incidence among adolescent children was found to be over 20% in many Western countries, while only about 2% in China. The highest levels of allergy and asthma around the world are found in Britain, Australia, New Zealand, Ireland, the U.S., and some countries in South America. The lowest rates of asthma are found in Indonesia, Greece, China, India, Ethiopia, Taiwan and Uzbekistan.

As some of these countries become westernized, however, their hay fever and asthma rates have been rising. In China and India, for example, hay fever and asthma rates have grown dramatically, especially among industrialized regions. In addition, regions of more affluence also predict higher hay fever and other allergy rates.

Then there is the hygiene issue. Children with more siblings, and those living in more crowded conditions have less allergies. Even amongst areas with significant environmental toxins such as smog, those living in more crowded conditions (greater family density) have less allergy incidence (Bråbäck et al. 1995). We'll be discussing these relationships in detail later.

Furthermore, among developed countries, those living in warmer, sunnier areas, with other factors controlled, have fewer asthma and allergies. In a large-scale international study, 17,280 adults between the ages of 20 and 44 from different countries were studied by researchers from Australia's Monash Medical School (Woods et al. 2001). Natives of Northern European countries such as Scandinavia or Germany had higher rates compared with Southern European countries such as Spain and Italy.

This geographical relationship has also been seen among urgent care facilities within the U.S. For reasons we will discuss in more depth later, those living in Southern states have lower incidence of allergic sensitivities and far fewer hospital room visits for allergy and asthma episodes (Rudders et al. 2010).

French researchers (Rancé et al. 2003) found that a child's first allergic sensitivity becomes evident at about two years old. This also depends, to some degree, on the type of allergy. It is also recognized that atopic dermatitis allergies and food sensitivities occur more frequently among infants and younger children. Hay fever, allergic rhinitis and allergic asthma tend to develop later in childhood, especially among children who are otherwise allergic during infancy.

Again, we'll dig further into these curious relationships in the coming chapters, as we uncover the real causes of allergic rhinitis.

Allergy Rates are Rising with Asthma Rates

While hay fever incidence has not been as closely monitored as asthma has over the past half century, correlations have found that hay fever incidence has increased in parallel with the astronomical growth in asthma incidence over the past few decades.

The research also indicates that allergy, hay fever and asthma rates have all been increasing primarily amongst the developed and developing world. As of 1980, about five million Americans had been diagnosed with asthma. Currently, asthma rates are close to 20 million Americans. This means that asthma levels have about quadrupled over the past thirty years: About a 400% rise in asthma incidence. And this is not due to population growth: The U.S. population has risen by only 30% or so over that period.

In terms of per-capita increases among children, U.S. National Center for Health Statistics data indicates that asthma occurrence among children rose an average of 4.6% each year between 1980 and 1996. Furthermore, childhood asthma rates grew by 3.5% in total over the next twelve years. In other words, growth rates might have slowed, but asthma incidence is still growing.

As of 2005, 6.5 million children had asthma, equating to 8.9% of children. Then in 2007, research from the National Center for Health Statistics, Centers for Disease Control and Prevention (Akinbami *et al.* 2009), estimated found that 6.7 million U.S. children suffer from asthma. This equated to 9.1% of all U.S. children. In other words, in the two years between 2007 and 2009, there were 200,000 more children suffering from asthma.

Furthermore, recent reports have estimated that about 7.1 million children currently have asthma, equating to about 9.6% of all U.S. children.

In research from the National Center for Chronic Disease and Prevention, asthma prevalence in 2006 among adults (over the age of 18) in their sampled communities ranged from 6.5% to 19%. In 2007, this range was found to be from 7.5% to 19% among the communities studied—an increase of 1% on the minimum side.

Meanwhile, rates in other developed or developing countries around the world have also continued to climb, with some at higher growth rates. This is supported by a number of international surveys.

For example, medical researchers from Sweden's Uppsala University (Uddenfeldt *et al.* 2010) studied 8,150 to 12,560 adolescents, adults and elderly adults between 1990 and 2003. They found that asthma incidence increased through the 13-year period among all ages. Asthma rose from 11% in 1990 to 25% in 2003 among the adolescents.

Scientists from Poland's Military Institute of Health Sciences (Bant and Kruszewski 2008) found that among people living in urban areas in Poland, IgE sensitivities to atopic allergens increased 52% in the 16 years from 1986 to 2002. This means that on the average, allergen sensitization increased at a rate of about 3.25% per year.

Australian researchers (Poulos *et al.* 2007) studied the prevalence of critical reactions including anaphylaxis and atopic asthma that resulted in hospitalization among developed countries. They analyzed data for three periods—1993-1994, 2004-2005 and 1997-2004. During the three periods, hospital admissions for angioedema (swelling of mucous membranes and submucosal tissues) increased an average of 3% per year. Allergic urticaria (skin rashes) increased an average of 5.7% per year. Hospitalizations for the sometimes-fatal anaphylaxis allergic response increased a whopping 8.8% per year in total. Increases in hypersensitivity hospitalization were highest among children under five years old.

Primary Signs and Symptoms of Allergic Rhinitis

First we should clarify that hay fever/allergic rhinitis is not a disease. Rather, allergic rhinitis is a symptom. It is a physiological response indicating a deeper, underlying condition. Due to this underlying condition, the mucous membranes of the nasal region, eyes and sinuses become hypersensitive to particular triggers. Once irritated by the trigger, the immune system launches an inflammatory response that enlarges the epithelia (cell surface) tissues and mucous membranes (thin layers of mucous) of these regions. They become filled with thickened mucous as a result, which further constricts the ability to breathe through the nose.

The most obvious symptom, then, is **nasal congestion**, also called a stuffy or even blocked nose. This can occur at any time, and can continue for days, depending upon the allergen, the type of response, and the condition of the immune system. If a stuffy nose completely blocks the nasal passages, it can completely restrict breathing out of the nose. Therefore, a common sign of allergic rhinitis is breathing in and out of the mouth.

The sinuses may also become congested. **Sinus congestion** is usually accompanied by an achy, congested feeling around the eyes and forehead. This can also cause a sinus headache, as the pressure in the sinuses changes the equilibrium of the blood vessels and tissues around the sinuses. A severe and enduring case of congested and painful sinuses may also indicate an infection within the sinuses. This often evolves not from an allergic reaction, but from an infection of the sinuses. Sometimes allergic rhinitis occurs together with **infective sinusitis**. We will briefly discuss some of the causes for infective sinusitis later.

Along with inflammation among the nasal passages and sinuses, allergic rhinitis also often is accompanied by **swollen, inflamed eyes** that may tear up and water. While these symptoms are also can be referred to as conjunctivitis, they occur very often with allergic rhinitis.

Sneezing may also occur in the beginning, or throughout an allergic episode. Sneezing is a reflex designed to remove foreigners from the nasal cavity and sinuses. Therefore, sneezing can be continuous, occur at the beginning of allergen exposure, or even not at all.

Itching can also accompany an allergic response. Itching may occur within the nose—sometimes causing sneezing—as well as around the mouth, palate, lips, and eyes. As the itchy area is rubbed, greater inflammation is often produced in the area, causing more redness and more discomfort. Itchiness often precedes a full-blown rhinitis attack. This is because the itchiness is usually the result of an initial release of histamine from mast cells.

Sometimes, especially for those with a sinus infection, the **Eustachian tubes may become clogged** with liquid or mucous. This can cause a dull ache under the ear, and even—in the case of a spreading bacteria infection—a middle ear infection.

As the thickened and loose mucous runs to the back of our palate and nasal cavity, it may run down the back of the throat and into the airways. This can cause **throat soreness, coughing,** and even **wheezing.**

For this and other reasons, allergic rhinitis is often accompanied by **asthma, eczema** and/or **urticaria**—also called **hives.** In addition, **headaches** and even **migraines** can accompany allergic rhinitis. In rare cases, **joint pains** can also come with a hay fever episode.

Nearly three-quarters of allergic rhinitis cases evolve into asthma, or are otherwise related to asthma.

Furthermore, research from the University of Copenhagen (Chawes *et al.* 2010) found that 66% of children with allergic rhinitis also had eczema.

What is Atopy?

Atopy is used frequently among doctors and scientists to describe allergy symptoms. What is atopy anyway? Atopy is derived from the Greek word meaning *"unusual"* or *"not ordinary."* Atopic is used to describe the condition where a person is reacting to a substance in a way that is unrelated to the contact with the substance.

For example, a normal response to breathing in some dust is to sneeze. A good sneeze should remove quite a bit of the dust from the nasal cavity. But if suddenly, rashes break out all over the body, the reaction becomes more than a normal response: It becomes atopic.

The atopic response is also a normal reaction that occurs with a severity outside the realm of a typical response for such an exposure. While a sneeze might be appropriate if we bring in some dust into our nose, sneezing for the rest of the day would be considered atopic.

In atopy, the immune system is triggered by antigens that engage antibodies such as immunoglobulin E (IgE). This engagement with IgE produces what is called a *mediated response*.

This type of IgE response is outside the ordinary IgA response, which expels foreigners before they penetrate the body's tissue systems. Once inside, the allergen interacts with IgE, stimulating the production of inflammatory mediators such as histamine, prostaglandins and leukotrienes. These in turn result in the atopic inflammatory response.

Atopic allergies will result in hives, rashes, itchiness, respiratory issues and/or allergic rhinitis. Atopic reactions are typically related to the mucosal membranes. These are expressed as asthma, allergic rhinitis, conjunctiva rhinitis, and even eosinophilic esophagitis. Some digestive symptoms are also considered atopic, but here again, the response is considered out of proportion with a typical response to the foreigner.

Eczema or dermatitis of the skin is considered atopic when the substance is not being consumed through the skin. While a skin response can appear anywhere on the skin, atopic skin rashes will often occur at the hands, elbows or knees. These areas can feel itchy and can be very uncomfortable in an atopic condition. Over a few days after an outbreak, they can become scaly and crusted. These lesions can also worsen with the use of chemical soaps or certain types of clothing.

On the other hand, a skin reaction to a chemical lotion we just spread onto the skin would not be considered an atopic reaction. This could be considered quite normal in the case of many chemical lotions on the market today, which contain what the body considers toxins.

With respect to pollens, most of the world's population—especially among less industrialized countries—have little or no reactions during even the heaviest part of pollen season. At worst, they might sneeze once or twice if a flurry of pollen enters the nose at once. Those with an atopic condition, on the other hand, will respond in an extraordinary way to even the slightest incoming pollen—with nasal blockage, watery eyes, itching and so on.

Asphyxia and Anaphylaxis

While anaphylaxis is more often seen in food allergies than hay fever/allergic rhinitis, it does occur in allergic rhinitis. An anaphylactic response is considered a severe response to an allergen. Practically any symptom of an allergy can become anaphylactic, and anaphylaxis is often life-threatening. The anaphylactic response can range from a skin response, a gastrointestinal response, a cardiovascular event, or most commonly, a respiratory event. In the latter, the throat constricts and reduces the ability to breathe.

A severe anaphylactic flare-up may cause a deprivation of oxygen to occur. This is called *asphyxia*. Asphyxia and anaphylaxis are difficult to differentiate from each other: They are for all tense and purposes, the same emergency event.

In the 12 years between 1993 and 2005, there were 17.3 million emergency room visits for acute allergic reactions in the United States. These represented 1.3% of all emergency room visits (Rudders *et al.* 2010). In other words, about 13 out of every 1,000 emergency room visits are for anaphylaxis.

There are generally three types of anaphylactic responses:
1) *Uniphasic*—a onetime rush of symptoms.
2) *Biphasic*—an initial reactive rush of symptoms, followed by another reaction later, sometimes several hours later.
3) *Protracted*—an ongoing rush of symptoms that do not abate for several hours. This is somewhat rare, but it does occur.

Those with allergic rhinitis have increased risk of anaphylaxis when their allergies are accompanied by asthma and/or food allergies (González-Pérez *et al.* 2010). About half of deaths from anaphylaxis come from allergic responses to tree nuts or peanuts.

Researchers from California's Kaiser Permanente (Iribarren *et al.* 2010) found that the incidence of anaphylactic shock among allergic responses occurred in about 109 person-years out of 100,000 person-years—primarily when allergies were associated with asthma.

Other population studies have found anaphylaxis/asphyxia occurs between one and 70 of every 100,000 people (Boyce *et al.* 2010).

It is also important to note that research has shown that death occurs in about 1% of all anaphylaxis episodes (Moneret-Vautrin and Morisset 2005).

Asthma and Allergic Rhinitis

The form of asthma that often relates to allergic rhinitis is called atopic asthma because it is typically triggered by environmental or allergen factors. These provoke the same type of immune system response that produces allergic rhinitis. For this reason, asthma and allergic rhinitis often occur simultaneously, or even alternatively.

Illustrating this, medical researchers from the University of Vermont (Dixon *et al.* 2006) studied the relationships between asthma, allergic rhinitis and sinusitis. The study included 2,519 asthmatics from three national asthma trials. Over 70% of the asthmatics had either allergic rhinitis or sinusitis in addition to their asthma symptoms. They also found that asthmatics with rhinitis and sinusitis had more severe asthma symptoms and more sleep difficulties, and more women had sinusitis or rhinitis.

Looking at the association between asthma and allergic rhinitis in the converse, researchers from the University of Copenhagen (Chawes *et al.* 2010) found that 21% of children with allergic rhinitis also had asthma.

In another study, researchers from the National Institutes of Health (Arbes *et al.* 2007) tested 10 allergens, and found that 56% of their asthma subjects were allergic to one of these allergens.

Nearly half of asthmatic responses are considered atopic. For example, researchers from the National Institute of Allergy and Infectious Diseases (Gergen *et al.* 2009) used the National Health and Nutrition Examination Survey (2005-2006) to determine the incidence of IgE-related asthma. Using this huge database of thousands of asthmatics, they found that IgE-related atopy was present in 42.5% of current asthmatics.

Atopy can also cause a variety of other hypersensitivity symptoms, including hives, rashes, itchiness and sinus congestion. Atopic reactions are typically seen among the epithelial layers and mucosal membranes. These are expressed as asthma, allergic rhinitis, conjunctiva rhinitis, and even eosinophilic esophagitis.

Again, these responses are all outside of what would be expected in a healthy immune system. For example, dust or smog might cause sneezing or mild coughing in a normal immune system, while a hypersensitive atopic response can invoke asthma symptoms along with allergic rhinitis.

Food Allergies and Allergic Rhinitis

Food allergies can occur before, after, or simultaneously to allergic rhinitis. For many allergy sufferers, food allergies appear to be the basis for their atopic asthma and/or hay fever. For others, it appears they are independent conditions.

In other words, a person who has become allergic to a food will typically be sensitized to the particular protein structure (remember the epitope) within the food. That same protein structure will often be evident among the pollen grains of the plant that food came from. This would make the same person theoretically sensitive to both the pollen and the food coming from that plant species.

Another event is cross-reactivity. Once the immune system becomes sensitized to one type of food or plant, it is more likely to become sensitized to another type of food or plant. This cross-reactivity can occur between different foods and pollens as well. We'll dig into this later.

University of Colorado medical researchers (Liu *et al.* 2010) determined from the 2005-2006 National Health and Nutrition Examination Survey data that about 2.5% of the U.S. population has a clinical food allergy. They also found that having a food allergy significantly increases the risk of contracting allergic rhinitis and asthma.

University of Copenhagen researchers (Chawes *et al.* 2010) found that 47% of children who have allergic rhinitis also have food allergies.

Researchers from the University of Delhi (Kumar *et al.* 2006) studied IgE levels in 216 asthmatic patients with an average age of 32 years old. Of the 216, they found that 172 had elevated serum IgEs that indicated allergies and hay fever. Of the total, 11% of the asthma patients were sensitized to rice, 10% were sensitized to black gram, 10% had IgEs specific to lentils while 9.2% were sensitive to citrus (some had multiple sensitivities).

Researchers from Poland's Medical University of Lodz (Krogulska *et al.* 2010) studied 54 children with food allergies and 62 without food allergies. Using methacholine provocation to test forced expiratory volume (FEV1), they found that the food allergic children had greater levels of airway hyperreactivity. Among the non-asthmatic children in the study, airway hyperreactivity was evident in 47% of the children with food allergies and only 17% of those without food allergies. Furthermore, bronchial hyperreactivity was found in 74% of those children who suffered from moderate anaphylactic reactions, and airway hyperreactivity existed among all of the children who had severe anaphylactic reactions.

Diagnosing Hay Fever/Allergic Rhinitis

There are a number of tests that physicians will initiate in order to first determine whether there is an allergy, and second, what the potential allergen is. Here are the major tests used:

Immunoassays

Blood may be drawn and submitted for testing to measure immunoglobulin levels. The most popular of these is the *radioallergosorbent test* (or RAST). This test is also called the *immunoassay for allergen-specific IgE*. The test measures the content of allergen-specific immunoglobulin Es in the bloodstream.

Because IgEs will specialize in responding to specific allergens, an IgE responsive to wheat protein will not be the same as an IgE that is responsive to dust mite endotoxins. This means that the immunoassay may determine not only whether an allergy exists. It can also determine what the allergen might be.

A well-respected immunoassay test for accuracy is the CAP-RAST test. Because CAP-RAST immunoassay tests determine the level of an allergen-specific IgE in the blood, they are considered more accurate. Typically the test comes with a level on a 1-to-100 scale, with 100 being the highest level and one being the lowest. A score of 75 will typically produce an allergy diagnosis. On the other hand, a level that is, say, 10 or

15, might be problematic to diagnose. At this level, there may be tolerance to something that was previously considered an allergen to the body.

Indeed, one of the problems of immunoassay testing is the fact that different people have different levels of tolerance at the same IgE levels. The immunoassay test also does little to indicate the severity or type of allergic reaction a person might have. A person, for example, might have a high immunoassay IgE number but have a strong immune system that manages the response quite well. On the other hand, an immunosuppressed person with a lower IgE level might have severe reactions.

On the other hand, one of the benefits of obtaining such a clear number is that from successive tests, a person and their physician can find out whether their sensitivity is dropping or increasing with time. A higher number can indicate increasing sensitivity, while a lowering number can indicate increased tolerance. This can be truly helpful with some of the strategies we'll discuss later on.

Skin Prick Tests

In skin prick testing (often referred to as SPT), a small amount of a substance the allergenist thinks we are sensitive to is inserted underneath the top layer of skin by a pricking of the skin. The skin is then monitored for response. If the skin responds with a *weal* (a small circular mark or welt), this indicates the existence of a sensitivity to that allergen.

There are typically three methods used to apply this skin prick test. A skin prick instrument may be soaked in the allergen before the skin is pricked with it. The diagnostician may also place a drop of the allergen onto the skin before pricking the skin underneath the drop with a needle or probe.

The diagnostician may also inject the allergen underneath the skin with a needle. This is also referred to as intradermal testing, and comes with a higher risk of anaphylaxis.

Once the prick is done, it usually takes about 10-15 minutes for the weal to come up in an allergic person. It will often look like a small pimple. It is the histamine response that makes this happen. A salt-water prick test is often deployed to test for skin sensitivity to the pricking alone.

Skin prick testing has proven to be one of the least accurate forms of testing, however. While a negative response (no weal) usually confirms no allergy, a positive response will not always indicate an actual allergy. Research shows that up to 60% of positive results can be false *(false positives)*.

Double-Blind Challenges

If there is a strong suspicion of an allergy, the allergist may invoke a challenge by having the patient consume first a tiny amount—and then increasingly larger doses of the allergen while they watch for reactions. This can be a painstaking and extensive test. And for someone who is showing signs of allergies, this test should only be performed by or in the presence of a trained health professional prepared to react with medical care should anaphylaxis result.

There are a number of different types of challenge tests, but the most employed method is giving the patient a capsule of the allergen (or a placebo). When a placebo is employed, it is called a *double-blind, placebo-controlled challenge*. In other words, neither the diagnostician nor the patient will know whether the capsule contains the allergen or the placebo. This can eliminate results produced through the inclinations of either the health professional or patient.

As mentioned earlier, the double-blind, placebo-controlled challenge is considered the gold standard among diagnostic tests for allergies.

Enzyme-linked Immunosorbent Assays (ELISA)

This test and its relative, the ALCAT test, have been met with significant resistance and criticism from conventional Western physicians. The complaint of some physicians is that ELISA testing has not been proven to be reliable for allergy diagnosis.

This was illustrated by researchers from India's Post Graduate Institute of Medical Education and Research (Sharnan *et al.* 2001). The scientists gave skin prick tests and ELISA tests to 64 children with food allergies previously confirmed through food challenges, along with 32 control subjects. They found that the ELISA tests had greater specificity than the skin prick tests (88% versus 64%). But while they found that ELISA provided reliability for a lack of allergy, the ELISA testing generally did not provide a reliable basis for determining an allergy was present. They concluded that ELISA provided no useful advantage over skin prick testing.

One of the issues with ELISA testing (and some say its advantage) is that it yields levels of other immunoglobulins such as IgG, IgG4 and IgA. Some research has indicated that IgG4 is indicative of a hidden food allergy (Shakib *et al.* 1986), but other research has shown that allergen-specific IgG4s can also simply indicate a recovery from a prior allergy (Savilahti *et al.* 2010).

One of the issues that some (including the author) have with ELISA is that some of the lab results can present an array of confusing and extensive sensitivity conclusions that may or may not apply to the patient. These often provide the patient with an overload of information about possible sensitivities (sometimes to hundreds of foods and substances) that may or may not exist. Talk about false positives.

Other (Some Questionable) Diagnostic Tests

There are other diagnostic tests that health care professionals may recommend. These include sublingual testing, immune-complex tests, cytotoxic tests, provocative tests, the Mediator Release Test, galvanometer skin testing and others. While some of these may have value in some instances, most have not been met with the rigor of definitive scientific study (Boyce *et al.* 2010).

Researchers from the Ospedale Civile Maggiore hospital in Varona, Italy (Senna *et al.* 2002) conducted a study of alternative allergy tests. These included the cytotoxic test, the sublingual provocation test, the subcutaneous test, the heart-ear reflex test, kinesiology, electro-acupuncture, the immunocomplex IgG test, and hair analysis. They concluded that none of these tests were reliable allergy diagnostic tests.

We might comment separately about applied kinesiology. This test is currently applied by many clinicians who subscribe to its accuracy. While not having been proven by significant research, it has a relatively low cost or risk to the patient. It can also be quite immediately verified through other testing methods, which can make the test results immediately verifiable to the clinician and patient.

In applied kinesiology, the patient's muscle strength is tested while the patient holds, touches or eats a suspect allergen. The practitioner may push against the arm of the patient before and after holding or touching the allergen, for example. A trained individual may also self-test, but this can be difficult, and blindedness is difficult.

Applied kinesiology has had a history of use among alternative practitioners, typically following special training through clinical mentorship. This is not atypical of other specialized medical treatments such as acupuncture or massage. Physicians also use mentorship. In other words, applied kinesiology should only be performed by someone properly trained in the procedure.

We should note that an allergic response is a type of kinesiological event, as nerves and muscles are typically involved in the atopic response.

Applied kinesiology is nonetheless still very controversial, as it has the potential of being highly subjective. Thus it requires a sensitive and knowledgeable practitioner. It should also be conducted using double-blind methods—where neither the patient nor practitioner knows what allergen is being held or touched.

Even with these in place, however, there is always the possibility of error. There can be a variety of environmental, muscle tension, mental or unseen influences that can skew the results. Therefore, while this test is relatively simple and inexpensive, it can also be unreliable. Results should therefore be confirmed with more established testing methods.

The Allergen Elimination Study

Even some of the more recognized tests discussed were no more reliable than a simple allergen elimination study. Furthermore, the allergen elimination study can be conducted at home by oneself if the symptoms are not severe. If the symptoms are severe, the elimination program should be supervised by a health professional or observed by someone prepared for anaphylaxis. This said, the only expense is time, patience, and careful record-keeping.

During the elimination study, the allergic person simply begins to eliminate suspect allergens from their environment one at a time. For dust mites or mold, this might require taking a trip to another location, or developing a clean room. We'll discuss this in more detail later. Or it might simply mean, in the case of pollen, closing windows and breathing only filtered indoor air for a few days. However the method, one or two allergens should be eliminated at a time if possible.

If symptoms subside after the allergen(s) are withdrawn, one can be fairly certain of the sensitivity. The period of elimination should be long enough to confirm the test, however. A good period is seven days without a symptom, but the longer the better. To provide confirmation, the patient can return to the environment with the allergen and then eliminate the allergen once more. Again, this assumes the symptoms are manageable and not severe, or there is supervision as mentioned above.

To confirm the sensitivity if need be, the allergen can be tested using the skin prick or double-blind, placebo-controlled allergen challenge tests.

Chapter Two

The Physiology of Allergic Rhinitis

What is going on inside the body with allergic rhinitis? In this chapter, we'll discuss the mechanisms at play that produce the characteristic symptoms of stuffy nose, watery eyes, itchiness and others discussed.

Understanding the mechanics of allergic rhinitis means gaining an understanding of the immune system. This is because, as we'll show, allergic rhinitis is an inflammatory condition.

Anyone familiar with the immune system will notice that there are a number of features we lay out here that aren't described in most other texts, websites and even standard physiology courses. This is because our understanding of the immune system has expanded greatly over the past few years. We'll cover them here.

Intelligent Recognition

In general, the immune system is an intelligent scanning and defense mechanism, combined with an efficient toxin removal process. There are, however, numerous systems in place to achieve these objectives.

The immune system has a number of intelligent abilities. The first is recognition. The immune system is set up to see, assess and memorize whether a particular molecule, cell or organism is healthy for the body. This requires a complex biochemical identification system and a process of memorization. It also means the immune system must monitor the health of the body's cells and tissue systems.

We might compare this recognition system to a criminal fingerprint search system. The computer maintains a database of fingerprints. The software searches for matches by breaking down elements of the fingerprints into a mapping system that classifies each section by type and position. When enough elements match a database record, the fingerprint is declared a match.

In the same way, utilizing a database of biochemical information, the immune system scans and checks molecular structures against its database of threat memory. If the molecular structure matches with the elements of something that threatened the body previously, the immune system begins to mobilize the appropriate mechanisms to block entry to the threat.

Now if the threat has already entered the tissues and gained access to tissue cells, the immune system will be forced to launch an inflammatory response to attack the foreigner and any cells the threat may have invaded.

When it comes to an allergen molecule, the immune system scans and remembers distinctive molecular sequences or combinations—these may be polypeptides, individual peptides or a portion of a peptide. Again, these molecular portions are epitopes. Epitopes are antigens that are also referred to as allergens, because they stimulate an allergic inflammatory response. They stimulate the inflammatory response because their epitopes are recognized by the immune system as threatening.

When the immune system first records an epitope, it also develops a special receptor for that epitope. This receptor might be compared to a lock, while the allergen epitope is a particular type of key that will only open that lock. These biomolecular 'locks' are the antibodies or immunoglobulins. The lock-and-key system of immunoglobulins provides a switch for the immune system to recognize an allergen and activate the immune system to remove it.

The immune system is located throughout the body. We find immune cells on the skin, in the blood, in the airways, in the bones and in every organ system. We also find the immune system within trillions of probiotic bacteria scattered around the body.

As we'll discuss, the body's probiotic bacteria are integral within the immune system. They also help the immune system recognize foreign entities or toxins. This information is invaluable to the rest of the immune system. Probiotic bacteria also have the ability to remember invaders and toxins. They can thus assist the body in the breakdown and ejection of foreign molecules and pathogens, and often do this before the rest of the immune system even has to get involved.

We might compare such a system to a castle from the middle ages. The castle typically has very tall walls and a moat surrounding it. It would most likely have a very large and heavy gate system. These together prevent attacking enemies from easily gaining access to the castle. But these systems would be easy to get through were it not for defending marksmen and spear-chucking warriors who stand guard in the towers and castle walls. These guards prevent enemies from climbing the walls, jumping over the moat, or setting fire to the gate. Without these living guards, the defense systems of the castle would be useless to any enemy with some conviction. In this chapter, we'll review all of these players and facilities.

The immune system is incredible in its ability to maintain specificity and diversity. These characteristics allow the immune system to respond to literally millions, if not billions of different antigens. Moreover, each particular antigen and epitope will require a distinct type of response to get rid of it. The immune system also remembers this particular response.

This issue of recognition brings up an important question to discuss in relation to hay fever: How does the body distinguish between "acceptable" things and "bad" (or threatening) things? And how does something become an allergen?

The body's databases are the key. The immune system accesses a variety of databases, including the T-cell, B-cell and antibody databases, the MHC database, our DNA, and the probiotic database. Like branches of a large but centralized database system, these memory systems interact and confirm the threat levels of particular antigens. This confirming process, of course, relies upon a balanced and strong immune system. A balanced and active immune system would readily remove pollens, molds and other foreigners as a matter of course.

If the system is overloaded or in emergency mode, it will easily become over-reactive. In this state, the body will likely react out of proportion for the type of foreigner.

As mentioned, one of the databases the immune system utilizes comes from the body's DNA. DNA sequences code the environmental issues our ancestors' bodies easily dealt with—such as pollens or molds—as well as those environmental issues that created problems for our ancestors—such as viruses and some bacterial infections. The DNA database is quite complex, but is generally a series of amino acid combinations that create a unique record. This unique record in turn stimulates the production of certain types of proteins and enzymes—which become or produce immune cells and general physiological responses to our environment.

For example, researchers from the Johns Hopkins Bloomberg School of Public Health (Liu *et al.* 2004) found that nucleotide polymorphisms among genes were associated with specific allergies. They found that a gene variant labeled C-1055T was associated with food or environmental allergies. They found that the variant Gln551Arg was associated with cat allergies. They also found that the variant C-590T was associated with dust mite allergies.

The immune system also 'remembers' the foods and environmental inputs our mother faced during pregnancy. Here we are sensitized to whatever comes along with our umbilical cord blood—the fluid mom provides, also containing nutrients and immune factors for our first nine months.

Our recognition process also records and responds to our changing environments. In other words, like a smart computer program, our immune systems learn as we go. We may have learned to deal with our mother's environment using our mother's immunity during pregnancy. Gradually, as we are weaned away from our mother's breast milk, our immune systems learn to stand on their own—to different degrees.

Once we have weaned away from our mother's immune responses, our immune system will mix the learning of our mother's recognition systems with our own. For example, our immune system, should it be healthy, may recognize that it does not need to respond in the same way our mother might have reacted. Our mother may have had allergies to certain environmental inputs, but our immune system could well also learn to tolerate those inputs in a more balanced way—ridding our body of those invaders without an allergic response.

In allergic rhinitis, foreigners identified as harmful will initially access the body via the mouth, nasal cavity, skin and/or eyes. There are four general facilities—or strategies—the healthy immune system's utilizes to recognize and keep foreigners out. Let's look at each.

Non-specific Immunity

The first layer of defense is called non-specific because it provides a barrier that doesn't differentiate well between the good and bad guys. This general defense utilizes a network of physical and biochemical barriers that work synergistically to block just about anything potentially threatening from getting into the body.

The barrier structures include the ability of our body to shut down its orifices. We can close our eyes, mouths, noses and ears to prevent foreigners from entering the body. Our skin is also a barrier. Within and around these lie further defenses: Nose hairs, eyelashes, tongue, tonsils, ear hair, pubic hair and hair in general are all designed to help screen and filter invaders before they enter the body.

These barrier structures utilize the body's refined autonomic systems, which automatically respond to even the slightest indication that there may be a threat to the body. For example, if there is a little smoke in the room, the eyes will become more watery to protect the eyes from the smoke.

Nearly every one of the body's passageways is also equipped with tiny cilia, which block but also assist the body in evacuating invaders by brushing them out. These cilia move rhythmically, sweeping back and forth, working caught pathogens outward with their undulations.

The surfaces of most of the body's orifices—including the mouth, nasal cavity, sinuses, esophagus, stomach and intestines—are also covered with mucous membranes. These thin liquid membrane films contain a combination of biochemicals (also called *mucin*) as well as immune cells, immunoglobulins and colonies of probiotics. While these immune cells and probiotics utilize other immune strategies, the mucin provides a non-specific barrier. Mucin contains biochemicals such as mucoproteins, glycoproteins, glycosaminoglycans, glycolipids, and various enzymes. These are designed to deter, stick to, alter and even break down foreigners.

The digestive tract is equipped with a similar type of sophisticated defense technology. Should any foreigners get through the lips, teeth, tongue, hairs, mucous membranes and cilia, and sneak down the esophagus and through the sphincter, they must then contend with the digestive fire of the stomach. Within a healthy stomach, this mucosal membrane also contains gastrin, peptic acid and hydrochloric acid that together maintain a pH of around 2.0. This is typically enough acidity to kill or significantly damage many toxins and pathogenic bacteria.

Unfortunately, many of us mistakenly weaken this protective stomach acid by taking antacids or acid-blockers. In this case, the stomach's ability to neutralize pathogens will be handicapped.

Humoral Immunity

The second layer of immune defense takes place when foreign entities (toxins, food molecules or pathogens) gain access to the body. "Humoral" originates from *"the body's humours,"* which Hippocrates and other Greek physicians used to describe the body's different physiological regions and tissue mechanisms. Allergies are most often humoral responses.

The humoral immune system involves a highly technical strategic attack that first identifies the invader's weaknesses, followed by a precise and immediate offensive attack to exploit those weaknesses.

The body can draw from more than a billion different types of antibodies, macrophages and other immune cells to execute specific attack plans. As an immune cell scans a particular invader, it may recognize a particular biomolecular or behavioral weakness within the toxin or pathogen. Upon recognizing this weakness, the immune system will devise a unique plan to exploit this weakness. It may launch a variety of possible attacks, using a combination of specialized B-cells (or B-lymphocytes) in conjunction with specialized antibodies—the immunoglobulins.

Cruising through the blood and lymph systems, the humoral system's antibodies and/or B-cells can quickly sense and size up foreigners. Often this will mean the antibody will lock onto or bind to the foreigner to extract and confirm critical molecular information. This process will typically draw upon the identity databases held within certain helper B-cells that recognize and memorize foreigners and their molecular vulnerabilities. In other words, the humoral immune system will either devise or draw from a memorized strategy for breaking down and ridding the body of particular invaders.

As mentioned, the specific vulnerability of the foreigner is typically revealed by its molecular structures or cell membrane structures. Each foreigner will be identified by these unique structures, called antigens. The B-cell then reproduces a specific antibody designed to record and communicate that information to other B-cells through biochemical signaling.

This allows for a constant tracking of the location and development of antigens.

Meanwhile, the B-cell's antibodies will lock on to the epitope of the antigen. This "locking on" is also called *binding*. When the antibody binds or locks on to a foreign molecule, inflammatory mediators such as histamine, prostaglandins and leukotrienes are released. This stimulates a systemic detoxification process, as we will discuss further.

An active humoral response can immediately produce a thickening of the mucosal membranes. This is seen in nasal congestion and watery eyes. Watery eyes—or conjunctivitis—results from an inflammatory response that swells up and clogs the tear ducts that drain the fluids in the eye. When the fluids can't drain, they can gush over the eyelids, causing the watery eyes often seen with rhinitis.

Cell-Mediated Immunity

The third defense process used by the immune system is the cell-mediated immune response. This also incorporates a collection of smart white blood cells called T-cells. T-cells and their surrogates wander the body scanning the body's own cells. They are seeking cells that have become infected or otherwise have been damaged by foreigners. Infected cells are typically identified by special marker molecules (also called antigens) that typically sit atop infected cell membranes. These cell antigens have particular molecular arrangements that signal to the roving T-cells that damage has occurred within the cell, or the cell is otherwise compromised.

Once a damaged cell has been recognized by the T-cell system, the cell-mediated immune system will launch an inflammatory response against the cell and its tissue system. This response will typically utilize a variety of cytotoxic (cell-killing) T-cells and helper T-cells—also called Th-cells. These immune cells will often directly kill the damaged cell by inserting toxic chemicals into it. Alternatively, they might send signals into the damaged cell, switching on the cell's own self-destruct mechanism.

The reader may wonder why this would be important to allergic rhinitis. T-cells also carefully scan the body's membrane cells, including those epithelial and submucosal cells that make up the sinuses, nasal region, eyes, mouth and throat. If the T-cells pick up that cells have been compromised somehow, they will stimulate an immune response against these cells. This immune response results in an inflammatory reaction within these regions. The type of inflammatory reaction is directly related to the invader and T-cell helpers, as we'll discuss further.

An inflammatory response of T-cells and T-cell helpers can greatly damage the tissues of that region. This is intentional, because the T-cells typically destroy cells that have been compromised. In other areas of the body, inflammation can cause arthritis, heart disease and a variety of other problems. In the nasal cavity, this T-cell inflammatory response can result in the swelling of those tissues, and the thickening of the mucous membranes that line those tissues. And if bacteria or other pathogens have infected the cells of the sinuses, this T-cell invasion can produce the inflammation of sinusitis.

Probiotic Immunity

The fourth and essential type of immune response takes place among the body's colonies of probiotics. The human body houses trillions of beneficial and harmful bacteria and yeasts at any particular time. When beneficial bacteria are in the majority, they can constitute up to three-quarters of the body's immunity. This takes place both in an isolated manner and in conjunction with the rest of the body's immune and digestive systems.

About one hundred trillion bacteria live just in a healthy body's digestive system—about 3.5 pounds worth. The digestive tract contains about 400-500 different bacteria species. About twenty species make up about 75% of the population. Many of these are our resident strains, which attach to our intestinal walls and swim within our intestinal mucosal membranes.

Healthy nasal cavities, oral cavities, sinuses and bronchial airways can also contain hundreds of probiotic species. Most people do not realize this, nor do they incorporate it into their health strategies.

These airway probiotics swim within the mucosal linings of those cavities. Here, they help stop foreigners, break down invaders, and in general, guard the castle.

Probiotics are critical to the body's recognition of foreign molecules. Remember the DNA memory system mentioned earlier? Well, probiotics also contain DNA, and this DNA have also cataloged the environments, foods and intruders our ancestors consumed and worked around for thousands of generations. If an incoming element is recognized by a probiotic as being typical of its historical environment, there is no problem. But if the molecules or microorganisms appear foreign or threatening, the healthy probiotic system will signal the immune system to launch an inflammatory response—while the probiotics launch their own responses to help get rid of the foreigners.

In other words, probiotic colonies work alongside and cooperatively with the body's immune system to organize strategies to prevent toxins and pathogenic microorganisms from harming the body.

Probiotics communicate and cooperate with the immune system through complex signaling systems. Probiotics utilize cytokine and immunoglobulin communication processes. These will stimulate T-cells, B-cells, macrophages and NK-cells with smart messages that coordinate specific immune responses. They can also activate phagocytic cells directly to mobilize an intelligent toxin-removal response.

Using this communication, probiotics can activate cell-mediated responses and humoral responses. Probiotics also organize and police the body's mucosal barrier mechanisms.

Probiotics can also quickly identify harmful bacteria or fungi overgrowths, and work directly to eradicate them. This process may or may not directly involve the rest of the immune system. Or the rest of the immune system may act in a supportive manner by breaking up and escorting intruders out after they are killed by our probiotics.

Probiotics produce many biochemical substances that kill and break down molecules and microorganisms. They also help digest food, and release biochemicals and nutrients that are healthy to the body.

For example, lactic acids produced by *Lactobacillus* and *Bifidobacteria* species set up the ultimate pH control in the gut to repel antagonistic organisms and other foreigners. These include a hydrogen peroxide complex called lactoperoxidase. They also include acetic acids, formic acids lipopolysaccharides, peptidoglycans, superantigens and heat shock proteins. These inhibit challengers to ultimately benefit the airways.

Probiotics police the mucosal membranes of the sinuses and respiratory tract. These membranes can easily become infected from a variety of viruses, bacteria and fungi. As we'll discuss further in detail, probiotics battle these infective microorganisms.

Some infective microorganisms are pretty smart. For example, pathogenic bacteria have been shown to stimulate the hypothalamus into increasing cortisol (hydrocortisone) production by producing more corticotropin-releasing hormone. This extra cortisol production—like cortisone—has the effect of suppressing populations of lymphocytes geared up for removing the bacterial infections and suppressing inflammation. This allows these crafty pathogen populations to grow unencumbered.

There is a lot of subtle intelligence going on within the body's biotic systems. For example, scientists now know that allergic children have different probiotic colonies and populations than do healthy children (Ozdemir 2010). Allergic children will also typically have insufficient colonies of probiotics.

Probiotics secrete a number of key nutrients crucial to their hosts' (our body) immune system and metabolism, including B vitamins pantothenic acid, pyridoxine, niacin, folic acid, cobalamin and biotin, and crucial antioxidants such as vitamin K. Research is increasingly finding that these critical nutrients are often lacking in modern society. The reason, of course, is the destruction of these important probiotic species within our intestines.

Probiotics also help the break down (or police the break down) of food molecules into useable nutrients. This is the case for the lactose in milk. Probiotics produce lactase, an enzyme that breaks down lactose into smaller, digestible sugars. The lack of this enzyme (and those probiotics) also causes people to become lactose intolerant.

Probiotics also produce antimicrobial molecules called bacteriocins. *Lactobacillus plantarum* produces lactolin. *Lactobacillus bulgaricus* secretes bulgarican. *Lactobacillus acidophilus* can produce acidophilin, acidolin, bacterlocin and lactocidin. These and other antimicrobial substances equip probiotic species with territorial mechanisms to combat and reduce pathologies related to *Shigella, Coliform, Pseudomonas, Klebsiella, Staphylococcus, Clostridium, Escherichia* and other infective genera. Furthermore, antifungal biochemicals from the likes of *L. acidophilus, B. bifidum, E. faecium* and others also significantly reduce yeast outbreaks caused by the overgrowths of *Candida albicans* (Shahani *et al.* 2005).

Furthermore, probiotics will specifically stimulate the body's own immune system to attack pathogens. For example, scientists from Finland's University of Turku (Pessi *et al.* 2000) gave nine atopic dermatitis children *Lactobacillus rhamnosus* GG for four weeks. They found that serum cytokine IL-10 levels specific to the infection increased following probiotic consumption.

In another study (Gill *et al.* 2001), the probiotic *Bifidobacterium lactis* HN019 (or a placebo) was given to 30 healthy elderly volunteers (average age 69 years old) for nine weeks. They found that the probiotic group had significantly greater levels of helper T-cells (CD4+), activated (CD25+) T-cells, and natural killer T-cells. The probiotic strengthened their immune response in general, and stimulated the production of communication cytokines.

The research confirming the role that probiotics play within the immune system is impeccable, consistent and undeniable. We will cover some of this research in this text, but for a more complete review of the research and practical application of probiotics, see the author's book, *Probiotics: Protection Against Infection.*

For now, let's discuss the other players among the body's immune system, and their relationships with allergic hypersensitivity.

The Immune Cells

The immune system is composed of a number of different cells, and most are referred to as white blood cells or leukocytes. There are at least five different types of white blood cells. Each is designed to identify and target specific types of antigens (or allergens). Most are also involved, either directly or indirectly, in the allergic rhinitis flare-up.

Once an antigen/allergen is identified, these immune cells will initiate an attack specific to the condition of the body and the weakness of the antigen: Generally, the weaker the condition of the body's immunity, the more systemic the response. The stronger the body's immune system is relative to the threat of the antigen, the more localized (and less systemic) the response will be. This is the reason why a high white blood cell count in a blood test will indicate that the body is fighting a big infection or toxin relative to its immune strength.

We might compare this to being bit by red ants as we walked by an anthill. The only reason the ants bit is because we threatened their ant colony and queen. The size of our foot was very large relative to the proximity of the anthill. If we were walking by a few of the same soldier ants further away from the anthill, being bit would be far less likely. They wouldn't feel as threatened because we weren't close enough to their ant colony and queen.

In the same way, the immune system kicks into high gear when it is most vulnerable. In the face of a less-threatening intruder, a strong immune system would not need to launch a full scale attack. It could easily take care of the invasion by less drastic means, and with fewer white blood cells. If the attack was a lethal virus, on the other hand, then even the strong immune system will kick into high gear and launch a systemic immune response.

The main types of white blood cells are lymphocytes, neutrophils, basophils, eosinophils, monocytes and macrophages. Each WBC plays an important role in the inflammatory process. WBCs are the body's immune response soldiers. They tackle invaders head on.

Monocytes

Monocytes are like the Neolithic ancestors of the attack soldiers. After being produced in the bone marrow, monocytes differentiate into either macrophages or dendrite cells. The macrophages are particularly good at engulfing and breaking apart pathogens. Dendritic cells are interactive cells that stimulate certain responses. They may, for example, isolate and present antigens to B-cells or T-cells. Dendritic cells also stimulate the production of those special communication proteins called cytokines.

Lymphocytes (T-cells and B-cells)

Lymphocytes are identification cells that code and target specific invaders. The primary lymphocytes are the T-cells (thymus cells) or B-cells (bone marrow cells). These cells and their specialized communication proteins work together to strategically attack and remove invaders. Then special memory helper cells memorize the strategy in preparation for a future invasion.

All white blood cells are initially produced by stem cells within the bone marrow. Following their release, T-cells undergo further differentiation and programming within the thymus gland. B-cells undergo a similar process of maturity before release from the spleen. Both T-cells and B-cells circulate via lymph, bloodstream, intercellular tissue fluids and mucosal membranes. Both T-cells and B-cells have a number of special types, including memory cells and helper cells to identify and memorize invaders.

B-cells, as mentioned earlier, look for foreign or potentially harmful antigens moving freely. These might include allergens, toxins or microbes. Once identified, B-cells will stimulate the production of a particular type of antibody, designed to bind to and neutralize the foreigner.

Most B-cells are monoclonal, which means they will adjust to a specific type of invader. Once they set up for a particular type of invader, they can make "clones" or copies that will launch an attack and bind to the foreigners.

Most B-cells are investigative and surveillance oriented. Once activated, they launch a variety of inflammatory responses through the release of mediators such as histamine and leukotrienes. This process allows them to interrupt foreigner activity. B-cells circulate throughout the body and mucosal membranes, but some are more specialized. For example, B-cells called plasma B-cells circulate and scan the bloodstream.

Other B-cells specialize in processes. For example, memory B-cells record and communicate previous invasions for future attacks.

B-cells typically work through legions of antibodies called immunoglobulins, which bind to antigens. As we'll discuss in a minute, immunoglobulins may be attached to B-cells or they may circulate independently. Once they bind to an antigen, inflammatory mediators are released.

T-cells, on the other hand, are oriented toward the body's own cells, and those foreigners who get mixed up with the cells' metabolism. This means T-cells are focused upon internal cellular and tissue systems. In other words, when antigens are absorbed by or invade cells, the cell becomes damaged. T-cells look for these damaged cells. Once found, the damaged cells will be destroyed or crippled by the T-cells.

There are different types of T-cells. Each is programmed in the thymus to look for different types of problems that may occur inside cells, such as infection or toxin contamination. This programming in the thymus is governed by the major histocompatibility complex, or MHC. See the Thymus section for more on MHC programming.

Many T-cells respond to a pathogen that has invaded the cell by destroying the cell itself—this is the killer T-cell. It does this by inserting deadly (cytotoxic) chemicals into the cell or by submitting instructions into the cell to kill itself. Cell death is called apoptosis, and those T-cells capable of killing our cells are called cytotoxic T-cells (*cyto* refers to cells) and natural killer T-cells.

T-cells work through the communication cytokines to relay instructions and information amongst the various T-cells. Prominent cytokine communications thus take place between helper T-cells, natural killer cells and cytotoxic T-cells.

The initial screening of an infected cell by a helper T-cell utilizes an electromagnetic scanning system not unlike the scanning systems airports use to screen passengers before they get on a plane.

Delta-gamma T-cells are especially good at scanning. Delta-gamma T-cells are sensitive to specific receptors on intestinal cell membranes. This means that delta-gamma T-cells are key to the body's tolerance to environmental inputs, as these molecules scan for foreign contact.

Helper T-cells record and communicate database information on previous invaders. They also communicate previous immune responses, memorize current ones, and pass on strategic information regarding the progress of pending attack plans.

The helper T-cell scan initially surveys the cell's membrane for indications of either microbial infection or some sort of genetic mutation due to a virus or toxin. This antigen scan might reveal invasions of chemical toxins or allergens that may have intruded or deranged the cell. The scanning helper T-cell immediately communicates the information by releasing their tiny coded protein cytokines. These disseminate the information needed to coordinate macrophages, NK-cells and cytotoxic T-cells.

B-cells and T-cells often coordinate their strategies through what is called *T-cell-dependent responses*. In other words, the B-cell is activated through cytokines after a T-cell recognizes the antigen among tissues.

Most healthy cells contain tumor necrosis factor or TNF—a self-destruct switch of sorts. When signaled from the outside by a cytotoxic T-cell, TNF will initiate a self-destruct and the cell will die. These "death-switch" communications will typically utilize intermediary cytokines.

Under some circumstances, entire groups of cells or tissue systems may become damaged. Macrophages may be signaled to cut off the blood supply to these deranged or infected cells.

The two primary helper T-cell types are the Th1 and the Th2. The Th1 T-cell focuses on the elimination of bacteria, fungi, parasites, viruses, and similar types of invaders. The Th2 cells stimulate more B-cell activity. This focuses the immune response toward antibody and allergic responses. The Th2 cells are thus explicitly involved in the inflammatory responses of allergic reactions. The Th2 response coordinates with the B-cell-antibody system that releases histamine, leukotrienes and other inflammation mediators.

This is important to note on a number of levels. Research has revealed that stress, chemical toxins, poor dietary habits and a lack of sleep tend to suppress Th1 immune responses and elevate Th2 levels. With an overabundance of Th2 cells in the system compared to Th1, the body is prone to respond more strongly to allergens and toxins, causing hypersensitive responses like hay fever and asthma. This is also why people under physical or emotional stress often also have hives, psoriasis and other allergic-type responses.

A weakening of the immune system leans the Th1/Th2 balance towards the Th2 inflammatory pathways, which encourages a heightened allergic response. Probiotics lean the Th1/Th2 balance the other way.

This was illustrated by Japanese researchers (Odamaki *et al.* 2007). Yogurt with *Bifidobacterium longum* BB536 or plain yogurt was given to 40 patients with allergies to Japanese cedar pollen. After 14 weeks, the peripheral blood mononuclear cell counts of the patients indicated that the probiotics reduced the body's Th2 counts and activity.

Granulocytes: Mast cells, neutrophils, basophils and eosinophils are called granulocyte white blood cells because they release "granules" of inflammatory mediators. They circulate within the bloodstream and lymph, looking for abnormal behavior or toxins. Once they identify a problem or are stimulated by B-cells and immunoglobulins, they will initiate a process to clean up the area. This invokes inflammation and allergic symptoms, as they work to remove toxins.

The significant players in this cleaning process are the inflammatory mediators histamines and leukotrienes. The release of these mediators in the case of an allergen is provoked by signals produced during the binding between immunoglobulins and allergen epitopes. Upon being signaled, the granulocytes release the mediators through their cell membranes.

Histamines are the primary mediators that produce allergy symptoms, while leukotrienes tend to produce asthmatic responses. Both are released by basophils, neutrophils and eosinophils. All four granulocytes also release prostaglandins and other inflammatory mediators.

As we'll discuss further, eosinophils in particular are associated with systemic inflammation, allergies and airway hypersensitivity.

Meanwhile, neutrophils have been associated with infective microorganisms, while basophils and mast cells have been associated with allergens. Furthermore, scientists have determined that neutrophils will also release histamine within the airways during allergic asthmatic responses (Xu *et al.* 2006).

Eosinophils have been linked to airway membrane leaking. Research indicates that a protein mediator released by eosinophils called eosinophil cationic protein (ECP) accumulates in the bronchial tissues of asthma sufferers and among the nasal tissues of allergic rhinitis sufferers. ECP has also been implicated in damaging bronchial and airway epithelial cells—stimulating more inflammation.

We'll discuss ECP in more detail in a bit.

The Communicators

Cytokines are the communicators that allow different immune cells to exchange information. Probiotics also utilize cytokines to communicate with the immune system's cells.

Well-known cytokines include interleukin (IL), transforming growth factor (TGF), leukemia inhibitory factor (LIF), tumor necrosis factor (TNF) and others. They are further complicated by the fact that there are multiple versions of each. In allergic rhinitis, for example, the more active cytokines include IL-17 and TGF-beta.

There are five basic types of cell communication: intracrine, autocrine, endocrine, juxtacrine and paracrine. Let's break these down:

Autocrine communication takes place between two different types of cells. This message can be a biochemical exchange or an electromagnetic signal. The other cell in turn may respond automatically by producing a particular biochemical or electromagnetic message. We might compare this to leaving a voicemail on someone's message machine. Once we leave the message, the machine signals that the message has been received and will be delivered. Later the machine will replay the message. The immune system uses this type of autocrine message recording process to activate T-cells. Once the message is relayed, the T-cell will respond specifically with the instructed activity.

Paracrine communication takes place between neighboring cells of the same type, to pass on a message that comes from outside of the tissue system. Tiny protein antennas will sit on cell membranes, allowing one cell to communicate with another. This allows cells within the same tissue system to respond in a coordinated manner.

Juxtacrine communications take place via smart biomolecular structures. We might call these structures relay stations. They absorb messages and pass them on. An example of this is the passing of inflammatory messages via immune cell cytokines.

Intracrine communication takes place within the cell. Or an external message may first be communicated into the cell through an antenna sitting on the cell's membrane. Once inside the cell, the message will be communicated around cell's organelles to relay internal metabolic responses.

Endocrine communication takes place between endocrine glands and individual cells. The endocrine glands include the pineal gland, the pituitary gland, the pancreas, adrenals, thyroid, ovary and testes. These glands produce endocrine biochemicals, which relay messages directly to cells.

Endocrine communications stimulate a variety of metabolic functions within the body. These include growth, temperature, sexual behavior, sleep, glucose utilization, stress response and so many others. One of the functions of the endocrine glands relevant to allergic rhinitis is the production of inflammatory regulators such as cortisol, adrenaline and norepinephrine. These coordinate and initiate instructions that inhibit and regulate inflammatory processes. Cortisol, for example, shunts or slows the inflammatory cascade by inhibiting interleukin. This is critical to the body's ability to control and contain the allergic immune response.

Another endocrine mediator to consider is GRMFT. The interleukin-blocking effects of cortisol are interfered by another element produced by the immune system—primarily in the spleen. This is called glucosteroid response-modifying factor, or GRMFT. GRMFT interferes with cortisol's effects, allowing the progress of inflammation to continue with little control.

Cytokines Associated with Allergies

T-cell cytokines: Allergic T-cell-dependent responses utilize specific cytokines to develop and communicate response strategies. Clusters of differentiation (CDs) are influenced and stimulated by cytokines.

For example, in studies of asthmatic children with and without food allergies, lymphocyte level changes indicated inflammatory responses. Among the allergic asthmatics, CD25+ T-cells and CD23+ B-cells increased substantially after food challenges in a classic inflammatory immune response. They also found that the inflammatory cytokines interleukin-4 (IL-4) and IL-5 were significantly increased among the asthmatics after the food challenges (Krogulska *et al.* 2009).

B-cell cytokines: Allergic responses tend to utilize the CD19+CD5+ stimulated cytokines to connect with B-cells. Then the allergen-oriented B-cells stimulate the allergic response by utilizing the IL-10 cytokine (Noh *et al.* 2010).

The Inflammation Mediators

Our body's immune system launches inflammatory cells and factors to rid toxins, heal injury sites and prevent bleed-outs. This process is stimulated by inflammatory mediators like histamines, leukotrienes and prostaglandins.

Histamine

Histamine is produced by mast cells, basophils, eosinophils and neu-trophils as mentioned earlier. Histamine is a key mediator in the allergic response because it serves to increase the permeability of blood vessels. This in turn allows white blood cells to spread out among the various tissues of the body. As the WBCs spread, they attack any kind of foreign molecule and produce widespread metabolic waste matter and dead cell parts—also referred to as phlegm.

As blood vessel permeability increases, the mucous membranes also become fuller with blood, lymph and fluid. These combined elements—increased waste matter and more blood, lymph and fluid—produce the congestion and excess fluids that fill up the eyes, nose and throat.

When histamine is released, it will bind with specific receptors located around the body. Depending upon the type of receptor, histamine will elicit a particular response.

For example, the H1 histamine receptor—located within the tissues of the lungs, muscles, nerves, sinuses, and other tissues—stimulates the allergic responses of congestion, watery eyes, sinusitis, skin rashes and so on. H2 receptors lie in the digestive tract and control the release of stom-ach acids and intestinal mucous membrane. H3 receptors stimulate the nervous system and the flow of neurotransmitters. H4 receptors involve the directional function of immune cells and intestinal cells.

While histamine might be considered a "bad guy" in the allergic proc-ess, histamine is actually critical for maintaining the body's natural equilib-rium. Histamine helps establish homeostasis among cells and tissue sys-tems. Without histamine to negotiate and communicate balance and imbalance, the body would have little reference to respond to threats. When histamine is released in abundance, this will often stimulate all four receptor systems, putting the body into hyper-vigilance mode. In this mode, the body can respond on a hair-trigger.

Leukotrienes

Leukotrienes are molecules that identify problems and stimulate the immune system. They are particularly important in allergic rhinitis. Leukotrienes pinpoint and isolate problems in the airways that require repair. Once they pinpoint the site of repair, one type of leukotriene will initiate inflammation, and others will assist in maintaining the process. Once the repair process proceeds to a point of maturity, another type of leukotriene will begin slowing down the process of inflammation.

This smart signalling process takes place through the biochemical bonding formations of these molecules. Leukotrienes are paracrines and autocrines. They are paracrine in that they initiate messages that travel from one cell to another. They are autocrine in that they initiate messages that encourage an automatic and immediate response—notably among T-cells, engaging them to remove bad cells. They also help transmit messages that initiate the process of repair through the clotting of blood and the patching of damaged tissues.

Leukotrienes are produced from the conversion of essential fatty acids (EFAs) by an enzyme produced by the body called arachidonate-5-lipoxygenase (sometimes called LOX). The central fatty acids involved of this process are arachidonic acid (AA), gamma-linolenic acid (GLA), and eicosapentaenoic acid (EPA). These are obtained from the diet. Lipoxygenase enzymes produce different types of leukotrienes, depending upon the initial fatty acid.

A key consideration with regard to fatty acids and leukotrienes is that the leukotrienes produced by arachidonic acid stimulate inflammation, while the leukotrienes produced by EPA halt inflammation. The leukotrienes produced by GLA, on the other hand, block the conversion process of polyunsaturated fatty acids to arachidonic acid. This means that GLA also reduces the inflammatory allergic response.

Prostaglandins

Prostaglandins are also produced through an enzyme conversion from fatty acids. Like leukotrienes and histamine, prostaglandins are mediators that transmit inflammatory messages to immune cells. Their messaging is either paracrine or autocrine. Prostaglandins, especially PGE2, are critical parts of the allergic process. They also initiate a number of protective sequences in the body, including the transmission of irritation and pain, and some of the swelling from inflammation.

Prostaglandins are produced by the oxidation of fatty acids by an enzyme produced in the body called cyclooxygenase—also called prostaglandin-endoperoxide synthase (PTGS) or COX. There are three types of COX, and each converts fatty acids to different types of prostaglandins. The central fatty acid that causes inflammation is arachidonic acid.

COX-1 converts AA to the PGE2 type of prostaglandin. COX-2, on the other hand, converts AA into the PGI2 type of prostaglandin.

The primary messages that prostaglandins transmit depend upon the type of prostaglandin. Prostaglandin I2 (also PGI2) stimulates the widening of blood vessels and bronchial passages, and pain sensation within the nervous system. In other words, along with stimulating blood clotting, PGI2 signals a range of responses to assist the body's wound healing at the site of injury.

Prostaglandin E2, or PGE2, is altogether different from PGI2. PGE2 stimulates the secretion of healthy mucosal membranes within the airways, stomach, intestines, mouth and esophagus. It also decreases the production of gastric acid in the stomach. This combination of stabilizing mucous and lowering acid production keeps healthy stomach cells from being damaged by our gastric acids and the acidic content of our foods. This is one of the central reasons NSAID pharmaceuticals cause gastrointestinal problems: They interrupt the secretion of this protective mucous in the stomach.

This means that the COX-1 enzyme instigates the process of protecting the stomach, while the COX-2 enzyme instigates the process of inflammation and repair within the body. The COX-2 process, along with the LOX process, often lies at the root of allergic airway responses.

Cyclooxygenase also converts ALA/DHA and GLA to prostaglandins. Just as lipoxygenase converts ALA/DHA and GLA to anti-inflammation leukotrienes, the conversion of ALA/DHA and GLA by cyclooxygenase produces prostaglandins that either block the inflammatory process or reverse it.

The arachidonic acid conversion process that produces prostaglandins also produces thromboxanes. Thromboxanes stimulate platelets in the blood to aggregate. They work in concert with platelet-activating factor or PAF. Together, these biomolecules drive the process of clotting the blood and restricting blood flow. This is good during injury healing, but the inflammatory process must also be slowed down as the injury heals. We'll discuss the role of fatty acids in the inflammatory process in more detail later on.

Acetylcholine

Acetylcholine is a key neurotransmitter within the nervous system, but it also stimulates muscle cells to contract. Most of our muscle cell membranes contain acetylcholine receptors. Once acetylcholine binds with one of these receptors, sodium channels on the cell membrane are opened. This is critical to the contraction of the smooth muscles that wrap around the lungs.

In other words, when acetylcholine production is increased, the smooth muscles around the airways are prone to tighten. In other muscles around the body, this is simply called *cramping*. But when it happens to the airways, it produces a tightening of the airways.

Epinephrine

Epinephrine counteracts the action of acetylcholine by blocking the acetylcholine receptors on the muscle fiber cells. This helps the muscles relax, and let go of the airways.

For this reason, epinephrine is often administered to a person who is having a severe allergic response or anaphylaxis. Epinephrine is also called adrenaline.

The body also naturally produces epinephrine in the adrenal glands. In a balanced body, epinephrine production is readily available to balance acetylcholine's effects. Assuming healthy adrenals and with a ready supply of amino acids phenylalanine and tyrosine, the body will readily make epinephrine as needed.

Epinephrine is a highly selective mediator, because while it relaxes the airway smooth muscles, it also constricts the blood vessels and stimulates the fight or flight physiology within the body. In other words, epinephrine is a stress mediator that helps the body respond to danger. When a person is constantly under stress, the adrenal glands may become overactive. This overactivity wears out the adrenal glands with continual stress.

This type of overload upon the adrenal glands is also called *adrenal exhaustion*. There is a significant amount of evidence showing that many hay fever sufferers have adrenal exhaustion caused by continual stress.

The bottom line is that these inflammatory mediators are not the bad guys. This type of isolation approach is what causes medications that target mediators to have so many side effects. The body is a smart organism, and it operates through a series of checks and balances that provide intelligent surveillance and appropriate response. The strategy of trying to shut off one process or another (such as histamines with antihistamines) with a single chemical can temporarily halt a few symptoms. But this cannot reverse or heal a condition caused by imbalance: It can only produce more imbalances, which in turn produces side effects.

The Immunoglobulins

Immunoglobulins are proteins that attach to the epitopes of antigens. They are released into the blood or lymph by B-cells; or they remain on the surface of B-cells—enabling B-cells to attach to antigens. The immunoglobulins secreted and released into the blood and lymph are called *antibodies*. Those that stay attached to the B-cells are called *surface immunoglobulins* (sIg) or *membrane immunoglobulins* (mIg).

Secretory immunoglobulins (SIgA) typically line the mouth, nose, ears, tears and digestive tract. Here they scan for pathogens or toxins that might harm the body. SIgAs look for initial tissue entry antigens. Most IgAs are SIgAs.

The other immunoglobulins reside mostly in the blood, lymph and among other tissues, targeting invasions within the body. Immunoglobulin Ds (IgDs) sense early microbial infections and activate macrophages. IgEs attach to early entry foreign substances (such as environmental toxins) and stimulate the release of inflammatory mediators—associated with most allergic responses. IgGs cross through membranes, responding to growing and maturing pathogens within the body. IgMs are focused on earlier (but not new) intrusions into cells and body fluids that have yet to grow enough to garner the attention of IgGs. The main immunoglobulin categories are summarized in the table below:

Type	Where located	Targets
IgA	Mucous membranes, saliva, tears, breast milk, intestines (SIg), also blood, lymph (serum IgA)	Prevent initial entry of toxins, allergens and microorganisms into tissues and bloodstream
IgD	Blood/lymph/B-cells	Detect initial microbial infections
IgE	Blood/lymph/B-cells/some mucous membranes, intestines	Detect early toxins and allergens in blood and tissues
IgM	Blood/lymph/B-cells	Detect infections and toxins that begin to damage cells
IgG	Blood/lymph/placenta	Detect mature infections that have damaged cells and invaded tissues

Each of these general immunoglobulin categories contain numerous sub-types geared to different types of pathogens and toxins. Other immunoglobulin proteins also exist. Some of these aid macrophages and lymphocytes in identifying specific pathogens.

The status of the body's immunoglobulins indicates the immune system's strength and health. An immune system with a large number of IgAs (SIgAs and serum IgAs) and healthy mucosal membranes will typically be more tolerant of all foods, toxins and pathogens; because intruders will typically be taken out before they can access the body's bloodstream and tissue systems. On the other hand, high IgE counts indicate a hypersensitivity mode for allergens and/or other toxins. Likewise, high IgM and IgG levels indicate a past infection or toxicity that is being increasingly managed or tolerated.

For example, Italian researchers (Fuiano *et al.* 2010) studied 192 sensitized patients who were either symptomatic or asymptomatic to allergies. While both were sensitized to allergens, only those who were symptomatic had allergen-specific IgEs within the nasal region.

This means that not only does the allergic person need to be sensitized to an allergen: They also need to have an immune system that is hyper-reactive to that specific allergen.

A key element of the immunoglobulins is the CD glycogen-protein complex. Again, CD stands for *cluster of differentiation*. CDs are molecules that sit on top of immune cells to navigate and steer their behavior. They will sit atop T-cells, B-cells, NK-cells, granulocytes and monocytes, identifying threats and infected cells. They will also sometimes negotiate with and bind directly to pathogens. This allows the lymphocytes to proceed to strategically attack the intruder.

Clusters of differentiation are identified by their bindable molecular structure: This is also referred to as a ligand. The specific molecular arrangement (or CD number) will also match a specific type of receptor at the membrane of the cell or pathogen. Each CD number maintains a bonding relationship with a certain receptor structure on the cell to allow the accompanying immunoglobulin or lymphocyte to have interactivity with the pathogen. This gives the immunoglobulin or lymphocyte an access point from which to attack the perceived threat, and a coding vehicle to remember the invader later on.

Immunoglobulins and CDs are also tools probiotics utilize to define or influence appropriate responses for the immune system. Probiotics stimulate IgAs through CDs, for example, when they discover a pathogen has invaded the body's mucous membranes.

CDs are also utilized by probiotics to alert the immune system to intestinal cells and tissues that have been damaged by toxins, bacteria, or viruses. Probiotics signal back and forth with the immune system to maintain a check and balance system among the intestines. This signaling process can stimulate particular immune responses as needed.

The Thymus

One of the most important players in the immune system is the thymus gland. The thymus gland is located in the center of the chest, behind the sternum. The thymus is one of the more critical organs of the lymphatic system. Some have compared the thymus gland of the lymphatic system to the heart of the bloodstream.

The thymus gland is not a pump, however. The thymus activates T-cells and various hormones that modulate and stimulate the immune and autoimmune processes. The thymus converts lymphocytes called thymocytes into T-cells. These activated T-cells are released into the lymph and bloodstream ready to protect and serve. Within the thymus, the T-cells are infused with CD surface markers—which identify particular types of problematic cells or invading organisms. Their CD markers define the mission of that T-cell.

In other words, the thymus codes the T-cells with receptors that will bind to and damage particular cells or toxins. The types of cells or toxins they bind to or identify are determined by the *major histocompatibility complex*, or MHC determinant. During the process of converting thymocytes to T-cells, their CD receptors are programmed with MHC combinations. This allows them to tolerate particular frailties within the body while attacking what the body considers to be true invaders (Kazansky 2008).

Therefore, it is the MHC that gives the T-cell the ability to identify the difference between the "self" and "non-self" parts of the body. A non-self identification will produce an immunogen—a factor that stimulates an immune response. Once the immunogen is processed, it stimulates the inflammatory cascade.

The thymus gland develops and enlarges from birth. It is most productive and at its largest during puberty. From that point on, depending upon our diet, stress and lifestyle, our thymus gland will shrink over the years. By forty, an immunosuppressed person will often have a tiny thymus gland. In elderly persons, the thymus gland is often barely recognizable. For many people today, the thymus is practically non-functional.

Throughout its productive life, the thymus gland processes T-cells with the appropriate MHC programming. If the thymus gland is functioning, it will continue to produce T-cells with MHC programming that reflects the body's current status. Its constantly updated programming will accommodate the various genetic changes that can happen to different cells around the body as we age and adapt to our changing environment. With a shrunken and non-functioning thymus, however, its ability to reprogram T-cells with a new MHC—enabling them to identify the body's cells that have adapted—is damaged. The T-cells will have to keep working from the old MHC programming. This means the T-cells will not be able to properly identify "self" versus "non-self" within the body's cells.

With this progression of thymus weakness and the resulting lack of updated MHC determinants, T-cells can begin attacking the body's own tissues instead of becoming tolerant to conditions created by new environments.

The Liver

The liver is the key organ involved in detoxification and the production of a variety of enzymes and biochemicals. The liver produces over a thousand biochemicals the body requires for healthy functioning. The liver maintains blood sugar balance by monitoring glucose levels and producing glucose metabolites. It manufactures albumin to maintain plasma pressure. It produces cholesterol, urea, inflammatory biochemicals, blood-clotting molecules, and many others.

These functions are major reasons for the liver's involvement in allergic sensitivities.

The liver sits just below the lungs on the right side under the diaphragm. Partially protected by the ribs, it attaches to the abdominal wall with the falciform ligament. The *ligamentum teres* within the falciform is the remnant of the umbilical cord that once brought us blood from mama's placenta. As the body develops, the liver continues to filter, purify and enrich our blood. Should the liver shut down, the body can die within hours.

Interspersed within the liver are functional fat factories called stellates. These cells store and process lipids, and fat-soluble vitamins such as vitamin A. The also secrete structural biomolecules like collagen, laminin and glycans. These are used to build some of the body's toughest tissue systems.

Into the liver drains nutrient-rich venous blood through the hepatic portal vein, together with some oxygenated blood through the hepatic artery. A healthy liver will process almost a half-gallon of blood per minute. The blood is commingled within cavities called sinusoids, where blood is staged through stacked sheets of the liver's primary cells—called hepatocytes. Here blood is also met by interspersed immune cells called *kupffers*. These kupffer cells attack and break apart bacteria and toxins. Nutrients coming in from the digestive tract are filtered and converted to molecules the body's cells can utilize. The liver also converts old red blood cells to bilirubin to be shipped out of the body. Filtered and purified blood is jettisoned through hepatic veins out the inferior vena cava and back into circulation.

The liver's filtration/purification mechanisms help clear our body of various infections and chemical toxins. After hepatocytes and kuppfer cells break down toxins and pathogens, the waste is disposed through the gall bladder and kidneys.

The gall bladder channels bile from the liver to the intestines. Recycled bile acids combine with bilirubin, phospholipids, calcium and cholesterol to make bile. Bile is concentrated and pumped through the bile duct to the intestines. Here bile acids help digest fats, and broken-down toxins are (hopefully) excreted through our feces. This is assuming that we have healthy intestines containing healthy mucous membranes, barrier mechanisms and probiotic colonies.

The liver's filtration and breakdown process is critical to allergic hypersensitivity. If a toxin gets through the mucous membrane IgAs, the liver gets a crack at removing it. If the liver is not able to metabolize and neutralize the molecule, the body must rely upon the inflammatory immune response to rid the body of the intruder.

In other words, a strong liver will reduce the body's dependence upon the inflammatory processes for removing intruders. If the hepatocytes and kuppfer cells are abundant and resilient, they can remove many toxins. Should those cells be damaged or overwhelmed by too many toxins at once, their ability to break down and remove toxins is diminished.

Subsequently, research and a wealth of clinical evidence tell us that the liver is damaged by an overload of chemical toxins. This is the very reason that alcohol (ethanol) and pharmaceuticals can cause liver disease: These chemicals overload and damage the liver's hepatocytes and kupffers.

The liver's health is specific to allergic hypersensitivity. Research from Britain's South Manchester University Hospital (Hassan 2008) investigated the reason why aspirin-allergic asthma patients continue to have asthma even though aspirin is avoided. They found that at the outset of the disease, aspirin stimulates an oxygen radical of arachidonic acid, 12-HPETE, which stimulates 5-lipoxygenase of leukotriene B4s. These mediators launch macrophages that produce the allergic and asthmatic episodes. They also noted that the liver antioxidant glutathione peroxidase, assuming healthy levels, can reduce 12-HPETE synthesis—halting or slowing the inflammatory process.

Today our diets, water and air are full of many other chemicals that produce the same result. These include plasticizers, formaldehyde, heavy metals, hydrocarbons, DDT, dioxin, VOCs, asbestos, preservatives, artificial flavors, food dyes, propellants, synthetic fragrances and more. Every additional chemical makes the liver work harder to break down these toxic chemicals.

Frankly, most modern livers—especially those in urban areas of industrialized countries—are now overloaded and way beyond their natural capacity. What happens then? Generally, two things. First, the hepatocytes collapse from toxicity, stimulating an overactive immune system—due to the additional burdens placed upon it. Second, liver exhaustion leads to increased susceptibility to infectious diseases such as viral hepatitis. The combined result is a downward spiraling of immunosuppression and hypersensitivity.

Liver disease—where one or more lobes begin to malfunction due to the death or dysfunction of hepatocytes—can result in a life-threatening emergency. Cirrhosis is a common diagnosis for liver disease, often caused by years of drinking alcohol or taking prescription medications combined with other toxin exposures. During this progression towards cirrhosis, the sub-functioning liver can also produce symptoms such as jaundice, high cholesterol, gallstones, encephalopathy, kidney disease, arthritis, clotting problems, heart conditions, hormone imbalances and many others. As cirrhosis proceeds, it results in the massive die-off of liver cells, and the subsequent scarring of remaining tissues, causing the liver to begin to shutdown.

As liver cells weaken and die, their enzymes flood the bloodstream. Blood tests for AST and ALT enzymes reveal this weakening of the liver.

We must therefore closely monitor the quantity and types of chemicals we put into our body. Eliminating preservatives, food dyes and pesticides in our foods can be done easily by eating whole organic foods. We can eliminate exposures to many environmental toxins mentioned above by simply replacing them with natural alternatives.

A number of herbs specifically help strengthen the liver. These include goldenseal, dandelion, milk thistle and others.

Probiotics play an important role in liver disease. When pathogenic bacteria get out of control in the intestines, they can overload the liver with endotoxins—their waste products. This bombardment of endotoxins onto the liver produces a result similar to alcohol or pharmaceuticals: During the putrefaction of pathogenic bacteria such as *Clostridium* spp., for example, one of the endotoxins is ammonia. Like ethanol, ammonia is toxic to the liver (Shawcross *et al.* 2007). Ammonia from pathogenic bacteria in the gut damages the liver, in other words.

Because probiotics reduce pathogenic bacteria, probiotics prevent these metabolites and endotoxins from reaching the liver. For example, researchers from the G.B. Pant Hospital in New Delhi (Sharma *et al.* 2008) gave 190 cirrhosis patients a combination of probiotics or placebo for one month. The probiotic group experienced an average of 52% improvement in cirrhosis symptoms and significantly lower blood ammonia levels.

The Adrenal Glands

The body's two adrenal glands are part of our endocrine system. The outer cortex is stimulated by master hormones from the hypothalamus and pituitary gland, while the inner medulla is stimulated directly with nerves. The adrenals produce an array of hormones, many of which are related to inflammation and stress. For example, the medulla produces epinephrine and norepinephrine, and other catecholamines. From our discussions earlier, we know that epinephrine (as well as norepinephrine) relaxes the smooth muscles of the airways, as part of a response to stress—more specifically in a fight-or-flight response. This allows the lungs to breathe deeper, so the body can respond and act faster.

At the same time, epinephrine constricts the blood vessels, increases the heart rate, increases metabolism, dilates the pupils and halts digestive activity, all in an effort to respond to stress.

This multi-organ adrenal stress response might seem beneficial to breathing, but it also comes with a double-edged sword: Epinephrine and norepinephrine also significantly slow the rate of mucous secretion by submucosal glands that feed the mucous membranes.

This effect can be quite dangerous to the highly-stressed individual, because the decreased mucous membranes also leave our airways and digestive tracts open to irritation from toxins and environmental changes. This, in fact—as we discussed in the mucous membrane section—is the likely reason why cold air (and other environmental changes) will often stimulate a rhinitis response in some hypersensitive people.

The adrenal glands also produce important steroids. Two of the most critical are cortisol and aldosterone.

Aldosterone is a mineralocorticoid. It and other mineralocorticoids are produced by the outer shell, or cortex, of the adrenal gland. Aldosterone and other mineralocorticoids adjust and balance the body's levels of sodium, potassium and other minerals; as well as alter sodium ion channels among various cells. These are critical to the acid/alkaline status of the blood and body fluids, and the body's ability to remove toxins through the kidneys, sweat glands and colon. Aldosterone is a critical player in maintaining blood pressure as well, and this affects the performance of respiration.

Aldosterone also balances the use and availability of cortisol and cortisone, because many aldosterone receptors also bind with cortisol. This means that a balanced production of these two steroids (cortisol is a glucocorticoid) by the adrenals is critical to the detoxification efforts of the body—along with the body's ability to balance inflammation with efforts to heal the body.

This means that adrenal glands stimulated by stress and inflammation repeatedly for long periods begin to wear down. As mentioned earlier, this is called adrenal exhaustion. When this happens, the adrenal glands produce inconsistently deficient levels of theses critical steroids and catecholamines.

This creates drastic imbalances within the body, affecting the body's ability to respond to toxins, inflammation and stress. Signs of adrenal exhaustion include being easily fatigued, overstressed and over-reactive to toxins and environmental changes. Adrenal exhaustion is typical in an immune system over-responding with hyper-inflammation: A condition typical of allergic metabolism.

The Intestines

What do the intestines have to do with allergic rhinitis? Plenty.

The health of the airways has everything to do with a healthy intestinal system. This relates to three mechanisms:

> ➢ When the body's mucous glands are not producing enough healthy mucous, the digestive system and the respiratory system are both affected.

> ➢ When the intestinal villi and their junctions are damaged by toxins and mucosal membrane deficiencies, endotoxins (the poop and byproducts of pathogenic bacteria) can get into the bloodstream—overloading the immune system and producing hypersensitivity.

> ➢ Increased intestinal permeability can also allow toxins and food macromolecules—undigested proteins—into the bloodstream. Once within the blood, an IgE allergic response can result. This can be expressed by an allergic rhinitis episode.

The intestines utilize non-specific, humoral, cell-mediated and probiotic immunity to protect intestinal tissues from larger peptides, toxins and invading microorganisms.

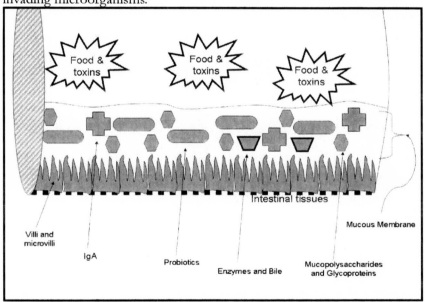

The Healthy Intestinal Wall

This is all packaged nicely into what is referred to as the *intestinal brush barrier.* The intestinal brush barrier is a complex mucosal layer of mucin, enzymes, probiotics and ionic fluid—sealed by villi separated by tight junctions.

The intestinal mucosal membrane forms a protective surface medium over the intestinal epithelium. It also provides an active transport mechanism for nutrients. This mucosal layer is stabilized by the grooves of the intestinal microvilli. It contains glycoproteins, mucopolysaccharides and other ionic transporters, which attach to amino acids, minerals, vitamins, glucose and fatty acids—carrying them across intestinal membranes into the bloodstream.

This mucosal layer is policed by billions of probiotic colonies, which help process and identify incoming food molecules; excrete various nutrients; and control toxins and pathogens.

The breakdown of the mucosal membrane causes it to thin. This depletes the protection rendered by the mucopolysaccharides and glycoproteins, probiotics, immune IgA cells, enzymes and bile. This thinning allows toxins and macromolecules that would have been screened out by the mucosal membrane to be presented to the intestinal cells.

In its entirety, the brush barrier is a triple-filter that screens for molecule size, ionic nature and nutrition quality. Much of this is performed via four screening mechanisms existing between the intestinal microvilli: tight junctions, adherens junctions, desmosomes, and colonies of probiotics.

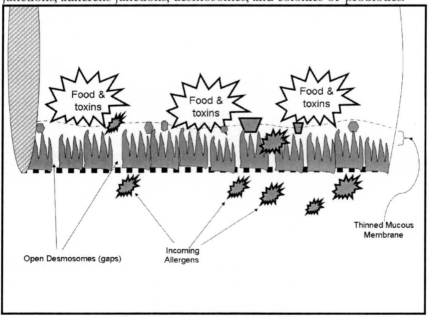

The Unhealthy Intestinal Wall

The tight functions form a bilayer interface between cells, controlling permeability. Desmosomes are points of interface between the tight junctions, and adherens junctions keep the cell membranes adhesive enough to stabilize the junctions. These junction mechanisms together regulate permeability at the intestinal wall.

This mucosal brush barrier creates the boundary between intestinal contents and our bloodstream. Should the mucosal layer chemistry become altered, its protective and ionic transport mechanisms become weakened, allowing toxic or larger molecules to be presented to the microvilli junctions. This contact can irritate the microvilli, causing a subsequent inflammatory response. Research illustrates that this is a contributing cause of irritable bowel syndrome (IBS).

Should the mucous membrane thin, these mechanisms become irritated, producing an inflammatory immune response that causes the desmosomes and tight junctions to open. These gaps allow toxins and food macromolecules to enter the blood, producing systemic inflammation.

Oral and Nasal Mechanisms

We find all four of the immune response systems active within the upper respiratory tract, which includes the oral cavity, the nasal cavity, the pharynx, and parts of the pleural cavity. This is because the mouth and nose provide one of the most accessible areas for microorganism and toxin entry.

Most of these systems require good probiotic colonies to be successful, however. This is because probiotics are not only part of the body's second line of defense: Their presence is essential for our immune response systems to work effectively.

The nasal cavity contains a labyrinth of various canals and chambers that allow any air we breath to have plenty of contact with the mucous membranes and cilia of the nasal cavity. Here the air is warmed and humidified as we breathe in. The mucous membrane-lined passageways of the nasal cavity, along with the larynx and pharynx warm and moisten the air. They are our body's natural humidifier system.

It was only until recently that researchers became aware that these various chambers housed more than mucous membranes and immune cells: They also hosted legions of probiotic colonies.

These probiotic colonies are saturated throughout the mucous membranes of a healthy person. Here they not only help identify invaders, but they launch their own attacks against invading bacteria, viruses and fungi. They will also translocate between different nasal cavities, the mouth, the pharynx and other regions of the respiratory system.

The ribs, or *concha*, of the nasal region also house olfactory bulbs. The bulbs are also positioned at the top of the sinus cavity on either side of the septum. They sit at the epithelium mucosa surface, where nerve fibers connect to the bulbs. These nerve fibers sense the waveform and polarity of odorous molecules traveling in the air as they interface with the mucosa of the nasal cavity. These 'odor-packets' traveling within and around gas and air molecules stimulate the nerves in the olfactory bulbs.

These olfactory nerve bulbs, collectively called the *vomeronasal organ* or VNO (also *Jacobson's organ*), may be stimulated on a more subtle level by pheromones. Pheromones carry and exchange information through the environment between living organisms. Pheromones have been shown to stimulate sexual and reproductive responses among animals, plants and insects. There is some debate as to whether humans also exchange pheromones. While humans have anatomical VNOs—known for pheromone exchanging in animals—significant nerve conduction has yet to be confirmed physically. The assumption has been that without obvious VNO nerve pathways there would be little chance of information conduction to responsive endocrine or cognitive mechanisms.

Consideration might be given to the work of a well-respected rhinologist Dr. Maurice Cottle. Dr. Cottle, known for his contribution towards the development of the electrocardiogram, invented a diagnostic machine in the mid-twentieth century called the *rhinomanometer*. Dr. Cottle wrote two books on the subject of rhinomanometry, and was a professor and head of Otolaryngology at the Chicago Medical School. Dr. Cottle was able to diagnose a number of ailments in other parts of the body simply by measuring the swelling or shrinking of the tissues and the airflow through the VNO.

The delicate turbinate membranes are more than mucous membranes: They are erectile, with thousands of tiny receptors. They respond to stimulation just as do other erectile regions. The turbinate erectile receptors respond to and coordinate airflow with the rest of the body. Clinical evidence demonstrated that Dr. Cottle's machine could accurately diagnose coronary heart disease, for example.

In reviewing the connection between oral bacteria and cardiovascular disease, we find that the inflammatory response stimulated by pathogenic bacteria through the NK-kappa mechanism could also be at the root of the phenomena Dr. Cottle observed. An inflamed turbinate and sinus area would likely be the result of an imbalance of pathogenic and probiotic bacteria, causing not only cardiovascular inflammation as has been shown in modern research, but the swelling of nasal membranes like the turbinates. This indicates a possible connection between turbinate responses and the body's various probiotic communications.

56

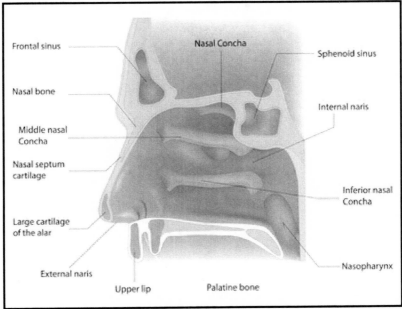

The Nasal Cavity and Sinuses (Illustration: Miro Kovacevic)

We can see the nasal concha and the turbinate regions from the rendering above. At the nasal entry, we see the atrium, then the middle and inferior meatus, separated by the concha inferior. Above these two chambers lie the septum meatus and then the sphenoidal sinus. These different passageways provide plenty of traps and filters to catch foreign particles and microorganisms. They also provide many warm and moist nesting areas for our probiotics.

Once foreigners such as pollens are trapped, these colonies of probiotics—along with our immunoglobulins and various immune cells—corner them and break them apart. Ths requires a vibrant, active immune system and strong probiotic colonies.

Within the mouth, we also find various chambers and traps. The entire oral cavity is lined with mucous membranes that help trap microorganisms. Instead of cilia, however, the mouth has teeth, gums, and a big wet, scaly tongue to trap and block particles and microorganisms. Once trapped, these foreigners can be taken apart or controlled by probiotics and immune cells in a healthy body. We can see all these crevices in the rendering on the next page.

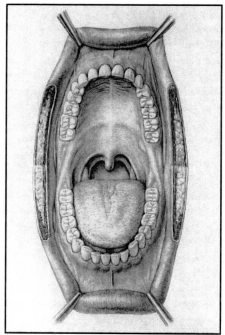

The Oral Cavity

Along with probiotic colonies, all of the oral, nasal and pharangeal mucosal membranes house immune cells and immunoglobulins Here we find legions of IgA and B-cells—along with IgE to a relative degree. These scan and identify particles and microorganisms that might slip past our probiotics and enter the body. When they discover potentially harmful organisms or toxins, they lock onto them in an attempt to break them apart and rid them from the body before they can penetrate our tissues.

Thus, we find, between the probiotics and immune cells, a 'drag net' of sorts within the oral and nasal cavities.

Under the tongue are salivary glands. They produce amylase. Amylase is an enzyme that breaks down starches into simple sugars. This is one reason the body is driven to eat starches. Taking our time and chewing a little more liquefies our food and mixes them with important mucus and enzymes. The mouth contains several parotid glands, located in the jaw behind the ears. As we chew, the parotid glands are stimulated, releasing B-cells and T-cells into the blood, mucous and lymphatic pathways. This gives the oral cavity and mouth more protection against foreigners that might try to slip in through our drag net.

58

Nasal Neuropeptides and the Stuffy Nose

The mechanisms for the stuffy, runny and blocked nose have eluded many physicians and researchers over the years. Recent evidence points to a collection of neuropeptides located among the sensory, sympathetic and parasympathetic nerves. These include tachykinins, substance P, neurokinin A, calcitonin gene-related peptides (CGRPs), vasoactive intestinal peptides (VIPs), and neuropeptide Y (NPY). These are primarily sensory neuron peptides.

Some of these are interactive. Substance P, for example, increases vascular permeability. Vascular permeability opens the tissues to a greater release of immune factors that cause inflammation. Substance P also stimulates the release of inflammatory factors. This has been seen following the binding to the neurokinin-1 receptor (NK-1R). Together, these responses increase swelling and restrict airflow.

Tachykinins are sensitive to allergen exposure, and they can stimulate the release of substance P. The other neuropeptides like VIPs and CGRPs can act similarly, but stimulating inflammation and vascular permeability.

Inflammation, Breathing and Atmospheric Pressure

A worsening of asthma and hay fever has been linked with what is termed *airway remodeling*. This is when the lungs become altered due to a continuing inflammatory event. Chronic allergic rhinitis has been shown to cause upper airway remodeling (Salib and Howarth 2003).

Healthy lung capacity is critical to immune function.

The average lung capacity of an adult is about 6,000 cubic centimeters. When we breathe unconsciously while relaxed, we might breathe 500 to 700 cc in and out. Typically, about 1,200 to 1,500 cc will be left in the lungs during this breathing. If we should completely exhale, we have the capacity to move out 4,800 to 5,200 cc of air.

These numbers indicate that we can utilize our lungs better than we typically do. With better breathing, we will not only bring more oxygen into the bloodstream. We will also push out more stale, acidic carbon dioxide as we exhale. This lowers the carbolic acid and carbon dioxide levels in the bloodstream, allowing more oxygen to associate with hemoglobin. By bringing in more oxygen, more acidified H+-hemoglobin is replaced with oxygenated, alkalized hemoglobin.

There are various negative consequences of having poorly oxygenated blood and/or highly acidic, carbon dioxide-rich blood. Poorly oxygenated blood can cause or contribute to brain fog, poor memory, fatigue, restlessness, nervousness, anxiety, indigestion, and cardiovascular diseases such as *cor pulmonale,* hypertension, atherosclerosis and angina. Poorly oxygenated blood can lead to low healing response, poor sleep, and increased inflammatory response—all of which are linked to a poor immune function, hypersensitivity and allergic rhinitis.

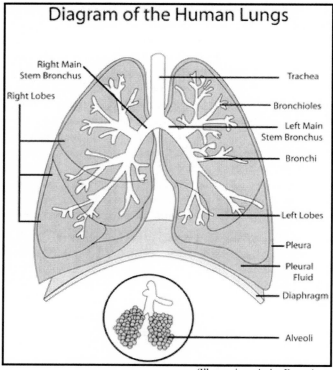

(Illustration: Anita Potter)

Oxygen is by far the greatest nutrient of the body. Oxygen is vital to the immune system and the operation of every organ and tissue system. Oxygen also helps provide an environment among the blood and tissues less hospitable to bacterial or viral invasion. With a poor supply of oxygen—whether caused by poor breathing habits, restricted airways, or contaminated air—the body operates at less than maximum efficiency, leaving our bodies subject to tissue damage resulting from acidosis.

Sinus, Nasal and Airway Mucosal Membranes

As we've mentioned, mucous membranes cover just about every region of internal epithelial cells. The mucosal membrane is a thin layer of glycoproteins (mucin), mucopolysaccharides, special enzymes, probiotics, immune cells and ionic fluid.

The ionic fluid provides a transporter medium, which escorts a host of elements back and forth between the epithelial cells and the surface of the mucosal membrane. These elements include chloride ions, sodium ions, oxygen, nitrogen, carbon dioxide, hydrogen carbonate and others.

Some of these—such as the sodium, bicarbonate and chloride ions—provide the transport mechanisms into the cells and tissues of the skin surfaces. These travel through openings or pores among the cells, attached to nutrients, oxygen and other elements—transporting them in, in other words.

Certainly, the body is choosy about what kinds of elements it will allow into the bloodstream and the epithelial cells of the airways. There are countless toxins, microorganisms, debris, allergens and other foreigners the body wants kept out of epithelial tissues.

So just how does the body keep these invaders out? The short answer is the mucosal membrane (along with cilia) that covers the cells. As mentioned, this membrane contains a host of immune cells. These include immunoglobulins such as IgA, B-cells, T-cells and others that are looking to trap foreigners before get any further. Once they find a foreigner, they will take it apart using a one of many immune system strategies.

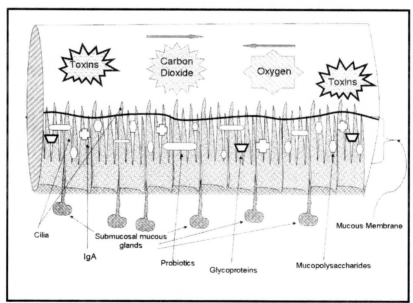

Airway Mucosal Membranes and Cilia

Probiotics are also an important part of this "wall" of protection. Tiny protective probiotic bacteria also inhabit a healthy nasal mucosal membrane. Like the immune system, these bacteria are trained to protect their territory. If an invading microorganism enters the mucosal membrane, they will face the immune system's process of breaking them down to be escorted out of the body.

The bottom line regarding the mucosal membrane is that the health of this membrane is crucial to the health of the airways. This is one of the prime reasons the airways become hypersensitive in the first place: Their protective coating has been diminished or altered in such a way that allows potential allergens to intrude upon the epithelial cells—stimulating the inflammatory response relating to IgE.

A healthy chemistry among our mucosal membranes buffers and calms immune response. Healthy mucosal membranes contains IgA that prevent foreigners from accessing our tissues and becoming marked as allergens by the immune system.

The mucosal membrane will also help transport components such as corticosteroids from the adrenals to squelch inflammatory immune responses. In other words, a healthy mucosal membrane is *calming* to the airways.

At birth, the mucosal membranes within our airways are raw and not well developed. Gradually, as probiotics begin to colonize the airways—along with the sinuses, mouth and intestines—the mucosal membrane begins to mature. This maturity, as we'll discuss in detail, requires a host of nutrients as well as stimulated probiotic populations in order to populate the mucosal membranes. As this colonization occurs, the body's epithelial cells and mucous glands provide a balance of chemistry.

We might compare this to how oil lubricates an engine. In a well-maintained car, good motor oil will be circulated through the rods and cylinders. The oil doesn't just allow the steel parts to move with minimal friction: The motor oil also helps keep the engine clean, and prevents dirt and other contaminants from clogging up the system. Imagine what would happen if a car were to run without oil for a few miles. The engine would surely seize up, and likely would break down completely.

While this is a crude example, there are several elements that are consistent. The lubrication ability of the mucous membrane allows the airways to remain flexible and responsive. This is accomplished by what is called the surfactant quality of mucous. This effectively reduces the surface tension of the epithelial cells.

Then there is the transporter mechanism. The mucous membrane utilizes this surfactant quality and ionic capabilities to transport nutrients among the airways epithelial cells, and the functional structures of the airways. It also transports toxins out of the area—assuming a healthy mucosal membrane.

Should this transport mechanism not be functioning properly, the respiratory airways will become laden with a thickened, toxic mucous.

Instead of the mucous membrane keeping the area clean, the mucous itself becomes toxic to the airways, because it has not only thickened, but it has also become full with toxins.

This thickened mucous membrane is typical in hyperreactive inflammatory conditions that include hay fever, sinusitis, colds, bronchitis, asthma and pneumonia.

Mucous is secreted by tiny mucous glands that lie within goblet cells scattered throughout the epithelia of the bronchi, sinuses and other parts of the airways. They are called goblets because they are shaped like little goblet glasses, except their upper surface extends out in tiny fingers called microvilli. In fact, goblet cells within the airways are practically identical with the villi and microvilli of the intestines. They function almost identically with respect to their production of mucous.

The goblet cells and villi both produce mucin through a process of contraction and glycosylation within the Golgi apparatus of the sells. This glycosylation of proteins produces the glycoproteins that are the mainstay in mucin.

The mucosal goblet cells of the respiratory tract are also similar to the gastric cells of the stomach and duodenum. The difference here is that these produce mucous fed by the pyloric glands in addition to the highly acidic gastrin. As we'll be discussing more at length throughout the remainder of the text, this similarity between the goblet cells, the villi and the gastric/pyloric cells facilitates an understanding of the mystery of GERD-related allergic asthma.

The mucous membrane fluids can also become dehydrated if the ions that open the pores are blocked. Here the pores may be blocked due to an imbalance of ion chemistry in the sub-mucosal membrane. Tests have shown that chlorine and bicarbonate anions stimulate the opening of the pores that bring liquids into the mucous membrane. The mucin proteins produced by the submucosal membrane glands have to be diluted with these ion fluids to give the mucous membrane the right balance of stickiness and fluidity.

In dehydrated mucosal membranes, the mucous is too thick and not viscous enough to provide its surfactant and transport functions.

In addition, exposure to allergens, toxins, cold air and any number of other triggers can stimulate the production of mucous by the goblet cells. In a healthy body, this stimulates the quick removal of the toxin or invader, as the excess mucous is swept out by the cilia.

However, should the body be immunosuppressed or otherwise overwhelmed by an invasion, the goblet cells will over-produce mucous, which can swamp the cilia along with dead cell parts and toxins. When the cilia are drowning in mucous, they cannot do their job. The lack of mucous transport, combined with the need to remove a toxin, is typically accompanied by the constriction of the airways, which may protect the airways from more toxins, but also further prevents the toxins in the mucous from being cleared out.

This combination of nasal airway constriction and mucous overload is the mainstay of the allergic rhinitis episode.

This link between the health of the mucosal membranes of the sinuses and airways was illustrated in research from Britain's National Heart and Lung Institute and the Imperial College and Royal Brompton Hospital (Niimi *et al.* 2004). Here 50 patients with chronic coughing, concurrent with asthma, postnasal drip, rhinitis and gastroesophageal reflux related to the coughing were studied. The pH and chloride levels of their condensed breathing were measured. The researchers found that compared with healthy subjects, all of these coughing patients had significantly lower pH levels, indicating an acidic condition among their mucous membranes, along with lower chloride levels. The researchers concluded: *"The epithelial lining fluid of patients with chronic cough has a reduced pH and reduced chloride levels which could contribute to the enhanced cough reflex."*

The Cilia

The cells of the airway passages are also equipped with microscopic hairs called cilia (see previous and next drawing). The cilia act like tiny brooms: They undulate towards the exits—the nasal cavity, mouth and pharynx. The little hairs "sweep" out the mucous, together with toxins and dead cell parts caught in the mucous membrane.

The ciliary hairs lining the airways beat rhythmically with the expansion and release of the lungs. This expansion and contraction increases the mucous surfactant as well.

Should toxin particles remain airborne, they will also likely be moved out through breathing and rhythmic ciliary hair undulations in healthy airways.

The membrane and ciliary hair move in slow waves—very similar to what we see among kelp beds as they move with undulating ocean waves. This wave-like action of the ciliary hairs acts as an effective transport system.

This transport mechanism—the clearing of toxins and cell parts out of the area by the cilia—is called the *mucociliary clearance apparatus*. This is a self-cleaning system of the airways: Should these 'automatic sweepers' become caught in the thick mucous of a toxin-rich and/or ionically imbalanced mucous membrane—they become ineffective.

The mucociliary clearance apparatus explains how we will gather an accumulation of phlegm within the throat and sinuses. Most of us clear our throats or blow our noses without a second thought. Little do we realize that much of that phlegm is the result of the cilias' self-cleaning undulations that sweep out toxins and mucous. This sweeping mechanism also helps prevent polluted air and particles from being absorbed into our blood. Those particles not tossed out with the breath or mucous get phagotized (broken down) and swept out. Or they may be transported to the blood or lymph and escorted out of the body through the colon, urinary tract or sweat glands.

However, should the mucosal fluid not be healthy and ionically balanced, thickened mucous will build up within the mucosal membrane. This will overwhelm and in effect *drown* the ciliary hairs—making them far less effective for removing toxins and toxin-rich mucous.

The cilia are stabilized by being seated in a thin pool of thicker mucous, with another layer of thinner mucous on top. The thinner mucous towards the surface of the mucous membrane allows the hairs to undulate faster near and at the surface of the mucous membrane.

It is essential that these cilia are healthy, vibrant, and free of toxin-debris. This is why, as we'll explain, that tar and soot from smoking and pollution can wreck such havoc on the airways. The tops of the cilia—and mucous—become jammed up with this gummy residue.

Cilia must also have a warm temperature in a moist atmosphere. Should cold, dry air get into the passages where these sensitive airway cilia dwell, they may shut down or become uncoordinated. The ultimate temperature for productive cilia is about 98.6 degrees F with 100% relative humidity. This doesn't mean that outdoor temperatures must be that. A temperature of nearly 100 degrees F with 100% humidity would be unbearable.

Rather, the cilia are kept warm and moist by the combination of body heat, the warming of the air as it travels through the sinus turbinates, and the secretion of warm mucous in the airways.

The Inflamed Airways

The inside lumen (or opening) of the nasal airways in a healthy person allows air to pass through unobstructed. In a person with allergic rhinitis, the epithelia tissues of the turbinates, sinuses and nasal cavity are in an inflamed condition. In this condition, even the slightest trigger can set off complete blockage of the nasal cavity and sinuses.

The evidence that allergic rhinitis is an inflammatory response is overwhelming. Leucocytes such as eosinophils, mast cells and neutrophils all release inflammatory mediators during allergic rhinitis. Histamine content, released through the IgE process described earlier is rampant. These, however, are only the byproducts of the inflammatory condition. They might be compared to seeing smoke rising from the fire.

Non-infection oriented inflammation typically involves reactive oxygen species. Indications of this during allergic rhinitis and asthmatic hypersensitivity include higher levels of superoxide anions and thiobarbituric acid-reactive products (TBARs), as well as hydrogen peroxide availability. One of the main inflammatory byproducts of superoxide reactions is hydrogen peroxide (H_2O_2).

Research has illustrated that people with allergies and asthma generate more hydrogen peroxide when they breathe out than do others. In one study, asthmatics breathed out 26 times the levels of hydrogen peroxide as healthy subjects did. They also found that TBAR levels among asthmatics were 18 times the levels of healthy subjects (Antczak *et al.* 1997).

Inflammatory eosinophils—evidenced by higher eosinophil cationic protein (ECP) levels—are also significantly higher in allergic rhinitis. This was confirmed in tests among 16 patients with allergic rhinitis at Turkey's Ege University School of Medicine (Sin *et al.* 1998). The researchers found that the higher ECP levels corresponded with high levels of allergic IgE levels in the bloodstreams of the patients.

While ECP can damage microorganisms such as viruses and bacteria, it can also damage and inflame our body's cells. ECP damages cells by forming pores in the cell membranes, which produce a type of cell membrane damage called *permeability alteration.*

The build-up of ECP is simply part of an inflammatory process that occurs as part of an immune response: A deranged immune response that medical researchers call hyperreactivity.

An Overview of Inflammation

Most people think of inflammation as bad. Especially when they hear that allergies involve inflammation.

Rather, inflammation simply coordinates the various immune players into a frenzy of healing responses. This is a good thing. Let's imagine for a moment that we cut our finger pretty badly. First, we feel pain—letting us know the body is hurt. Second, we will probably notice that the area has become swollen and red. Blood starts to clot around the area. Soon the cut stops bleeding. The blood dries and a scab forms. It remains red, maybe a little hot, and hurts for a while. As the healing proceeds, the cut is soon closed up, leaving a scab with a little redness around it. The pain soon stops. The scab falls off and the finger returns to normal—almost like new and ready for action.

Without this inflammatory process, we might not even know we cut our finger in the first place. We might keep working, only to find out that we had bled out a quart of blood on the floor. Without clotting, it would be hard to stop the bleeding. And without some continuing pain, we would be more likely to keep injuring the wound, preventing it from healing.

Were it not for our immune system and inflammatory process slowing blood flow, clotting the blood, scabbing and cleaning up the site, our bodies would simply be full of holes and wounds. Our bodies simply could not survive injury.

The probiotic and immunoglobulin immune system work together to deter and kill particular invaders—hopefully before they gain access to the body's tissues. Should these defenses fail, they can stimulate the humoral immune system in a strategic attack that includes identifying antigens and recognizing their weaknesses. B-cells and probiotics coordinate through the stimulation of immunoglobulins and clusters of differentiation (CDs).

This progression also stimulates an activation of neutrophils, phagocytes, immunoglobulins, leukotrienes and prostaglandins. Should cells become infected, they will signal the immune system using paracrines located on their cell membranes. Once the intrusion and strategy is determined, B-cells will surround the pathogens while T-cells attack any infected cells. Natural killer T-cells may secrete chemicals into infected cells, initiating the death of the cell.

Leukotrienes immediately gather in the region of injury or infection, and signal to T-cells to coordinate efforts in the process of repair. Prostaglandins initiate the widening of blood vessels to bring more T-cells and other repair factors (such as plasminogen and fibrin) to the infected or injured site. Histamine opens the blood vessel walls to allow all these healing agents access to the injury site to clean it up.

Prostaglandins also stimulate substance P within the nerve cells, initiating the sensation of pain. At the same time, thromboxanes, along with fibrin, drive the process of clotting and coagulation in the blood, while constricting certain blood vessels to decrease the risk of bleeding.

In the case where the foreigner is an allergen, the inflammation process will also accompany an H1-histamine response. As mentioned earlier, histamine is primarily produced by the mast cells, basophils and neutrophils after being stimulated by IgE antibodies. This opens blood vessels to tissues, which stimulates the processes of sneezing, watering of the eyes and coughing. These measures, though sometimes considered irritating, are all stimulated in an effort to remove the toxin and prevent its re-entry into the body. As histamine binds with receptors, one of the resulting physiological responses is alertness (also why antihistamines cause drowsiness). These are natural responses to help the body and mind remain vigilant in order to avoid further toxin intake.

At the height of inflammation, swelling, redness and pain are at their peak. The T-cells, macrophages, neutrophils, fibrin and plasmin all work together to purge the allergen from the body and repair the damage.

As macrophages continue the clean up, the other immune cells begin to retreat. Antioxidants like glutathione will attach to and transport the byproducts—broken down toxins and cell parts—out of the body. As this proceeds, prostaglandins, histamines and leukotrienes are signaled to reverse the inflammation and pain process.

One of the central features of the normalization process is the production of bradykinin. Bradykinin slows clotting and opens blood vessels, allowing the cleanup process to accelerate. A key signalling factor is the production of nitric oxide (NO). NO slows inflammation by promoting the detachment of lymphocytes to the site of infection or toxification, and reduces tissue swelling. NO also accelerates the clearing out of debris with its interaction with the superoxide anion. NO was originally described by researchers as endothelium-derived relaxing factor (or EDRF)—because of its role in relaxing blood vessel walls.

The body produces more nitric oxide in the presence of good nutrition and lower stress. Probiotics also play a big role in nitric oxide production in a healthy body. Lactobacilli such as *L. plantarum* have in fact been shown to remove the harmful nitrate molecule and use it to produce nitric oxide (Bengmark *et al.* 1998). This is beneficial to not only reducing inflammation: NO production also creates a balanced environment for increased tolerance.

Low nitric oxide levels also happen to be associated with a plethora of conditions, including diabetes, heart failure, high cholesterol, ulcerative colitis, premature aging, cancers and many others. Low or abnormal NO production is also seen among lifestyle factors such as smoking, obesity, and environmental air pollution.

Cough Reflex

The cough reflex is complicated. Irritated sites in the airways and lungs stimulate coughing, but this is also attenuated by a neural cough center located within the brainstem and within the cerebral cortex, where coughing is often initiated, suppressed or modified by consciousness. The cough reflex is, as put by Dr. John Christopher, *"a result of nature's effort to expectorate mucous from the lungs, after which breathing becomes easier."*

In other words, the stimulus for chronic coughing is the build-up of inflammatory mucous. While incidental coughing might follow the inhalation of some smoke or other toxin, a chronic cough is stimulated by a build-up of this thickened mucous in the airways.

And why is there this build up of mucous? Because the immune system is undergoing the inflammatory process by flushing out broken-down cells, broken down toxins, and even live infections. This thickened mucous is like the composition of toilet water after a bowel movement: *it is full of crap*.

The Allergic Response

There are several kinds of hypersensitivity responses within the body. These might sound similar but they are actually different in many ways and yet share common traits. Let's review these:

Atopic Hypersensitivity

This response occurs when IgE antibodies bind to an allergen. Antigens include air pollutants, pollen, dust mite allergens, and dander. An allergen can also be any food the immune system has become sensitized to. When this binding between an antigen and IgE takes place, the bound IgE will set off the release of inflammatory mediators from white blood cells called mast cells, basophils and/or neutrophils. The mediators released by these immune cells include histamine, prostaglandins and leukotrienes. Depending upon the location and type of mast/basophil/neutrophil cells, these mediators can spark an inflammatory response within the airways, and/or other tissues, including the sinuses, skin, joints, intestines and elsewhere.

This response can be further broken down into two stages: sensitization and elicitation.

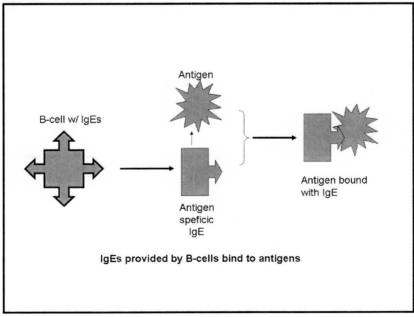

IgEs provided by B-cells bind to antigens

Sensitization: As illustrated on the previous page, the allergen sensitization process takes place when a potential antigen comes into contact with a type of immune cell called a progenitor B-cell. As part of their immune system responsibilities, these B-cells will break apart the allergen proteins into smaller parts—often called *epitopes*. These will become attached to hystocompatibility complex class II complex molecules.

The T-cell hystocompatibility complex is transferred onto the surface of the B-cell, which binds to a particular allergen. Once upon the B-cell surface, T-helper cells take notice of this foreign particle stuck to the B-cell. The T-helper cell cytokine CD4 receptors trigger a response, and this stimulates the production of the IgE immunoglobulins. These particular IgE immunoglobulins are now sensitized to the particular epitope of the antigen in the future.

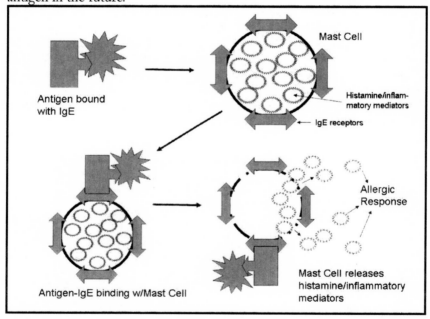

Elicitation: Once sensitized, the IgE associates with the specific IgE receptors that lie on the surface of the neutrophil, basophil or mast cells. Within these cells are packages called granules. The above diagram illustrates elicitation.

The granules are stock full of a variety of inflammatory mediators. The most notorious of these are the histamines and leukotrienes as we've mentioned. As the allergen-specific IgEs connect with the IgE receptors on these immune cells, the immune cells will release these inflammatory mediators into the bloodstream and lymph. This is what drives much of the symptoms of an allergic attack, including but not limited to watery eyes, blocked nose, scratchy throat, itchiness, sinusitis and others.

Cytotoxic Responses

In this type of immune response, antigens have penetrated the tissues, and the immune system is on a state of alert as it responds to kill these cells. This typically takes place through an antigen binding to IgG or IgM immunoglobulins in a delayed immune and inflammatory response. This response can happen concurrently to allergic responses; though it is most often a delayed response. It is this type of response that can cause an allergic episode that lasts over several days.

Should the red blood cells be involved in the antigen absorption, hemolysis (the destruction of red blood cells) and anemia (a lack of red blood cells) may result. These can in turn cause more severe allergic rhinitis responses.

Systemic Inflammation Responses

Systemic and chronic inflammation creates hypersensitivity of the airway passages due to the immune system being stressed and on high alert status. In this situation, the immune system is overloaded by infection(s), chemical toxicity, or a diet that constantly exposes the body to toxins. One or a combination of these effects generally produces a whole-body diseased state. In such a state, the body will overreact to an exposure. These triggers can be as simple as exercise, cold air, smoke or fragrances.

This type of systemic inflammatory status is evidenced by high C-reactive protein in the body. CRP levels are easily determined through blood analysis. We'll discuss some of the research that illustrates this later.

Immune Complex Responses

Here the allergen-bound antibody complex actually penetrates cell tissues and injures them. This can occur within the airway epithelial cells, intestinal cells, liver, or virtually anywhere around the body. Here the damage to the cells immediately stimulates the inflammatory response, regardless of whether there is an allergen trigger involved or not. Whatever is damaging the cells is considered a direct threat.

In some instances, these immune complexes can severely change alveoli permeability, vascular permeability and/or intestinal permeability, producing imbalances in respiration, circulation and digestion—sometimes even simultaneously.

This type of response is also often a delayed response, occurring hours or even a day or two after exposure to the allergen or trigger.

This alerted immune complex condition will also stimulate mast cells, basophils and/or neutrophils, resulting in continued degranulation of

71

histamine, prostaglandins and leukotrienes, which in turn produce ongoing allergic hypersensitivity.

Delayed T-Cell Responses

While the immune complex response may generate an immediate T-cell response once cells and tissues are damaged, a delayed T-cell response will occur over a period of time—as T-cells continue to destroy damaged airway cells. Here airway epithelial cells become damaged, and the T-cells are removing those damaged cells with an inflammatory response.

This type of response is the driving factor behind airway remodeling. In airway remodeling, the epithelial cell network that lines the airways become inflamed, damaged and chronically irritated. They are swollen and hyperreactive on an ongoing basis, in other words.

This same general condition can exist within the epithelial layers of many parts of the body. On the skin, this is seen as eczema. In the intestines, it is seen as colitis or Crohn's disease. In the sinuses, it is called sinusitis. In the urinary tract, it is called interstitial cystitis. In the stomach and lower esophagus, it is called GERD. Whether involving microorganisms or not, the irritation is the inflammatory hypersensitivity response.

This response is also often attributed to autoimmunity, which is explained as the immune system attacking healthy cells. This notion is incorrect, however, because the immune system is not attacking healthy cells. The immune system is removing cells that have been damaged. Once these epithelial cells are damaged, T-cells stimulate the immune response to clear out the damaged cells. In other words, our immune system is simply trying to do its job.

Airway Remodeling

Allergic asthma—especially for a young person—can cause the airways to undergo what is often described as remodeling. In airway remodeling, the bronchi and their mucosal membranes undergo structural changes. This typically means that the walls of our airways—made up of epithelial cells and cilia—become thicker. The smooth muscles surrounding our airways also become dense and thick—much as weight-lifting muscles can thicken. Our mucous membrane chemistry also changes, and the vascular-capillary system around our airways changes.

Airway remodeling is the primary reason given for the irreversibility of asthma. This is despite the fact that airway remodeling often is reversed, and many children with remodeled airways outgrow asthma. The basis for this is that epithelial cells live for a few weeks and then die, to be replaced by newly divided epithelial cells. Cells are also constantly recycling nutrients and fluids. This means that while the DNA of the new cells may respond similarly for a few generations, should the conditions change for these cells (including nutrition, mucous membrane health, environmental conditions and so on) they will adapt to the new conditions and gradually become healthy cells.

Probiotics and Inflammation

Yes, we did discuss probiotics earlier. But this section will specify the roles that probiotics play in the inflammatory process. They temper and balance the inflammation process, reducing hypersensitivity responses. This needs elaboration because this information is not readily considered in allergic rhinitis and hay fever.

Probiotics increase IgA levels and reduce IgE allergic response. Finnish scientists (Ouwehand *et al.* 2009) gave healthy elderly volunteers *Lactobacillus acidophilus* or a placebo. The probiotics improved anti-allergic IgA and PGE2 levels. The probiotics also improved spermidine levels—an enzyme involved in DNA synthesis. The researchers concluded that these improvements suggested increased mucosal and intestinal immunity among the probiotic group.

In a study of 105 pregnant women, University of Western Australia scientists (Prescott *et al.* 2008) found that *Lactobacillus rhamnosus* and *Bifidobacterium lactis* stimulated higher levels of cytokine IFN-gamma, higher levels of TGF-beta1, and higher levels of breast milk IgA. Plasma of their babies had lower CD14 levels, and greater CB IFN-gamma levels. These indicated that the probiotics strengthened immunity and moderated hypersensitivity.

Researchers from the Teikyo University School of Medicine in Japan (Araki *et al.* 1999) gave *Bifidobacterium breve* YIT4064 or placebo to 19 infants for 28 days. IgA levels significantly increased among the probiotic group.

Researchers from the Turku University Central Hospital in Finland (Rinne *et al.* 2005) gave 96 mothers either a placebo or *Lactobacillus rhamnosus* GG before delivery and continued the supplementation in their infants after delivery. At three months of age, immunoglobulin IgG-secreting cells among breastfed infants supplemented with probiotics were significantly higher than the breastfed infants who received the placebo. In addition, the non-hypersensitivity IgM-, IgA-, and IgG-secreting cell counts at 12 months were significantly higher among the breastfed infants who supplemented with probiotics, compared to the breastfed infants receiving the placebo.

Probiotics help modulate the inflammatory processes. In research from Poland's Pomeranian Academy of Medicine (Naruszewicz *et al.* 2002), scientists found that giving *Lactobacillus plantarum* 299v to 36 volunteers resulted in a 37% decrease in inflammatory F2-isoprostanes. Isoprostanes are similar to prostaglandins, formed outside of the COX process.

Probiotics also stimulate a healthy thymus gland. Illustrating this, medical researchers from the University of Bari (Indrio *et al.* 2007) gave a placebo or a probiotic combination of *Bifidobacterium breve* C50 and *Streptococcus thermophilus* 065 to 60 newborns. The thymus glands of the probiotic group were significantly larger compared to babies who consumed the standard (placebo) formula.

Scientists from the Nagoya University Graduate School of Medicine (Sugawara *et al.* 2006) found in a study of 101 patients that supplementation with probiotics increased NK activity and lymphocyte counts. Pro-inflammatory IL-6 cytokines also decreased significantly among the probiotic group. Serum IL-6, white blood cell counts, and C-reactive protein also significantly decreased among the probiotic group.

Furthermore, probiotics have the ability to *uniquely* modify cytokines—relative to the condition of the person. Illustrating this, a probiotic drink with either placebo or a probiotic combination of *Lactobacillus paracasei* Lpc-37, *Lactobacillus acidophilus* 74-2 and *Bifidobacterium animalis* subsp. *lactis* DGCC 420 (*B. lactis* 420) was given to 15 healthy adults and 15 adults with atopic dermatitis. After eight weeks, CD57(+) cytokines levels increased significantly among the healthy group taking probiotics, while CD4(+)CD54(+) cytokines decreased significantly among the atopic patients taking the probiotics (Roessler *et al.* 2008).

Researchers from Poland's Pomeranian Academy of Medicine (Naruszewicz *et al.* 2002) gave *Lactobacillus plantarum* 299v or placebo to 36 healthy volunteers for six weeks. Monocytes isolated from probiotic subjects had significantly reduced adhesion to endothelial cells, and the probiotic group had a 42% reduction in pro-inflammatory cytokine interleukin-6. No changes were observed among the placebo group.

Probiotics are often involved in the production of critical intermediary fatty acids used in LOX and COX enzyme conversions, producing anti-inflammatory effects. To illustrate this, scientists from the University of Helsinki (Kekkonen *et al.* 2008) measured lipids and inflammation markers before and after giving probiotic *Lactobacillus rhamnosus* GG to 26 healthy adults. After three weeks of probiotic supplementation, the subjects had decreased levels of intermediary inflammatory fatty acids such as lysophosphatidylcholines, sphingomyelins, and several glycerophosphatidylcholines. Probiotics also reduced hyper-inflammatory markers TNF-alpha and CRP in this study.

The bottom line is that our body's probiotics and our immune system are interconnected. They are inseparable. At least 70% of the immune system *is* probiotic. Consider this carefully: If our probiotic populations were decimated by either a lethal bacteria infection or a course of antibiotics, *we would lose nearly three quarters of our gut's immune system.*

The Role of Genes in Allergic Rhinitis

Research has confirmed that the risk of contracting allergies is greater amongst those with family members who have or have had allergies. The question is, what are the mechanics for this? Is it a simple matter of inheriting certain DNA sequences? And do these genetic sequences cause allergies? In a word, no. Let's look at the science on the relationship between genetics and allergies:

First, let's be clear. A multitude of research has shown that having one parent with allergies increases the risk of getting allergies to about one in three, and having two parents with allergies increases the risk by about seven times. There is no question about this. Yet there are still a lot of children of one or two parents with allergies who do not have allergies—and even more that do not have allergies as adults.

And yes, there appears to be some genetic similarities between allergic people. Researchers have seen a common genetic variation among the Charcot-Leyden crystal protein (CLC) in allergic rhinitis patients. This showed a recessive inheritance potential (Bryborn *et al.* 2009).

We must remember that prior to two centuries ago, hay fever was virtually unknown. Furthermore, the dramatic explosion of allergies over the past century clearly indicates that their origins could not be genetic.

We should also clarify that during pregnancy, a child shares hypersensitivities with mama. Through the umbilical cord, the blood is shared. This means that the immunoglobulins, cytokines, T-cells and B-cells are all distributed through the baby's body. Whatever mother is sensitive to, the baby—at least during pregnancy—is also sensitive to.

Now once the baby is born, it begins to develop its own immunity. Its immune system begins to directly identify threats. But this doesn't mean it leaves behind what the immune system learned while sharing mama's blood. The immune system can learn to deal with foreigners differently than mama's body did, but this will need to be developed—and developing tolerance is something the healthy body knows how to do.

For this very reason, many people outgrow their allergies after childhood.

For example, research from the North West Lung Research Center at Wythenshawe Hospital in Manchester (Frank *et al.* 2008) studied 628 children who developed wheeze (often from allergies) over a five-year period, from 1993 and 2004. They found that having a family history of asthma did not predicate lifelong asthma or allergies among those children who developed wheeze during their preschool years.

Genes do not influence the body in isolation. They typically need to be triggered in order to be expressed. For example, the toll-like receptor 2 and 4 genes (TLR2 and TLR4) appear to influence the body's response to the toxins brought on by air pollution. The presence of these two genes increase the likelihood of a hypersensitive response to smog, but the smog must be present for the gene to be expressed (Kerkhof *et al.* 2010).

Other genes, such as IL2RA, TLR2, TGFBR2, and FOXP3, may also predispose a person to allergies and asthma. These are involved in the production and operation of regulatory T-cells. However, multiple gene-gene interactivity is required for this to occur (Bottema *et al.* 2010). A gene-gene interactivity would require multiple relationships outside of heredity, including toxin overloading, which would switch on that interactivity.

Researchers from the Department of Medical Genetics at Japan's University of Tsukuba (Matsumoto *et al.* 2011) studied 32 seasonal allergic rhinitis patients with 25 healthy control subjects. They found that three genes were significantly altered during allergen exposure. These included the expression of interleukin-17 receptor beta (IL17RB). In the allergic group, the IL17RB gene was "upregulated" during allergen exposure. This genetic expression is an illustration of the epigenetic process: The interaction between the environment and hypersensitive persons.

In other words, when *epigenetics* are considered—which we'll explain shortly—we can better understand the relationship between genes, toxins and disease conditions from both perspectives.

Consider the impact of farm animals on reducing allergies and asthma. Swedish researchers (Bruce *et al.* 2009) studied the relationship between living on farms and lower allergy and asthma incidence together with the gene neuropeptide S receptor 1 (NPSR1). Triggering this gene receptor appears to modify certain genes (polymorphism), and those modifications have been shown to accompany reduced airway hypersensitivity. These also exist amongst those from family farms—notably those who work with farm animals.

NPSR1 polymorphisms and the farming lifestyle were also linked using laboratory models (*in vitro*). The researchers then examined 3,113 children from the PARSIFAL European cross-sectional study on lifestyles and childhood allergy. They found that NPSR1 polymorphisms were obvious and measurable among those children who had regular contact with farm animals—specifically among SNP546333, rs740347, rs323922 and rs324377—which are implicated in modifying allergies. This illustrated that contact with farm animals produced *epigenetic changes* among farm family children that protected them against hypersensitivities.

These relationships are also evident from allergy research.

Researchers from the Department of Pediatrics of Brazil's State University of Campinas (López *et al.* 1999) studied allergies among 114 newborns (including three twin pairs) starting at birth through one years old. They measured IgE levels of the umbilical cord blood, and again after three months, six months and at 12 months. They also correlated the relative influences of race, sex, family income, birth month, family allergy history, breastfeeding, parents' smoking, and symptoms. At one year, they found *no association* between IgE (allergy) levels and a family history of allergies. They concluded that, *"immune response for atopy was in a large degree influenced by environmental factors and serum IgE at 12 months was a good marker for identifying infants with risk of atopic disease in early life."*

Researchers from Germany's Philipps University of Marburg (Pfefferle *et al.* 2008) found that 24% of newborns had allergen-specific IgE antibodies when they tested blood samples from 922 infants and mothers. The only allergen-specific IgEs found to be common between mother and infant were for milk, eggs, and soybeans IgE. Note also that these three types of allergies are often outgrown during the first few years of childhood.

Our understanding of genetics is still in its infancy. This is indicated by the progress of our genome research. Over the last two decades, geneticists have focused on assembling a catalog of gene combinations that together classify the genome of particular organisms. Genome research has expanded into a worldwide focus on establishing the genome of humans and other species.

The assumption in the beginning of the genome research project—which has involved hundreds of scientists from different specialties over two decades—was that we would find within the genome the answers to all the mysteries of nature. In other words, we'd find out the cause for every disease—and why people die when they do.

The hypothesis that the genome would provide these answers has proved to be erroneous. The first invalid assumption was that the combination of genes in humans would uniquely indicate the occurrence of disease pathologies. And yes, preliminary research seemed to connect certain gene combinations to particular diseases. It was assumed that every disease came with a particular genetic sequence. This worked out pretty well in the beginning, until researchers began discovering that many people with gene sequences associated with a particular disease never contracted that disease. And sometimes multiple diseases were associated with the same genetic trait. For example, Angelman syndrome and Prader-willy syndrome both occur with the same chromosome 15 deletion.

These and other problems revealed that perhaps our understanding of the genetics of disease etiology was not as advanced as we'd like to think.

Consider obesity. It was assumed by geneticists that obesity was a genetic disorder that could be cured by switching off a particular gene sequence. However, researchers from the Massachusetts General Hospital (Ashrafi *et al.* 2003) went through 16,757 worm genes (most of which are common with humans), and found that 303 switched on genes reduced fat and 112 switched-on genes increased fat storage. This means that at least 415 genes are involved in obesity.

This complexity is confirmed when we consider two groups of Pima Indians, one living in Arizona, U.S. and the other living in the Sierra Madre region of Mexico. While these two groups are genetically identical—as confirmed by testing—the Arizona group has one of the highest rates of obesity and diabetes in the world. The Sierra Madre group, meanwhile, has extremely low rates of obesity and diabetes.

According to a study by University of Wisconsin researchers (Schulz *et al.* 2006), 38% of the U.S. Pimas suffer from type 2 diabetes, compared to 7% of the Mexican Pimas. Obesity was ten times more prevalent among the U.S. Pima men than among the Mexican Pima men. The central difference between the groups? Diet and lifestyle. The Sierra Madre Pima get plenty of physical activity and eat a traditional diet, while the Arizona group gets significantly less physical activity and eats more of a western diet.

This is further evidenced by research on monozygotic twins—which share the same DNA at conception. They do not necessarily develop the same diseases. In other words, identical twins often have very different pathological outcomes throughout life. How could this be if diseases were genetically derived?

Among autoimmune diseases, for example, genetic associations among twins and families do exist, but the stronger factor is also related to environmental issues. For example, a study from the University of Western Ontario's Clinical Neurological Science Department (Ebers *et al.* 1996) reviewed the research on twins and autoimmune complexes such as multiple sclerosis. They also conducted a genome search of 100 sibling pairs, looking for MS gene markers. Their research concluded that while monozygotic twins showed higher concordance levels (matching pathologies) than dizygotic twins and siblings (25-30% versus 4%); they found that *"environmental factors strongly influenced observed geographical differences."* They also concluded: *"Studies of candidate genes have been largely unrewarding."*

This of course is because twins make different choices and have different behavior; and behavior directly relates to their intake and management of toxins. Twins also have physiological differences despite their genetic similarity.

In a study of genetically identical twins and lung capacity from Pennsylvania State University (Whitfield *et al.* 2004), lung expiration capacity was only 14% attributable to genetic factors. About 30% was found to be due to shared environments and 56% was due to non-shared environmental effects. These and other studies confirm that our environments, lifestyles, and diets have much greater effects upon our health than do genetic factors.

But don't twins also maintain similar environmental conditions? Certainly they do. Especially during childhood. They also share the same mother and the same breast milk. They also share the same birthing canal, where they receive similar doses of immunoglobulins and probiotics—just as they receive in breast milk.

However, depending upon how much time they spend together, they will typically make distinctly different choices in life. In general, they display significantly unique and often diverse behaviors. Hur and Rushton (2007) studied 514 pairs of two- to nine-year-old South Korean monozygotic (identical) and dizygotic (non-identical) twins. Their results indicated that 55% of the children's pro-social behavior related to genetic factors and 45% was attributed to non-shared environmental factors. It should also be noted that shared lifestyle and environmental factors could not be eliminated from the 55%.

The lifestyle/environmental issues versus genes association could well be higher if the twins' early shared environments had been removed. In another study (Forget-Dubois *et al.* 2007), an analysis of 292 mothers demonstrated that maternal behavior only accounted for a 29% genetic influence at 18 months, and 25% at 30 months.

In a study done at the Virginia Commonwealth University's Institute for Psychiatric and Behavioral Genetics (Maes *et al.* 2007), a large sampling revealed that individual behavior was only about 38-40% attributable to genetics, while shared environment was 18-23% attributable; and unshared environmental influences were attributable in 39-42%. This illustrates the independence of twins' lifestyles.

Studies of arthritis—another inflammatory disorder—have revealed a range of only 12-15% concordance between monozygotic twins for rheumatoid arthritis (RA). This indicates an even weaker connection between genetics and RA exists—contradicting a decades-old assumption that RA was generally a genetic disease. If RA were significantly genetic, then we would see that among twins with the RA genetic traits, both twins would contract the disease at least more than 50% of the time, instead of 12-15% of the time (Silman *et al.* 1993, Jones *et al.* 1996; Aho *et al.* 1986).

Rather, 12-15% indicates other factors, such as shared diets and shared toxin loads.

To further close the door on the genetic-arthritis association, the *British Medical Journal* (Swendsen *et al.* 2002) published a nationwide study from Denmark on RA among monozygotic twins and dizygotic twins. This concluded no significant difference between monozygotic twins and dizygotic twins with regard to 1) onset of RA; 2) presence of RA factor; or 3) any other RA association. In other words, RA occurrence was no more shared between genetically identical twins than non-genetic identical twins—the opposite of what should happen if RA was genetic.

At the same time, this does not mean that genetic disposition has nothing to do with the development of allergies and many other diseases. A genetic disposition can increase the likelihood of contracting the disease *given susceptibility genes are switched on.*

We might compare this to automobile ownership. Say two people purchase the exact same make, model and year automobile at the same time. Comparing the two cars in the future will reveal the cars had vastly different engine lives and mileages. They each had different types of breakdowns, and different problems. This is because each car was driven differently. One was likely driven harder than the other was. One was likely better taken care of than the other was. They may have been the same make and model, but each had different owners with different driving and maintenance habits. While the model might have a particular weakness in its design, this weakness may only affect performance if the car is pushed in a way that exploits this weakness—and is not maintained correctly.

Because twins have the same genetics—just as the cars shared the same make, model and manufacturer—their unique disease factors stem from the fact that each body is operated differently by a different individual under different conditions.

This distinction between inherited genes and continued environmental inputs is a realm that scientists are just beginning to explore. Realizing that even the same genes or the same genetic abnormalities will not render the same pathologies, researchers want to better understand the full matrix of causation in differentiated gene expression. Even twins who shared the same diet and environment will still have vastly different disease pathologies. This means there are missing elements that future research must take into consideration.

These missing elements have forced a re-calibration of the genetic theory, and the rise of the concept of *epigenetics*—as we hinted at earlier. In general, epigenetics is the acceptance of lifestyle, environmental and/or dietary factors that *switch off and on* the expression of our genes. In other words, it has been hypothesized—and confirmed by the research—that ones DNA is not as important as how gene expressions—or *phenotypes*—are switched on or off. If the genes are expressed, particular metabolism consequences result. If they are not expressed, there are different consequences. Furthermore, even if the susceptibility gene is not present, certain activities can *create* the epigenetic sequences that switch a particular disease event on (and often produce the susceptibility for future generations). It is for this reason alone that even a person with no family history of allergies may become allergic during their lifetime.

The original concept of epigenetics was penned by geneticist Conrad Waddington in the early 1940s to explain in general how environmental circumstances could affect ones genetic instructions. The concept, however, got lost until the 1990s and early 2000s, as scientists discovered the many gaps in their genetic assumptions.

The biochemical relationships of gene expression have focused upon the action of DNA histone regulation. These biochemical messengers have been observed switching gene alleles on or off. For example, cruel mice experiments at McGill University's Douglas Hospital Research Center (Szyf *et al.* 2008) found that phenotype switching could be turned on and off with increased nurturing from the mother. Those baby mice receiving affectionate nurturing from mama would switch on genes differently than those mice that received less nurturing.

Epigenetic mechanisms for allergies and asthma are now starting to become accepted by medical researchers. Dr. Rosalind J. Wright a leading researcher and professor at Harvard Medical School, has illustrated that maternal stress can help "program" the physiology of newborns, including their nervous systems, endocrine systems, and immune systems. The mother's physiological responses to stress can be passed on to the child through behavior, in other words. This programming may also occur within the household, according to Dr. Wright, as families adapt to stress in their particular manner. These are all *"learned"* by the physiologies of the infant, enabling the passing on of allergy and asthmatic reflexes (Wright 2011).

Biochemical mechanisms like phosphorylation, sumoylation, acetylation, methylation, and ubiquitylation appear to show some of the mechanics responsible for phenotype expression—which connect gene expression to the availability of nutrients like oxygen, water, vitamin B, Co-Q-10 and so on. This of course confirms the link between genes and our particular diet and toxin exposures.

Researchers from France's INSERM Genetics and Epigenetics of Metabolic Diseases Division (Gabory *et al.* 2009) have found that the overall phenotype of a person is derived from *"complex interactions between genotype and current, past and ancestral environment leading to a lifelong remodeling of our epigenomes."*

The researchers also pointed to recent studies that have suggested epigenetic programming can be transmitted to subsequent generations through what is called transgenerational effects or TGEs. Transgenerational effects allow epigenetic programming changes to be passed on, tying the epigenetic changes of ancestors to affect the sensitivities of later generations. Sometimes this transfer is solely single generational, although it has been repeatedly seen among research as multi-generational.

In other words, the diet or lifestyle of our grandmother, grandfather or further up the line may affect our body's susceptibility to certain sensitivities.

As stated clearly by esteemed nutrition researcher Dr. T. Colin Campbell:

> *"Genes do not determine disease on their own. Genes function only by being activated or expressed, and nutrition plays a critical role in determining which genes, good and bad, are expressed."* (Campbell 2006)

As we review allergy sensitivity research, it becomes evident that even if a parent has had allergies, the child's lifestyle/environmental factors play a stronger role. These lifestyle factors switch on, or express a particular genetic trait.

The prime example often missed in the genetic discussion is the common diet and common living environments between parents and their children. With rare exception, children consume the foods and diets chosen by their parents. Recipes and cooking methods, for the most part, are passed down from generation to generation. As a result, the diet the children have may be practically identical, with the exception of brand names and packaging, to the diet the parents, grandparents and great-grandparents ate. While this succession of dietary choices may not always follow once the child is an adult, at least during the formative years of the child—their diets are practically identical.

In the case of mothers who provide the womb, the birthing canal and breast milk to their children, their lifestyle and diet choices become part of the baby's environment.

Again, the pregnant mother and the infant share the same food and blood for nine months. This means that whatever the mother eats directly affects the child via the umbilical cord. It also means that whatever toxins the mother consumes will also be consumed by the baby. This has been supported by research testing umbilical cord blood.

Furthermore, the house and those environmental toxins present in its furniture and building materials are presented equally to the parents and the children. The outside environment—automobile pollution, pesticides and so on—is also mutually presented to parents and children. And because they are developing, children are more sensitive to environmental conditions. Children are also more vulnerable to the influences of their parents' diets and lifestyles.

Even if the child does not assume the lifestyle choices of the parent as an adult, the environmental exposure has already been accomplished. In other words, we can prevent further exposures to our bodies and to the next generation's. But our bodies will have to deal with our childhood exposures.

This "passing" of lifestyle habits is undoubtedly more important than the genes parents pass on to their children. Why? Because even if the children received the genes predisposing some weakness towards a particular issue such as allergies—those genes still have to be switched on in order for the sensitivity to be expressed. And how do we switch on the genes? By our environment and lifestyle choices—including diet, air, water consumption and exercise.

As we'll discuss further, chemical and environmental toxins become potent free radicals once inside the body. Here they can damage cell membranes, overloading the immune system and producing systemic inflammation. They can also damage the mucosal membranes and expose the airway epithelia to additional toxins.

In such exposure sequences, the immune system must use whatever available resources it has to try to correct the damage. Sometimes this means putting the body on a high-scale alert—called hypersensitivity. Once this inflammatory status is in place, the body is more likely to respond with allergic symptoms.

This effect is now prominent as researchers look at the dramatic rise of allergies among the developed world. This relates directly to the diet of the child and the diet of the mother. This is called the "maternal diet," as the physiological effects of the mother's diet directly affect the risk of allergies for the child.

This epigenetic conclusion was confirmed by researchers from China's Sun Yat-Sen University (Fu *et al.* 2010) who studied late embryo maturation among peanut allergy children. They found that an epigenetic change took place during the developmental stages related to the environment. Their nucleosomes on the assigned match for the *Ara h3* peanut protein were depleted. Histone H3 levels were significantly reduced. Because these factors changed during development, they were determined not to be genetic: They were epigenetic. Gene developmental changes that evolve during embryo maturation are responses to environmental changes. This relates to the diet of the mother and the mother's environment.

83

Another important element to consider is the genome of our probiotic colonies. A thriving population of more than three trillion organisms renders the conclusion that our bodies have ten times more bacteria than cells. This resounding fact has led scientists to the concept of the *microbiome*—an extended genome of the genetics of our resident microorganisms. Recent research indicates that our probiotics' genes better reflect our body's predispositions and pathologies than does our own cellular DNA (Kinross *et al.* 2006).

Margaret McFall Ngai, Ph.D., microbiome researcher and professor of microbiology and immunology at University of Wisconsin's School of Medicine told the author:

> *"Understanding the human microbiome may be as or more important to understanding human health than mapping and understanding the human genome."*

Chapter Three

The Prime Suspects

Hay fever and allergic rhinitis are symptoms of allergic hypersensitivity. Once a person has allergic hypersensitivity, their symptoms can be triggered by an immediate response to an allergen or a hypersensitive response to a trigger that is not necessarily an allergen.

In other words, the hypersensitive metabolism is on high alert, and many things can trigger an out-of-proportion response. Thus, there are two sorts of rhinitis triggers:

The atopic trigger: This is when the body's immune system has produced an IgE antibody specific to a certain allergen. The body can maintain a host of different specific IgEs, which can also cross over and become sensitive to other allergens.

The non-atopic trigger: A non-atopic trigger is any environmental exposure that stimulates hypersensitivity outside of the IgE-antibody system. Here a rhinitis episode might be triggered by a sudden change in temperature. It might be a warm fall one day, and the next day a cold front moves in. This might trigger a hypersensitivity response in a hypersensitive person. It is not as if we have formed IgEs to cold temperatures. The cold temperature simply stimulated a physiological response out of proportion with the situation. In a healthy person, for example, cold weather may simply cause some shivering—muscle contraction to help keep the body warm.

Interestingly, some triggers that are atopic in one person can be non-atopic in another. This is can happen with mold. A person can become sensitive to mold without developing IgE sensitivity. Another person might have or develop a severe IgE sensitivity to mold spores.

Regardless of whether we have non-atopic or atopic-triggered rhinitis flare-ups, chronic rhinitis is still a defective inflammatory response—as we've shown. Let's review some of the main allergens/triggers:

Pollen

In the first chapter, we discussed some the history and research associating pollen with many cases of hay fever and allergic rhinitis. Does this mean that hay fever/allergic rhinitis is pollen-induced? Not necessarily. A bout of rhinitis can be triggered by pollen even if there is no pollen allergy. However, having a pollen allergy is typical among those who respond to pollens with rhinitis.

Regardless of whether there is an allergy, pollen hypersensitivity is an inflammatory condition.

Illustrating this, University of Chieti researchers (Di Gioacchino *et al.* 2000) studied the relationship between pollen allergies and inflammation factors. Testing 28 asthmatic and allergic farmers, they were able to correlate bronchial allergy symptoms with specific-IgEs and the pro-inflammatory eosinophil cationic protein (ECP). They tested the farmers for IgE levels and ECP levels before, during and after pollen season. They found that bronchial symptoms of cough and wheezing continued 41 days through the fall, well after the pollen season ended. They found that IgEs were moderately high, while grass pollen IgEs actually remained fairly consistent before and during the pollen season.

This and other research provides strong evidence that pollen allergies are inflammatory processes. The pro-inflammatory eosinophil cationic protein levels of the farmers increased significantly during pollination season, and fell off afterward. They also found that the number of after-pollen season asthma symptom days related with eosinophil cationic protein levels.

As we discussed in the first chapter, plants use pollens to stimulate the sexual activity that results in seeds being produced. Without seeds, plants cannot prosper, and we'd starve. Seeds directly and indirectly provide us with nutrition.

Pollens are all around us, and they are necessary for life. Most plants pollinate periodically, and many do at the same time each year—during the springtime. Springtime, however, depends upon the location and the plant. The arrival of spring depends on the latitude and location. Furthermore, some plants push out pollen for much of the summer, and into the fall. Heck, a few will push out their pollen over the winter.

Anyway, it is not the pollens themselves that rhinitis sufferers become sensitized to. It is the epitope portions of their proteins. The protein epitope responsible for allergies to *Artemisia vulgaris*, for example, is Art v1, while ragweed (*Ambrosia artemisiifolia*) allergies are primarily caused by the 29-31 kDa protein. These two proteins are common allergens (Léonard *et al.* 2010).

The vast majority (about 70%) of hay fever in the United States is related to ragweed pollen. The grass and tree pollens follow in prevalence. Here are the major pollen-producing plants associated with hay fever/allergic rhinitis:

Common Pollen Allergy Sources

Weeds	Trees	Grasses
Burning bush	Alder	Bahia
Careless weed	Beech	Bermuda
Dandelion	Birch	Bluegrass
English plantain	Cottonwood	Brome

86

Firebush	Elm	Common reed
Goldenrod	Eucalyptus	Johnson
Lamb's quarters	Hazel	Meadow fescue
Mexican fireweed	Hickory	Meadow foxtail
Nettle	Maple	Orchard
Ox-eye daisy	Mountain cedar	Redtop
Pigweed	Oak	Ryegrass
Ragweed	Poplar	Sweet vernal
Russian thistle	Sycamore	Timothy
Sagebrush	White ash	
Sheep sorrel	White pine	
Spiny amaranth	Willow	

(Adapted from Faelten 1983)

When an immunosuppressed person (notably a person with weakened mucosal membrane immunity) breathes in pollen, should the pollen escape the mucosal membrane shield within the sinuses and respiratory tract, the pollen may penetrate the epithelial layer and reach the body's tissues and bloodstream. When this happens, especially among the immunosuppressed, the immune system can overreact with hypersensitivity. The immune system will also remember the pollen protein as an invader for the next exposure.

Note that hyperreactivity responses to pollens are mostly limited to plants that carry their pollen through the air by wind. Those plants that pollinate strictly through insect pollination, such as dandelion, goldenrod and similar flowering plants, do not typically cause pollen allergies. This, however, does not mean that hypersensitive people do not become allergic to these pollens. This may occur through direct contact (such as rolling in a field of these plants) or via a crossover reaction for someone allergic to a relative of the plant.

Because pollen release is seasonal, allergic hypersensitivity responses to pollen typically occur during the pollen-release season. For example, researchers from Italy's G. D'Annunzio University (Di Gioacchino *et al.* 2001) studied 20 farmers who had pollen (Graminae and Parietaria) allergies with bronchial hyperreactivity. Their bronchial symptoms progressed with the pollen seasons. They were worse in the summer, followed by spring and autumn. Winter had the fewest symptoms.

Here is a short table with some common pollen allergens and their typical seasonal release, given a Northern latitude (well north of the equator). Southern hemisphere locations should have opposite seasonality, and locations nearer the equator can have variable pollen seasons, depending upon the plant, weather (Hawaii, for example, has grass pollens nearly all year long). Also, keep in mind that seasonal weather patterns have been significantly changing over the past few years, which has produced variable pollen seasons:

Common Name	Family	Pollen Season
Acacia	Acacia	January-October
Alders	Alnus	December-June
Amaranths	Amaranthaceae	May-October
Ashes	Fraxinus	April-May
Aspen	Populus	April-May
Bayberry	Myrica	February-June
Beeches	Fagus	April-May
Birches	Betula	April-Sept
Bulrush	Scirpus	August-Sept
Chestnuts	Castanea	June-July
Cypresses	Cupressaceae	September-June
Dandelion	Asteraceae	April-Sept
Docks/Sorrels	Rumex	April-August
Elders	Sambucus	May-July
Elms	Ulmus	March-May
Eucalyptus	Eucalyptus	December-March
Goldenrod	Compositae	April-Sept
Goosefoot	Chenopodiaceae	May-October
Grasses and Sedges	Gramineae, Poaceae	April-September
Hazel	Corylus	February-April
Heathers	Erica/Calluna	April-October
Hickories	Carya	March-May
Hops	Humulus	July-August
Hornbeam	Carpinus	February-April
Horse chestnuts	Aesculus	April-May
Ironwoods	Carpinus	April-May
Japanese Cedar	Crypomeria	February-April
Junipers	Cupressaceae	February-June
Lindens	Tilia	June-July
Maples	Acer	March-Sept
Mesquite	Prosopis	May-July
Mugwort/Wormwood	Artemisia	July-Sept
Nettles	Urtica	May-September
Oaks	Qercus	February-June
Olives	Olea	May-June
Osage	Maclura	April-June
Pecans	Carya	March-May

Pellitories	Parietaria	May-August
Pigweeds	Amaranthaceae	June-October
Pines	Pinaceae	April-July
Planes	Plantanus	March-May
Plantains	Plantago	July-October
Poplars	Populus	March-May
Privet	Ligustrum	May-June
Ragweeds	Amrosia	April-December
Sagebrush	Artemisia	May-September
Spruces, Firs	Pinaceae	July-August
Walnuts	Juglans	April-June
Willows	Salix	March-May
Yews	Taxus	March-April

(Adapted from Bostoff and Gamlin 2002)

This table expands the various regional seasons. Your local season may be shorter, and within this range.

As mentioned, in recent years, as the weather has become quite variable, and as a result, pollen seasons have been expanding. Plants become more tolerant to weather changes by loosening up their seasonality.

Illustrating this, researchers from Poland's Adam Mickiewicz University, (Stach *et al.* 2007) studied the relationships between pollen severity and meteorological conditions during the pollen year and the previous year. They found that pollen severity correlated with weather conditions during the year before pollination relating to the phases of the North Atlantic Oscillation (NAO)—a current and weather system pattern that flows across the North Atlantic Ocean and Northern Europe.

Remember that allergic rhinitis may not be the only symptom of a pollen allergy. This is evidenced by the fact that many pollen-allergy sufferers have respiratory asthma-like symptoms, and some have eczema. Some pollen allergy sufferers will not even exhibit rhinitis.

Pollen-Related Food Sensitivities

When foods containing those sensitized proteins found in pollen are eaten, the immune system may again respond in the same way it overreacted to the pollen. This becomes a pollen-related food sensitivity. Often the combination also produces more severe symptoms.

For example, Spanish researchers (Cuesta-Herranz *et al.* 2010) found in a study of 806 patients from eight hospitals that people suffering from both pollen and pollen-related food allergies have significantly more respiratory symptoms than pollen-only allergies.

Researchers from the Institute of Internal Medicine at Italy's University of Ferrara (Boccafogli *et al.* 1994) studied 169 allergic patients who were sensitized to grass pollen. They compared them to a 50-patient control group who were sensitized to dust mites. The grass pollen allergy sufferers reported more adverse food reactions than did the dust mite group.

The pollen-sensitive group reported sensitivities to peanut, garlic, tomato, onion, and some fruits. They also reported sensitivities to egg whites and pork. The researchers concluded a cross reactivity between pollen and food allergens.

Researchers from Japan's Yokohama City University Hospital (Maeda *et al.* 2010) studied food allergies and pollen allergies among adults. After studying IgE antibodies for five pollens among 622 allergy sufferers with an average age of 37 years old, they found twice as many of those allergic to pollens having food allergies than the general population.

However, when considering the rare types of allergies of the subjects—apples, peaches and melons—the increase in rates was significantly higher. Cedar, ragweed, orchard grass, mugwort, and alder pollen were the most common pollen allergies. Apple allergies correlated more with alder pollen allergies. Peach allergies correlated with alder and orchard grass sensitivity. Mellon allergy correlated with alder, orchard grass and ragweed sensitivity. The researchers commented that allergies relating to trees in the Betulaceae family (alder, birch, hazel, hornbeam and some tree nuts) are implicated with similar food allergies.

Pollen allergies affect different people differently, however. Italian researchers (Asero *et al.* 2009) studied 25,601 allergy clinic patients throughout Italy, and found that pollen-related food allergies were the most prevalent, at 55% of all allergies. Of those pollen-related food allergies, 45% had atopic IgE allergies, and the majority (72%) of those had allergies to fruits and vegetables.

Of the pollen allergy group, 96% of those with IgE food allergies lived in Southern Italy, and most of these were related to lipid transfer protein (LTP) sensitization. The researchers indicated a link between diet and pollen exposure because of this geographical trend. Most Italians understand that the diet of Northern Italy is typically healthier and more traditional, with less fried and fast foods, as compared to the typical diet of the primarily urban Southern Italy population. Pollen type can also have an effect between regions.

Here are a few pollen allergy-related foods and some of the research evidence linking some of these associations:

Peaches: Spanish researchers (Fernández-Rivas *et al.* 2003) studied peach and related Rosaceae fruit allergies. They found that cross-reactivity of IgE antibodies to lipid transfer proteins (LTPs) were prevalent among the subjects.

The scientists studied 98 people with peach sensitivities. IgE allergies were found among 77% of the patients. Furthermore, 76% of the peach allergy subjects also had allergies to pollens. Furthermore, all of the 22 subjects not IgE allergic to peach also had pollen allergies.

The proteins most sensitized to were *Pru p3, rBet v1,* and *rBet v2.* IgE responses to *rBet v2* were greatest among pollen allergy sufferers. They concluded that *Pru p3* is the major protein allergen in peach.

Peach allergy sufferers in the north of Spain are sensitive to different allergens than sufferers from the South of Spain (Gamboa *et al.* 2007). Those from the north have more systemic responses, with the protein *Pru p3* being the key allergen mixed with a *profilin-Bet v1* protein sensitivity. This is often referred to as an *LTP-profilin-Bet v1* sensitization—also common in Northern and Central Europe.

Apples: Apple sensitivity is quite common in some parts of Europe due to cross-reactivity. Research has established that about 2% of people who live in Northern and Central Europe are sensitive to apples.

Danish researchers (Hansen *et al.* 2004) found that among 74 patients allergic to birch pollen, 69% were also allergic to apples.

Denmark National University Hospital researchers (Skamstrup *et al.* 2001) tested the seasonal occurrence of apple sensitivity among 27 patients allergic to birch pollen. They were tested for reactions to apples before and during the 1998 birch pollen season. The results of their oral challenge testing concluded that sensitivity to apples significantly increases during birch pollen allergy season, and decreases or disappears after the season is over.

However, while birch pollen can cross-react and cause apple and other fruit allergies, it can also significantly reduce allergies among certain fruits, including some varieties of apples (Bolhaar *et al.* 2004).

In other words, not every apple variety has the same allergic potential. Some apples produce more sensitivity than others do. For example, researchers at Groningen University Medical Centre found that among three different apple cultivars—Santana, Golden Delicious, and Topaz—a majority (53%) of the allergic patients were not sensitive to the Santana apple variety. Those who were sensitive were far less sensitive to the Santana apple than to the other two. After the study, 73% of the participants said that they would eat Santana apples in the future.

Cherries: While cherry allergies occur throughout Europe, they occur with more severity and more systemic reactions in Southern Europe. Cherry allergy sufferers among the Central and Northern European countries have primarily oral responses. This appears related to the sensitization to LTP, which occurs more in the Northern countries, and sensitivity to cherry proteins, such as *Pru av3,* which occurs primarily in Southern locations such as Spain and Italy (Reuter *et al.* 2006).

Figs: Fig allergies can occur among those also allergic to both rubber latex and birch pollens.

In an Austrian study (Hemmer *et al.* 2010) of 85 patients with birch pollen allergies, 78% of them were also sensitized to fresh figs and (interestingly) only 10% were sensitized to dried figs. In addition, 91% were sensitive to mulberries, 91% to jackfruit, 77% to Rosaceae fruits (which include almonds, apples, apricots, cherries, peaches, pears, plums, raspberries, strawberries as well as ornamentals such as firethorns, hawthorns, meadowsweets, photinias and roses).

The researchers concluded that other fruits of the Moraceae family should also be cross-reactionary with fig allergies. These include breadfruits and many other trees.

Kiwifruit: Kiwis may be an exception to pollen allergies in some cases. In a study of 33 people with kiwi allergy symptoms, food challenge was positive in 23 patients. Twenty-one percent were not allergic to pollen, however. Twenty-eight percent of the kiwifruit allergy sufferers had sensitivities to latex (Alemán *et al.* 2004).

Kiwifruit's main allergens are *Act d1, Act d2, Act d4, and Act d5, Bet v1, Act d8* and *profilin rAct d9* (Bublin *et al.* 2010). Italian researchers (Fiocchi *et al.* 2004) found that children allergic to fresh kiwifruit were by and large not allergic to steam-cooked (100 degrees C for five minutes) and homogenized kiwifruit. Twenty kiwi-allergic children were tested. Only one child reacted to the cooked kiwi food challenge.

Melon: Spanish researchers (Rodriguez *et al.* 2000) found in testing 53 patients complaining of melon allergies that only 42% had IgE allergy and 42% were positive using the skin prick test. Eighteen of these confirmed melon-allergy patients were also allergic to up to 15 other foods. The most prevalent included banana (39%), kiwi (33%), watermelon (33%), and peach (28%).

Melon allergies first occurred among the patients at an average age of 20, with a range of six years old to 45 years old. In addition, 88% had seasonal rhinitis (sinus issues, watery eyes and so on) and/or asthma symptoms.

The chart below summarizes foods and types of pollens:

Pollen Type	Food Allergy Associations
Birch	almonds, apples, apricots, avocados, bananas, carrots, celery, cherries, chicory, coriander, fennel, figs, hazelnuts, kiwifruit, nectarines, parsley, parsnips, peaches, pears, peppers, plums, potatoes, prunes, soy, strawberries,

	wheat, walnuts
Ragweed	banana, cantaloupe, cucumber, honeydew, watermelon, zucchini, echinacea, artichoke, dandelions, hibiscus, chamomile
Alder	almonds, apples, celery, cherries, hazel nuts, peaches, pears, parsley, strawberry, raspberry
Grass	figs, melons, tomatoes, oranges
Mugwort	carrots, celery, coriander, fennel, parsley, peppers, sunflower

(Adapted from Zarkadas *et al.* 1999)

Lipid Transfer Proteins

While many LTPs relate to pollen, we've separated a section on LTP to dig deeper. The reader might have noticed that many of the foods listed above included LTP as an allergen. This includes apples, peaches, kiwifruit, melon, cherries and many other fruits and vegetables. As we'll see, LTPs are even more pervasive among allergies than this indicates.

Italian researchers (Asero *et al.* 2002) selected 20 patients who were lipid transfer protein allergic out of 600 Rosaceae (apples and related fruits) allergic patients. They found that all the patients also had allergic reactions to a large number of other plant foods, including nuts, peanuts, legumes, celery, rice, corn and others. The researchers concluded that LPT was a *"pan-allergen."*

As discussed earlier, Spanish researchers (Palacin *et al.* 2010) discovered that increasing wheat allergy rates likely relate to increased sensitivity to LTP. The wheat flour lipid transfer protein, *Tri a14,* appears to be the key allergen responsible for baker's asthma and wheat food allergy. Bakers sensitized to this LTP will often also become allergic to eating bread at some point, illustrating the LTP syndrome, as mentioned earlier. The Spanish research found that LTP syndrome was the likely issue among eight adults who had suffered anaphylaxis after eating wheat foods.

Researchers (Hartz *et al.* 2010) have discovered that allergies to hazelnuts and cherries are mediated by non-specific lipid transfer proteins and often stem from an initial sensitization to the *Pru p3* protein from peaches. They found that sensitization occurred with nsLTPs in 88% of peach allergies, 85% of hazelnut allergies and 77% of cherry allergies.

Corn allergies with anaphylaxis have been found to be mostly in response to the IgE reaction to alpha-amylase inhibitor and a *9-kDa* LTP. The *9-kd* lipid-transfer protein (LTP) is the major allergen of corn. The binding capacity to IgE was tested among different corn hybrids, and all showed about the same sensitization rates. Furthermore, cooking did not seem to affect this LTP allergen content in corn (Pastorello *et al.* 2003, Pastorello *et al.* 2009).

The major allergen of green beans (*Phaseolus vulgaris*) is the non-specific lipid transfer protein called *Pha v3*. This was confirmed in tests of 10 Spanish allergic patients (Zoccatelli *et al.* 2010).

About 1.1% of children with food allergies have allergies to mustard (Morisset *et al.* 2003). Researchers have found that nsLTP and profilin are the allergens in mustard seeds (Sirvent *et al.* 2009).

Researchers from Japan's Hiroshima University (Ibrahim *et al.* 2010) found a Japanese cedar pollen protein called CJP-8 had the genetic traits of a lipid transfer protein. This means that there is a likely crossover between sensitivities to LTP food proteins and various pollens.

The bottom line is that LTP is now being considered by a growing legion of researchers as the allergen most responsible for a majority of plant sensitivities, especially those with multiple cross-reactive food allergies. In most of these cases, a weakened immune system is involved in the sensitization. This is evidenced by the fact that we all breathe the same air, yet only a few of us become allergic to LTPs. Once an LTP breaks through normal mucosal immune barriers, sensitization occurs. The LTPs are then recognized by the weakened immune system as being antigens, or invaders—effectively stimulating an allergic reaction every time there is a similar LTP exposure. Worse, becoming sensitized to one type of LTP can also cross over to becoming sensitized to other LTPs in our environment.

Insect Endotoxins

Many believe that the dust mite—a tiny arachnid in the spider family—triggers allergies. This is not the whole story: the allergens are actually the mite's endotoxins. Their waste matter or byproduct streams trigger allergic hypersensitivity. Within their waste exist certain proteins, which can become allergens if the body becomes sensitized to them.

Many other insects also produce endotoxins that one may become sensitized to. These include cockroaches, ladybugs, aphids and other household pests. We should be clear that insect endotoxins are practically everywhere. They are unavoidable. They are in our water, air, foods, carpets, seats, floors… practically everywhere we live.

While insects are ubiquitous, dust mites are especially insidious because they are so tiny and hardy. They can live on practically any surface, especially beds, pillows, carpets, and other fabrics, and their favorite food is dead skin cells that slough off our bodies and those of our pets.

There are two prevalent household species: The American house dust mite (*Dermatophagoides farinae*) and the European house dust mite (*D. pteronyssinus*). Storage mite species include the *Acarus spp.* and *Tyrophagus spp.*

Dust mites feed on organic matter—meaning organism byproducts. The primary allergens these mites create are the skin moltings they shed as they grow, and their feces. Because of their propensity for eating skin, mites are usually not found in vents or ducts.

Many health experts have advised that dust mites like warm and humid places, so they suggest placing a dehumidifier in the house. University of Cambridge researchers (Hyndman et al. 2000) tested this theory. They investigated 76 households given a dehumidifier, a behavior program, or nothing for one year. Other trap measures were also instituted to reduce dust mites. Every three months they tested each house for humidity, temperature, dust mite counts, dust mite allergens, and several other environmental elements. The houses with dehumidifiers had no fewer dust mites than did the other more humid houses.

Confirming this, researchers from New Zealand's Wellington School of Medicine (Crane et al. 1998) studied lowering humidity levels in heat-exchanger systems (MVHE) units. They tested ten buildings in Wellington, NZ. Again, lowering the humidity in these buildings did not reduce concentrations of the Der p1 dust mite allergen.

German researchers (Kroidl et al. 2007) found, in a study of 132 patients with allergic asthma, over half were sensitized to either storage mites or house mites. Only three patients were allergic to storage mites and not household dust mites. Farm workers, bakers, forestry and paper mill workers had the most risk of storage mite allergies.

Researchers from Italy's G. D'Annunzio University (Riccioni et al. 2001) studied the seasonal nature of mite and pollen sensitivity among 165 allergic patients. They found that pollen symptoms increased with pollen seasons as expected. However, symptoms among patients allergic to dust mites increased in the fall—seemingly as mites or their endotoxin populations also increase.

Researchers from the UK's Imperial College (Atkinson et al. 1999) studied the relationship between allergen exposure and subsequent asthma among infants. They collected and analyzed dust samples from 643 homes. They coupled this with surveying each house and studying each infant. They found that higher dust mite allergen content was seen among houses that were carpeted, had double-glazed windows and less ventilation. Houses sampled in the winter had more dust mites than those sampled in other parts of the year. These conditions did not produce greater levels of cat allergens, however. Homes with more occupants had more dust mites and fewer cat allergens, regardless of cat ownership. Homes with smoking inhabitants had significantly fewer dust mites, but again had no difference in cat allergens.

More importantly, the researchers found no meaningful differences between allergen content in the homes between those sensitive to dust mites and those not sensitive.

This study and others have countered the hypothesis that allergies are predicated by homes with greater exposure to allergens.

This conclusion (that exposure does not cause allergies) is also quite simply determined by observation: Very few people have hay fever, despite the fact that pollens are ubiquitous.

Animal Dander

This naturally leads us to the topic of animal dander. Animal dander can come from any number of animals, including pets, farm animals, zoo animals and wild animals. This means that sources for animal dander include pet stores, zoos, vet clinics, farms, barns, and just about anywhere else animals may occupy for extended periods.

The allergic or sensitive element of animal dander is not necessarily their hair, however. It is typically the shedding of their skin as it flakes off their bodies. This can resemble dandruff, but may also be invisible to the naked eye. Dead skin or waste matter excreted by their skin is included in this. In other words, we are talking about animal waste matter.

Yet while both dog and cat ownership are ubiquitous in the United States, dog allergies are rare.

Furthermore, cat allergens (such as protein *Fel d1*) are found virtually everywhere. Scientists from New Zealand's Canterbury Respiratory Research Group and Christchurch Hospital (Martin *et al.* 1998) tested a variety of public places to understand exposure levels for the *Fel d1* cat allergen. They tested 203 floors, 64 beds and 24 seats in hotels, hospitals, rest homes, churches, schools, daycare centers, ski lodges, movie theaters, banks and airplanes. They found that 95% of the floors, 91% of the beds, and 100% of the seats maintained exposure levels of *Fel d1*. Furthermore, they found that theater seats and airplane seats contained the greatest levels, with more cat allergens than other public places, and most floors. Not surprisingly, cat allergen levels were greater on carpeted floors than on hard floors.

New Zealand has relatively high rates of asthma and allergies. About half of Kiwi households also have a cat, according to the research. To test the relationship between cat allergens and hypersensitivity, Wellington School of Medicine researchers (Patchett *et al.* 1997) tested the cat allergen (*Fel d1*) levels within schools and the clothing of children. They analyzed the clothing of 202 children and floors of 11 school classrooms. They found cat allergen practically everywhere—and (duh) highest on the clothing of children from homes that had cats. They also found a significant amount of cat allergen among the carpeted classes, significantly more than the floors without carpets.

While the researchers concluded that carpeting should be discouraged from schools and daycare centers, they could not correlate allergies and asthma frequency with increased cat allergens.

While this and other studies have confirmed that greater levels of pet dander do not necessarily produce allergies, pet dander is one of the most prevalent rhinitis triggers for those who have hypersensitivity.

Dairy Sensitivities

Hay fever, allergic rhinitis and asthma often develop among those who were or are allergic to milk as infants. Medical researchers from Rome's University La Sapienza (Cantani and Micera 2004) followed 115 infants with milk allergies for up to eight years starting at six months old. They found that while 57% eventually achieved tolerance of milk and other food allergens, asthma and hay fever later occurred in 54% of the milk-allergic children—many after becoming tolerant of milk.

Researchers from Portugal's Coimbra Pediatric Hospital (Santos *et al.* 2010) studied milk-allergic children in under-two-year-olds at their Pediatric Allergy Clinic between 1997 and 2006. Among the 139 children tested, 74% suffered from more than one symptom. Over time, 32% developed asthma.

Milk contains three principle parts: whey, butterfat and milk solids. The whey is the major protein component, while the butterfat contains several fatty acids, including butyric acid, palmitic acid, myristic acid, stearic acid, caproic acid, oleic acid, conjugated linolenic acid and linoleic acid (Månsson 2008). Milk solids contain proteins and various sugars such as lactose.

Research has found that the proteins casein and beta-lactoglobulin are the primary allergens in milk. However, lactose is the primary cause for milk intolerance.

About 2.5% of young infants among industrialized countries have allergies to cow's milk, including the United States (Schouten *et al.* 2010). Not surprisingly, milk allergies are highest among countries with more milk consumption. For example, University of Helsinki researchers (Salmi *et al.* 2010) found that cow's milk allergy is the most common form of food allergy in Finland.

This and other research has determined that most children are not born with milk allergies. Rather, milk allergies usually appear within the first few months after birth, and sometimes even later.

Research from Finland's National Institute for Health and Welfare (Metsälä *et al.* 2010) found in studies of children born between 1996 and

97

2004 that Cesarean section increased the risk of cow's milk allergies by 18%. Mothers being over 35 increased the risk by 23%. On the other hand, low socioeconomic status, several previous children and multiple pregnancies significantly decreased the risk of the child having milk allergies.

While wheezing and skin rashes are prevalent, other symptoms of milk allergy are often overlooked. Acid reflux is one example. Researchers from Denmark's University of Southern Denmark (Nielsen *et al.* 2004) studied 42 patients with cow's milk allergies. Eighteen of the 42 had severe acid reflux (GERD).

Helsinki University Central Hospital researchers (Suomalainen and Isolauri 1994) found that IFN-gamma levels were low in active milk allergy but higher among those who were recovering from milk allergies. After over a year on a milk elimination diet, IgA response to milk had increased among those who became tolerant to milk.

Japanese researchers (Nakano *et al.* 2010) found that casein and beta-lactoglobulin were the main allergens in cow's milk—as confirmed by other research. They also found that 97% of 115 milk allergy children had casein-specific IgE antibodies, while 47% had IgE antibodies against beta-lactoglobulin (beta-LG).

Oslo researchers (Sletten *et al.* 2006) found that beta-LG is resistant to enzymatic breakdown. This makes it available for non-immunoglobulin-mediated gastrointestinal symptoms should it be presented to intestinal tissues and bloodstream. Furthermore, patients tested for serum levels of beta-LG IgG and IgE levels were found to have delayed gastrointestinal food sensitivity symptoms.

The LG-immunoglobulins in this study were about 40 times lower in milk-tolerant people compared to milk-allergic patients. This was accompanied by a 90-fold increase in IgA-dominated immune responses in tolerant persons as compared with active-allergy patients. This of course means that those who are tolerant of milk still respond to the beta-LG molecule. They simply respond differently (without a hypersensitivity response) than those with active allergies. Milk-tolerant people respond with more mucosal membrane-IgA response initially—keeping beta-LG from invading the body.

This, by the way, is the normal way to respond to molecules not considered nutritious to the body. There are innumerable molecules like this in every meal. Our bodies respond quite normally, by simply preventing their inclusion into our tissues.

Italian researchers (Paganelli *et al.* 1985) found beta-lactoglobulin-specific antibodies within the blood of patients with ulcerative colitis and Crohn's disease. The IgG and IgM antibodies to beta-LG were found to be significantly higher compared to non-allergic individuals. This indicated prior immune system sensitivity to beta-LG.

Researchers from the University of Helsinki (Salmi *et al.* 2010) studied the urinary concentrations of 37 organic acids in 35 infants under one years of age with atopic eczema. Sixteen of the infants also had diagnosed milk allergies. The milk allergy infants had different urinary levels of hydroxybutyrate, adipate, isocitrate, homovanillate, suberate, tartarate, 3-indoleacetate and 5-hydroxyindoleacetate. This indicates that milk-allergic children metabolize milk components substantially differently. Why? We'll discuss this further in the next chapter.

Food-induced Allergic Rhinitis

Food-induced allergic rhinitis can be provoked via crossover or multiple allergies to pollens, dust mites or other airborne allergen producers. Or allergic rhinitis may be stimulated directly from the dust of grain flours, rice or other foods. These may be the initial sensitivity, or in some cases—as was found by Ajou University School of Medicine researchers (Kim *et al.* 2010)—be combined with other allergies. The allergic response may also be the result of a cross-reactivity with a similar pollen protein.

In the case of airborne flour allergies—also called baker's asthma or baker's allergies—the protein that produces the sensitivity is the LTP protein and the thaumatin-like protein (Lehto *et al.* 2010). These common proteins are often present in many of the grass pollens.

The thesis rising to the top among allergy researchers is the notion that many pollen allergies got their start from an initial allergic sensitization to larger food proteins that snuck into the bloodstream (hint: intestinal permeability). After all, we often eat the same basic proteins that exist within the plant's pollen. Let's discuss a few of these protein sources:

Wheat and Grains

Gluten is actually not a single protein. It is a category of proteins. Rather, the proteins in wheat are primarily either *gliadins* or *glutenins*. Within these two types are many different specific proteins. Furthermore, the types of glutinous proteins in wheat are not like the glutinous proteins in most other grains. In fact, between these two types, gliadins are considered the most prevalent allergen—common in both baker's asthma and wheat allergies (Ueno *et al.* 2010).

There also many other possible wheat allergens. They include *alpha-amylase inhibitor, peroxidase, thaumatin-like protein* (TLP) and *lipid transfer protein 2G* (LTP2G) and low-molecular-weight glutenins. These allergens are heat resistant and do not readily cross-react with grass pollen allergens (Pastorello *et al.* 2007).

From this information, we can know we can cross-react to proteins in wheat and other grains when our bodies have sensitivities to similar proteins to airborne allergens such as pollens.

While the full proteins (complex strings of hundreds of amino acids) will be different between wheat, barley and oats, for example, they will share similar peptide strings. These are also sometimes referred to as protein fractions.

French researchers (Bodinier *et al.* 2007) found that hydrolyzed omega5-gliadin fractions and lipid transfer proteins were detected within the epithelial layers after wheat consumption. We've discussed the repercussions of macromolecule intestinal wall contact in the previous chapter, and we'll dig into this topic further later.

These common protein fractions may be present in wheat, rye and barley. They may also be present in oats, corn and rice, although to a far lesser degree. However, these latter three grains have significantly different protein fractions, so it is less likely that a wheat protein sensitivity will cross over to oats, rice and corn.

Even so, a full carryover of gliadin or glutenin sensitivity may leave one sensitive to other foods that can contain wheat proteins. These include blue cheese, bouillon cubes, chocolate, curry, food colorings, starches, grain alcohols (including beer, ale, rye, scotch, bourbon or grain vodka), gum base, hydrolyzed vegetable protein, malts, marshmallows, modified food starches, monosodium glutamates, non-dairy creamers, processed meats, pudding, wheat/soy sauce, and even distilled vinegars.

This of course significantly changes the perspective that most people have as they consider "gluten sensitivities." In fact, gluten-free is somewhat of a misnomer, because nearly every grain elevator and trucking company transports or holds a variety of grains, which include those fractions considered "glutens." In these facilities, there is a strong likelihood of cross-contamination between grain proteins because the same bins and trucks will shift variably from one type of grain to another.

This doesn't mean that there aren't facilities dedicated to non-gluten-type protein grains. These may not mix bins and may carefully wash trucks. However, the risk of cross-contamination is still there, because grains can also cross-pollinate via the wind.

Thus, practically any grain can have some level of a protein fraction that can cross over with a pollen allergy. Most grains do come from grasses that indeed also produce pollen. But it is a very hard road to hoe, as it were.

For example, in a study published in the *Journal of the American Dietetic Association* (Thompson *et al.* 2010), 22 grains, seeds, and flours that were supposedly inherently gluten-free (but not labeled gluten-free)—including flours from sorghum, buckwheat and millet—were analyzed for gluten-type protein fraction content in a laboratory in June of 2009. The lab found that nine of the 22, or 41% of the supposedly gluten-free samples contained more than the limit considered as quantification for gluten-free, of five ppm (parts per million). In addition, seven of the 22 samples, or 32%, contained gluten levels that averaged more than 20 ppm. Under the FDA's proposed rule for gluten-free labels, these would not qualify to be labeled as "gluten-free."

Baker's asthma is a condition often experienced by food workers who become allergic to one or more of these wheat proteins. Spanish researchers (Palacin et al. 2010) found that the wheat flour lipid transfer protein (LTP) Tri a14 is the key allergen responsible for baker's asthma and wheat sensitivities among their test population. And because cross-reactivity is common among the LTPs, bakers who become sensitive to flour particulates at the workplace will or have already become allergic to eating bread at some point.

Many children with wheat allergies become tolerant as they get older. In the Cantani and Micera study mentioned earlier, the average age for becoming tolerant to wheat was seven years and two months.

Eggs

While egg allergies may not be connected with pollen allergies, they may be connected with feather and bird dander allergies.

Egg allergies are the second-most prevalent allergy in most Western countries behind dairy. They occur primarily among children, but also occur among adults. Egg allergies typically involve the OVO proteins ovomucoid, ovotransferrin, ovomucoid, or apovitillin, vosvetin, livetin, and/or ovalbumin.

Asthma and allergic rhinitis symptoms are prevalent among egg allergies. Researchers from Malaysia's Kebangsaan University (Yusoff et al. 2004) found that the removal of eggs and milk significantly improved wheezing symptoms and lung function of 22 allergic asthmatic children.

Australian researchers (Palmer et al. 2005) found that when lactating mothers ate cooked eggs, OVO concentrations within their breast milk increased substantially. The researchers concluded that this was the primary pathway for egg allergy development among infants who contract egg allergies prior to eating any eggs.

Contrary to what many believe, egg whites also contain egg allergens. Researchers from South Korea's Chung-Ang University's College of Pharmacy (Lee and Kim 2010) tested various products for egg allergens, and found the same allergens among egg whites, egg yolks, ovomucoid, alpha-livetin, ovalbumin, votransferrin, and lysozyme portions of eggs.

Furthermore, it is difficult to differentiate between egg protein allergens and chicken protein allergens. This is not surprising, since eggs are essentially the fetuses of unhatched chickens. This is confirmed by testing with the DNA-based PCR method of protein analysis, which cannot distinguish egg protein from chicken meat protein.

In addition, researchers (Swiderska-Kiełbik *et al.* 2010) have found that people regularly exposed to birds—which include zookeepers, pet shop workers, food industry employees and even pet bird keepers—have an increased risk of allergies to feathers, egg proteins, latex and even disinfectant chemicals.

Peanuts

Peanuts are not nuts. Really. Peanuts are legumes. They are closer relatives to beans and potatoes than to nuts, which typically grow on trees. Thus while peanut allergies don't directly crossover to pollen sensitivities, they can indeed crossover to a variety of sensitivities.

Peanut allergies are primarily a concern among developed countries of the Western world. Major studies have shown that developing countries exhibit far less prevalence of peanut allergies among their populations (Yang 2010).

Researchers from France's Allergology University Hospital (Morisset *et al.* 2005) calculated that peanut allergies are one of the most prevalent food allergies among Western countries, and third or fourth in prevalence in the U.S., the U.K. and Canada. In these countries, peanut allergy rates range from about 0.8% to 1.5% of the population. This calculates to nearly 20% of all food allergies in these countries.

This research also found that the peanut allergy rate in France was between 1% and 2.5% of the French population—the highest rate globally.

Furthermore, peanut allergy rates have been rising dramatically.

In a large epidemiological study, researchers working with the David Hide Asthma and Allergy Research Centre and St. Mary's Hospital on the Isle of Wight (Venter *et al.* 2010) studied the incidence of peanut allergies between 1994 and 2004 in thousands of children. The first group, born in 1989, was studied at four years old. The second group, born between 1994 and 1996, was studied between three and four years old. The third group, born between 2001 and 2002, was studied at three years old. Peanut sensitization levels increased from 1.3% in the first group to 3.3% in the second group. In the third group, sensitization to peanuts reduced to 2%. Peanut allergies were 0.5%, 1.4% and 1.2% respectively among the three groups.

It should be noted that peanut allergies often occur between three and four years old, so the third group in this study would still represent significant growth from the second group, as the second group included four-year-olds while the third group did not.

Peanuts are one of the most severe allergies in terms of potential anaphylaxis and asthmatic symptoms. Researchers from the Alfred I. DuPont Hospital for Children in Wilmington, Delaware (Simpson *et al.* 2010) studied children with peanut allergies older than three years old. They found that children with peanut allergies had more than double the chance of hospitalization than other children, and 1.6-times the risk of being prescribed systemic steroids. They also found that peanut allergies are often a predictive factor for death from anaphylaxis.

At the same time, research has illustrated that about 20% of young people with peanut allergies outgrow them. On the other hand, about 8% of those who outgrow a peanut allergy experience a recurrence. This is more significant among those who completely abstain from eating peanuts or only rarely eat them. Several studies have shown that a recurrence is less likely among those who consistently eat at least small amounts of peanuts periodically (Byrne *et al.* 2010).

The proteins in peanuts most known to cause allergies are the *Ara* protein epitopes. Specific IgE and IgG antibody levels (PN-IgE and PN-IgG) are prominent in most peanut allergies. Allergies to other peanut proteins have also been found, however (Lewis *et al.* 2005).

Research shows that the large increase in peanut allergies coincided with the mass distribution of roasted peanuts in the 80s and 90s. Many researchers are now concurring with this hypothesis, as we'll discuss further later.

As with eggs, many children have peanut allergies though they have not eaten any peanuts yet. Others have peanut allergies when they just begin to eat peanuts. How do these children contract their allergies if they have yet to be exposed to them?

Researchers from Montreal's Immunology-Allergy Department at Sainte-Justine's Hospital (DesRoches *et al.* 2010) tested 403 infants with peanut allergies under the age of 18 months, together with their mothers. Their focus was on exposure: How did the child gain exposure? Was it from the home? Or possibly from the mother or her breast milk?

They found that infants of mothers who consumed more peanuts during breastfeeding were over four times more likely to have peanut allergies than infants with mothers who did not eat peanuts during breastfeeding. They also found that mothers of infants with peanut-allergies were over twice as likely to eat more peanuts during pregnancy as mothers of non-allergic children. Outside of this exposure from their mother, the peanut-allergic children were no more exposed to peanuts in their environments than were the non-allergic children—who were, according other research, considerable.

Tree Nuts

While real nuts all grow on trees, most people refer to real nuts as tree nuts to avoid any confusion with peanuts. That said, nut sensitivities typically appear later than most other sensitivities. Nut allergies also tend to have a high risk of anaphylaxis. A good number of nut allergy sufferers will also be allergic to more than one nut. Crossover allergies between nuts and peanuts are less likely, but they do happen.

Tree nut allergies are also known to crossover with allergies to the tree pollens of those nut trees—walnuts, for example. Also, birch allergies have been associated with tree nut allergies.

Walnuts

The two allergens thought to cause most walnut allergies are *2S albumin* and *vicilin-like* protein. However, Italian researchers (Pastorello *et al.* 2004) studied 46 people with walnut sensitivities, and found that the allergens that caused sensitization were 9-kd lipid transfer protein—which affected 37 patients—and two vicilin proteins. Interestingly, the IgE response to walnut LTP was halted by LTP from peaches.

Cashews

Among cashew nut allergy sufferers, French researchers (Rancé *et al.* 2003) found that the average age of diagnosis was 2.7 years old. Out of these, only one in five, or 12% were exposed to nuts prior to their diagnosis. They also found that 56% suffered from skin symptoms. A quarter had respiratory issues and 17% had digestion issues. Many also had food allergies for other nuts, eggs, mustard, shrimp and milk.

Pistachios

The same researchers found that nearly one-third of those children allergic to cashews are also allergic to pistachios—which belong to the same botanical family as cashews.

Manganese superoxide dismutase (MnSOD) may be the allergen most responsible for allergic responses to pistachios, however. Iranian researchers (Noorbakhsh *et al.* 2010) found that MnSOD had the greatest potential for cross-reactivity as well.

Hazelnuts

Hazelnut's allergens include homologues to *Bet v1* and *Bet v2* proteins, a sucrose-binding protein, a legumin, a *2S albumin*, and a lipid transfer protein.

Research has confirmed that those allergic to hazelnuts are most sensitive to lipid transfer proteins *rCor a1.04, rCor a2, rCor a8* and *rCor a11.*

Spanish researchers (Hansen *et al.* 2009) also found that where a person lived often determined which type of LTP the person was allergic to. In other words, Italians and Spaniards were allergic to different LTPs than most of the Swiss or Danish allergic subjects.

Furthermore, some sufferers of hazelnut allergies are not allergic to roasted hazelnuts. Researchers from Denmark's National University Hospital (Hansen *et al.* 2003) found that roasting hazelnuts reduced their allergenicity in a majority of cases. They tested 17 confirmed hazelnut food allergy sufferers with roasted hazelnuts, and found that twelve were not sensitive to roasted hazelnuts. However, five of the 17 tested sensitive to the roasted nuts. That is still significant enough to be concerned.

Soy

Researchers from Johns Hopkins University School of Medicine (Savage *et al.* 2010) studied 133 soy-allergic patients. Of the 133, 71% had allergic rhinitis.

The *Gly m4* protein is considered soy's central allergen. However, the content of the soy allergen *Gly m4* in soy foods depends on the amount and type of processing, and whether it has been fermented. Fermenting reduces *Gly m4* levels. This means that someone allergic to soy flour or raw soybeans may not be very sensitive to tempeh or tofu.

This said, soy and a number of other beans also contain a particularly difficult saccharide called *raffinose*. Many people who are intolerant of soy cannot digest this saccharide well. Raffinose requires a special enzyme termed by some as raffinase, but its more technical name is *alpha-galactosidase*. Alpha-galactosidase is not produced by the human body.

However, alpha-galactosidase *is* produced by probiotic bacteria. For this reason, a person with healthy colonies of probiotic bacteria in their intestines should have no problem breaking down raffinose into sucrose and galactose. We should note that other foods, such as broccoli, beans, cabbage and Brussels sprouts, also contain raffinose.

Another complex saccharide in soybeans is stachyose. Stachyose contains similar properties as raffinose. Broccoli, Brussels sprouts, cabbage and other plant foods contain stachyose as well.

Alternatively, the probiotics used to produce fermented soy foods will also break down much of the raffinose and stachyose. See the section on fermented foods in the last chapter.

The incomplete breakdown of raffinose from beans into sucrose and galactose also has an interesting byproduct: flatulence. Many choose to add alpha-galactosidase with over-the-counter supplement solutions. Supplementing with probiotics is another possible strategy.

Back to soy allergies: Swiss researchers (Ballmer-Weber *et al.* 2007) have found that only 10 mg to 50 grams of soy will produce symptoms recognized by the allergic person. They also showed that it would take from 454 mg to 50 grams of soy to produce *"objective symptoms"* (symptoms recognizable by health professionals). This number decreases dramatically when soy isolates are considered.

It also should be noted that IgE sensitization to soy is rare, particularly during early infancy. It is more frequently seen following pollen sensitization contracted during school-age childhood. Birch pollen allergies have been known to cross-over to soybean allergies.

Seafood

Researchers from Canada's McGill University (Ben-Shoshan *et al.* 2010) surveyed nearly 10,000 people in 2008 and 2009, and found that seafood allergies were greater than any other food allergy, with a 2.1% total between fish (.5%) and shellfish (1.6%).

Parvalbumin is the central protein allergen among fish seafood. Cod seems to be one of the more allergic fish, as it contains significant parvalbumins. Often cod brings on the initial sensitivity, and other fish such as carp, salmon, tuna, halibut, flounder and others become cross-reactive as they are consumed. Once sensitive, even inhaling cooked fish vapors can set off a significant reaction (de Martino *et al.* 1993; O'Neil *et al.* 1993).

Fish allergies often come with severe reactions, which include severe skin rashes and anaphylaxis. This means that bronchospasm, wheezing, and choking can arrive almost immediately after eating seafood or breathing fish cooking fumes.

Mollusk allergies include squid and other cephalopods. The *36 kDa* protein from squid tropomyosin (muscle) has been shown to be a significant allergen. The heat-sensitive protein is *50 kDa*. This can cause increased sensitivity when squid is eaten raw (Yadzir *et al.* 2010).

Tropomyosin is also suspected as the major source of crab allergies (Liu *et al.* 2010). It is resistant to stomach pepsin, but trypsin and chymotrypsin enzymes can break it down if available (Ueno *et al.* 2010).

Meat

Despite the lack of attention, meat allergies do exist. Researchers (Theler *et al.* 2009) from Zürich's University Hospital found people with IgE allergies to pork, beef and chicken. Those with meat allergies complained of skin rashes, nausea, diarrhea, vomiting and/or abdominal pain.

Other research has confirmed that beef allergies can have other symptoms such as skin rash, artery inflammation, digestive difficulties and anaphylaxis. Basophil testing can expose immunoglobulin E-mediated allergies for beef protein (Kim *et al.* 2010).

Albumin is often the central allergen in meat. This protein is contained in most animal foods. Albumin-specific IgE antibodies are frequently found. Bovine serum albumin (or BSA) is often the culprit (Fiocchi *et al.* 1995).

Food Trigger Doses

Most IgE-mediated food allergies require a specific range of dosage before sensitivity symptoms will result. Foods will require anywhere from five to 5,000 milligrams to produce a clinical response. For oils including peanut, sesame, sunflower, and soy oil, up to 30 milliliters can cause a response for those sensitive. Here is a chart based on the research:

Food	Respiratory Symptoms	Reaction at 65mg/.8mL	Lowest Reactive Dose
Eggs	12%	16%	2 mg
Peanuts	20%	18%	5 mg
Milk	10%	5%	0.1 mL
Sesame	42%	8%	30 mg

(Morisset *et al.* 2003)

Foods Containing Histamine

Foods like cheese, sausage, sauerkraut, tuna, tomatoes, and alcohol can contain up to 500 mg/kg of histamine. Eating foods that contain high levels of histamine may sometimes trigger allergies.

To test this, researchers from the Floridsdorf Allergy Center in Vienna, Austria (Wöhrl *et al.* 2004) gave 75 mg of liquid histamine dissolved in tea or the tea alone to ten healthy non-allergic females between the ages of 22-36 years old. After testing with a standardized symptom protocol over 24 hours, they found that five of the ten subjects experienced reactions to the histamine. These included tachycardia, mild hypotension, sneezing, runny nose and itchy nose, most within the first hour. Four of the five also had diarrhea, flatulence, headaches and other delayed symptoms that began after three hours of consuming the histamine.

French INSERM researchers (Kanny *et al.* 1996) also studied histamine levels in food and intestinal permeability. They had previously demonstrated that ingested histamine could promote or stimulate chronic urticaria (hives). The researchers fed seven urticaria patients with 120 mg of histamine. They found that histamine stimulated diarrhea, urticaria, headaches, increased heart rate and a drop in blood pressure among five of the seven within an hour of the histamine exposure. The researchers performed intestinal biopsies on the urticaria patients before and after the histamine. They found that the histamine also caused inflammation within the intestinal intercellular regions.

These studies gave pure liquid histamine to their subjects. The question of course is whether eating otherwise healthy foods high in histamine, such as tomatoes and sauerkraut, will necessarily produce these reactions.

We should remember that healthy foods also contain a variety of nutrients (tomatoes contain over 10,000 healthy constituents, for example) that are anti-inflammatory. These buffer histamine reactions and balance the activity of histamine within the tissues.

However, an unhealthy source of histamine, such as sausage or alcohol, may be another matter altogether, because these sources contain other elements (nitrites, ethanol and so on) that can stimulate inflammation in considerable amounts because of their radical-producing abilities. These foods have been associated with damaged livers and an increased risk of cancer.

Food Additives

Many commercial foods contain numerous synthetic chemical additives. These include hundreds of artificial food colors, preservatives, stabilizers, flavorings and a variety of food processing aids. A number of these additives have been found to cause sensitivities in some people.

Food additives that have been particularly suspected to trigger allergies include preservatives such as sodium benzoate, 4-hydrooxybenzoate esters, BHA, BHT, aspartame, MSG and sulfites.

Suspected colorings include FD&C Yellow #5 (tartrazine), FD&C Red No. 40, FD&C Yellow #6, FD&C Red No. 3, FD&C Blue No. 1, FD&C Blue No. 2 and FD&C Green No. 3.

Clinical experience has confirmed that azo dyes, sulphur dioxide and benzoates have triggered allergy and asthmatic episodes in children (Freedman 1977; Novembre et al. 1992).

Illustrating the effects that food additives can have, Australian researchers (Dengate and Ruben 2002) studied 27 children with irritability, restlessness, inattention and sleep difficulties. The researchers saw many of these symptoms subside after putting the children on the *Royal Prince Alfred Hospital Diet*, which is absent of food additives, natural salicylates, amines and glutamates.

Using preservative challenges, the researchers were also able to determine that preservatives significantly affected the children's behavior and physiology adversely.

Researchers from Britain's University of Southampton (Bateman et al. 2004) screened 1,873 three-year old children for hyperactivity and the consumption of artificial food colors and preservatives. They gave the children 20 mg daily of artificial colors and 45 mg daily of sodium benzoate, or a placebo mixture. The additive group showed significantly higher levels of hyperactivity than the group that did not consume the artificial colors and preservative.

Once an additive has caused intolerance symptoms such as those from the research above, the immune system may begin to become sensitive to some of the foods these additives are combined with. This likelihood increases should the immune system become continually exposed to the foods and additives over a considerable period.

Note also that many pharmaceuticals also contain significant trigger-suspect colors—such as FD&C yellow No. 5 (tartrazine).

Sulfites

The sulfite ion will aggressively preserve a food. Sulfites can also produce wheezing, tightness of the throat and other symptoms almost immediately after eating foods preserved with them. There is sufficient evidence to point to sulfites as a potent allergy and asthma trigger (Schroecksnadel *et al.* 2010).

Researchers from the University of Cape Town (Steinman *et al.* 1993) studied sulphur dioxide reactivity among 37 asthmatic children. They were challenged with sulphur dioxide in apple juice (at levels common among soft drinks with sulphur dioxide) or apple juice without the SO2. Among the SO2 group, 43% reacted with reductions in forced expiratory volume (FEV1) by greater than 10%. None of the only apple juice group suffered a fall in FEV1.

The alcohol levels may also contribute to this effect when wine is being considered. Illustrating this, researchers from Australia's Centre for Asthma (Vally *et al.* 2007) tested eight wine-sensitive subjects with sulfite wine and non-sulfite wine. The researchers found that the wine sensitivities were unlikely caused by the sulfites in the wine.

Today, sulfites are used to preserve many wines, dehydrated potatoes and numerous dried fruits. Sulfites include potassium bisulfite, sulfur dioxide, potassium matabisulfite and others. Often labels do not disclose the use of sulfites, because the preservative may have been used early in the processing of the raw ingredients instead of added into the finished product. In addition, under current U.S. labeling laws, if an ingredient such as sulfite is less than 10 parts per million, there is no requirement for putting the ingredient on the panel.

Sulfite sensitivity may also be a result of B12 deficiency. In a study presented to the American Academy of Allergy and Immunology, 18 sulfite-sensitive persons were given sublingual B12. The B12 effectively blocked adverse reactions to sulfites in 17 of the 18 (Werbach 1996).

Monosodium Glutamate

Monosodium glutamate also gets a lot of attention for triggering allergic rhinitis symptoms. This assumption, however, has been largely unconfirmed in controlled research.

In research from the Scripps Research Institute in La Jolla, California (Woessner *et al.* 1999), 100 asthmatics were double-blind challenged with 2.5 grams of MSG. Thirty of the test subjects had a history of asthma attacks during Oriental restaurant meals. The research found that none of the patients suffered from any asthma symptoms after receiving the MSG challenge, regardless of whether they had perceived they had an MSG-sensitivity or not.

To better understand this, Harvard researchers (Geha *et al.* 2000) set out to study the effects of MSG sensitivities in a multi-center study. They found that of 130 human volunteers who thought they were sensitive to MSG, 38% physically responded to MSG with allergic symptoms. However, 13% also responded to a placebo (they thought contained MSG). Subsequent retesting continued to show inconsistent responses among some of those who thought they were MSG-sensitive.

This led the researchers to conclude that people who believe they are sensitive tend to react more strongly to MSG, but their responses were not always consistent. This of course may be the result of differing levels of tolerance and periods of sensitivity—again depending upon immunity.

This research still confirms that MSG can cause sensitivity responses, but there is a strong possibility of a placebo effect in some. There may also be a stress-related relationship between MSG and the allergic rhinitis episode.

Pesticides/Herbicides

Fumigant residuals can remain in our foods long after spraying. Foods with thin or no peels, and animals—which bioaccumulate chemicals—have the most risk. Pesticide residues have been observed in bloodstreams and even the umbilical cords of mothers. While they might be considered toxins rather than allergens, they can still trigger hypersensitive responses.

Yeast, Molds and other Fungi

Microorganisms and their endotoxins can also trigger allergies. These are collectively called *biological pollutants*. These microorganisms include bacteria, viruses, fungi and mold.

Bacteria can come from rotting food, plants, people and pets. Dander also can carry these creatures. Viruses can trigger inflammation initially, or once they infect the body's cells. Viruses damage DNA within the cells, and reproduce through the body via the DNA damage. Once the inflammation grows, the body's immune system can become suppressed.

Microorganisms can grow on anything wet, because like most living organisms, they need water to stay alive.

Yeasts

There are a variety of different species of yeasts. Some of these are pathogenic and will stimulate allergic responses, while still others are probiotic at controlled population levels.

Yeast (*Saccharomyces cerevisiae*) is a type of fungus considered by researchers to be harmless and even probiotic among most people. Yeast is commonly used to prepare a variety of foods, including breads, pizza and other baked goods. Yeast is also found within the colons of healthy people. For this reason, this species of yeast is considered either safe or having probiotic functions within the body.

As we'll discuss in detail in our chapter on nutrition, the *Saccharomyces cerevisiae* yeast is also the subject of a nutritional supplement. Here the yeast is stressed, and this stimulates its production of a number of nutrients and immune factors, both of which will assist our bodies.

Like any microorganism, however, there must exist a balance between the different probiotic species and strains within the gut in order the maintain health. Persons without that balance, or who have become infected with overgrowths of other not-so-probiotic yeast colonies such as *Candida spp.*, may become sensitive to foods containing yeast. Yeast sensitivities may also yield or be a symptom of other intestinal problems.

Molds

Yeasts and molds are both members of the fungi family. While many fungi such as mushrooms are protective to the immune system, an overburdened immune system can become sensitive to microorganism yeasts and molds. Yeasts can become infective and can directly overload the immune system. Molds and their airborne spores can also overload the immune system.

Mold spores float through both the outdoor and indoor air. Should they land on a hospitable locale, they begin multiplying into larger cultures. Almost all molds require moisture to grow and populate. A concentration of spores riding the indoor air currents can land in the airways, causing allergic responses in vulverable people (Sahakian *et al.* 2008).

Mold spores also produce a number of byproducts called mycotoxins, which can create health concerns if inhaled.

This was confirmed by researchers from the National University of Singapore (Tham *et al.* 2007), who found that home dampness and indoor mold is linked to an increase in asthma and allergy symptoms among children. They studied 4,759 children from 120 daycare centers. After eliminating other possible effects, home humidity was significantly associated with increased rates of allergic rhinoconjunctivitis. As discussed earlier, allergic rhinoconjunctivitis is the inflammation of the conjunctiva and sinuses as a result of histamine release following an allergic immune response. As mold burdens the immune system, the body can respond with allergic inflammation.

In a study of school buildings (Sahakian *et al.* 2008), 309 school employees in two older elementary schools were tested. Excess dampness produced increased incidence of respiratory irritation, wheezing and rhinitis symptoms among the employees. The older, damper school of the two also produced more allergic asthma symptoms.

Homeowners and renters should be aware of this, and make sure the houses they live in have no water entry into the basement. Moist appliances like air conditioners, bathtubs, bathroom carpets, and air ducts can also grow mold.

For these reasons, we might want to frequently check the various corners and dark places in our houses and workplaces for moisture, because the fungal or bacterial populations growing on these surfaces will only get bigger with time—disbursing toxins into the air as they grow. Once found, the area should be dried, the mold or bacteria should be cleaned up (water with a few drops of rubbing alcohol, vinegar or chlorine will kill most mold or bacteria) thoroughly. If a mold growth is significant, a mold specialist may need to be called in to eliminate the mold.

Overgrowths of yeasts like *Candida albicans* can also contribute to or be a primary cause for asthma and allergies. A 1987 study (Gumowski *et al.*) found that among 64 cases of asthma or rhinitis, 52 had formed hypersensitivities to *Candida albicans*—meaning they were likely infected now or in the recent past.

Candida albicans can grow conjunctively with *Staphylococcus aureus,* resulting in the accelerated growth of both microorganisms. This can result in a tremendous burden for the immune and probiotic systems as they try to defend against the incursion of combined yeast and bacteria infections.

As the immune system becomes overloaded with a microorganism invasion, it will often respond with an acute inflammatory response, simply because the system is already on alert mode. This produces a system-wide pattern of inflammation responses—which can produce allergies.

Bacteria

Bacteria also produce endotoxins that hypersensitive people may become allergic or sensitive to. Lipopolysaccharides are a class of bacteria endotoxins found to cause sensitivities. Lipopolysaccharides make up the cell membranes of gram negative bacteria, so they slough off in the course of their tiny lives. Lipopolysaccharides have shown in research to produce inflammation and asthma symptoms. Their ability to cause allergy symptoms is still being debated.

Illustrating this, researchers from the Britain's Imperial College School of Medicine (Nightingale *et al.* 1998) gave lipopolysaccharide or placebo (saline) to eight allergic-asthmatics, seven allergic but not asthmatic people, and eleven healthy subjects. The lipopolysaccharide or placebo was inhaled through the nostrils. Post-inhalation tests revealed that the asthmatics—but no other group—experienced a rise in fever temperature after inhaling the lipopolysaccharides. Differential neutrophil counts were also heightened in the asthma group compared to the others after lipopolysaccharide inhalation.

Delayed (24 hours) interleukin 8 (IL-8) levels also significantly increased among the asthmatic group. These results indicated that asthmatics had greater levels of inflammation, and this made them more sensitive to these bacterial endotoxins. In other words, they were already immunosuppressed.

Parasites

An analysis of the Third National Health and Nutrition Examination Survey sponsored by the Centers for Disease Control (Walsh 2008), which included 18,883 participants, found that helminth infection was associated with lower forced expiratory volumes (FEV1). This was more specific among those who had an infection of *Toxocara spp*. It should be noted that *Toxocara spp*. is a parasite typically infecting cats—often without obvious symptoms.

The study found that those with current or former *Toxocara* infections had FEV1s an average of 105.3 mL lower than those who had not been infected with *Toxocara*. Other associations were removed to establish the link.

There is little indication that *Toxocara* and other parasites produce allergies or asthma. However, they burden the immune system, and their endotoxins can provoke inflammation.

Positive Ions and Allergens

Research has indicated that for many, atmospheric conditions related to positive ions trigger allergic hypersensitivity episodes.

The electromagnetic interaction between water, atmospheric elements, and geomagnetism produces polarity within our local environment. Positive ions attract dust, pollens and endotoxins, while negative ions repel them (Soyka and Edmonds 1978).

Atmospheric ions are suspended in our atmosphere. They provide stability among the elements and their atmospheric effects. Humidity, smog, cities, buildings, wind and weather storms all affect our local ion levels.

Outdoor ion counts in rural areas in good weather conditions can range from 200 to 4,000 negative ions and 250 to 1500 positive ions per cubic centimeter. Positive ion count can increase to over five thousand ions per cubic centimeter ahead of an incoming storm front. This is due to the sudden increase in humidity within the storm front. Once the storm front hits, the level of positive ions falls quickly, and negative ion levels dramatically rise.

Smog and other pollutants dramatically reduce total ion count. This is thought to be because both positive and negative ions will attach to unstable pollutant particles.

Natural settings containing moisture can contain dramatically more negative ions. For example, a waterfall might have as much as 100,000 negative ions per cubic centimeter. Negative ion levels around crowded freeways tend to be quite low, on the other hand—often below 100 negative ions per cubic centimeter.

Numerous trials have indicated that indoor negative ion levels are slightly lower than outdoor levels in most areas. This is thought to be because outdoor ions tend to interact with greater levels of moisture, and thus last longer than do their indoor cousins. This also correlates with the existence of the various electromagnetic fields existing within the home due to the use of various electronic appliances.

Negative ions can form easily. One pass of the comb through the hair can create from 1,000 to 10,000 ions per cubic centimeter. The living organism is a tremendous ion producer. Assuming adequate grounding onto the earth or a grounding metal, a typical human exhalation will contain from 20,000 to 50,000 ions per cubic centimeter. This correlates with the fluid levels in the body.

Positive ions are typically generated with a decrease of atmospheric pressure; an increase in wind and temperature; a decrease in humidity and a decrease in elevation. This is particularly noticeable in *Foehn winds*— warm winds that descend from mountainous areas down to areas of lower elevation.

Wind patterns considered Foehn include the dry southerly wind blowing through the Alps, Switzerland and across southern Germany. The Sharav or Hamsin winds blowing though the desert of the Middle East are also Foehn winds. The Sirocco winds that blow through Italy and the Mistral winds that blow through southern France are both considered Foehns. The Chinook winds of western Canada and NW United States, and the Santa Ana winds that blow through southern California from time to time are also considered Foehn winds. Foehn winds have also been occasionally registered around various mountain ranges such as the Colorado Rocky Mountains and Tennessee's Smokey Mountains. Foehn winds tend to funnel between mountain ridges, which accelerate their gusting speeds to an excess of 50 miles per hour.

Foehn winds are known for their heat and ultralow humidity, and their propensity for causing erratic fires. They also can cause a number of negative physical and emotional effects in both humans and animals. For these various reasons, the Foehn is often referred culturally as an 'ill wind.' While some have disputed the effects of Foehn winds, both research and observation has indicated otherwise. Research performed by Sulman, et al. (1977; 1980) has indicated that these winds are associated with headaches, heat stress, and irritability. Others have documented an increase in allergies and sinus ailments during Foehn winds.

Positive ions are thus associated with immediate changes in temperature, pressure, and humidity. Because positive ions are linked to Foehn winds, it is safe to assume that the various effects related to positive ions are also connected with the environmental effects of Foehn winds.

Not surprisingly, ions' effects upon health and behavior have been the subject of scientific study for the past eighty years. This began in 1926, when Russian scientist Alexander Chizhevsky exposed animals to air ionized with negative ions and/or positive ions. In these studies, he found—as have many others such as Krueger and Reed (1976)—that living in positive ion conditions is associated with more illness and shorter life duration when compared with those living in areas with greater negative ion conditions.

In Sulman's 1980 study, daily urine samples were taken from 1,000 volunteers one to two days before a storm's arrival during Foehn winds, and then during normal weather conditions. The samples were analyzed for neurotransmitter and hormone levels, including serotonin, adrenaline, noradrenaline, histamine, and thyroxine metabolites. The results concluded that during positive ion conditions, an overproduction of serotonin levels resulted in irritability. In positive ion conditions, Sulman found increases in adrenal deficiency and early exhaustion. Positive ions were also associated with hyperthyroidism and subclinical "apathetic" thyroid symptoms.

There are a number of ways we can temporarily increase our negative ion count in our home. These include salt lamps, small indoor waterfalls, and house plants. Some new ionizing machines will apparently increase negative ions as well.

Beyond this, living in a rural or natural environment or at least frequenting such an environment can surround us with greater levels of negative ions.

Multiple Sensitivities

Remember the research from the National Institutes of Health (Arbes et al. 2007) that used the Third National Health and Nutrition Examination Survey to study allergens and asthma. They found that most of the asthmatics in this huge study were allergic to multiple triggers. Of the allergens tested, cat dander was found to be the most prevalent allergen, at 29%.

Combinations of allergens can overwhelm the immune system and provoke inflammatory response. Researchers from the University of North Carolina's School of Medicine (Eldridge and Peden 2000) illustrated this effect when they tested twelve allergic asthmatic subjects with a combination of inhaled endotoxins and allergens. They gave subjects nasal lavages with saline, *E. coli* endotoxin, and/or dust mite allergen. Those subjects receiving both the endotoxin and dust mite allergen responded with asthmatic reactions, while those receiving saline or one of the other two alone did not have the response.

The researchers also found that the post-response for the combination of endotoxin and allergen produced increased levels of inflammatory cells. In other words, the immune system is more reactive when it was burdened with multiple toxins.

Multiple triggers are typically prevalent among hypersensitive people. Early food triggers, for example, often lead to other allergies later, and vice versa. Significant research has confirmed that most hay fever sufferers develop multiple allergies.

Illustrating this, researchers from UK's Heartlands Hospital (Tunnicliffe *et al.* 1999) studied indoor allergens among 28 people with severe asthma and 26 people with mild asthma. They tested sensitivities to dust mites (*Der p1*), dogs (*Can f1*) and cats (*Fel d1*). Every severe asthmatic subject was sensitive to at least one of the allergens, and 20 of the 28 severe asthmatics were sensitive to all three of the allergens.

Of the mild asthmatics, only 14 of the 26 were sensitive to any of the three allergens, and only one was sensitive to all three.

When children present with multiple asthma triggers, doctors will often attempt to find which trigger was primary to the others. The primary allergy is thought to be the one that the child became sensitized to first. The primary allergen is also thought to produce the cross-reactivity that caused the second sensitivity. In other words, once there is an initial allergy, subsequent allergies can follow the primary one.

To explain this relationship, researchers from Germany's Charité University Medical Center (Matricardi *et al.* 2008) followed 1,314 children for up to thirteen years from birth. They found that sensitization to milk and eggs decreased over years, from levels of 4% at two years old to less than one percent at ten years old. On the other hand, allergies to soy and wheat increased as the children got older: From about 2% at two years old to about 7% at 13 years old for soy; and from 2% to 9% for wheat allergies.

When the children were ten years old, confirmed allergies to grass pollen were from 97% to 98% of those children who were allergic to soy and wheat. In addition, allergies to birch pollen among the soy and wheat allergy children occurred in 86% and 82%, respectively.

The researchers concluded that the pollens must be the primary allergens in most of these cases. They found that soy or wheat allergies were primary to grass or birch pollen in only 4% and 8% of participants sensitized to soy and wheat, respectively.

University of Chicago researchers (Sahin-Yilmaz *et al.* 2010) found that when peanut, shrimp, and milk allergies are compared, peanut is associated with multiple allergies, and milk is more associated with later asthmatic symptoms. In 283 allergic adults, they found that peanut and shrimp sensitivities are most commonly symptomized by allergic rhinitis.

The bottom line is that multiple triggers are frequent among allergy sufferers. This illustrates that it is not the particular allergy that makes a person have hay fever or allergic rhinitis: There is an underlying condition. many allergy triggers are also toxins to the body. They are not welcomed by the immune system. For some reason or another, the immune system considers them threatening to the body's tissues, organs or cellular processes. As we'll discuss further in the next chapter, this is the product of the immune system being deranged and overloaded, and hypersensitive to a fault. As we've shown, the human body under normal circumstances should easily become tolerant to those allergens produced by other living organisms. At any rate, the chart below provides a short list of the major allergen sources:

Major Allergen Sources

Source	Allergen-Supplier
Animals	Dried skin, bacteria, waste excreted from animal (dander)
Carpets, rugs	Molds, dander, lice, PC-4, latex
Foods	Dairy, eggs, glutens, pollen-foods, seafood, meats, peanuts, tree nuts, etc.
House and Garden	Pollen, dust mites, mold, dander, insect endotoxins
Insects	Endotoxins from mites, cockroaches and other insects
Microorganisms	Mold, sometimes bacteria
Mattresses/pillows	Endotoxins, molds, dust mites
Pets	Dander, up to 240 infectious diseases & parasites (65 from dogs/39 from cats)

Pollinating plants	See pollen list in pollen section
Work and school environments	Practically all of the above

Strategies to Reduce Allergen Exposure

From the research discussed, allergen exposure does not necessarily cause the allergy, but for someone with an underlying disposition, exposure can increase allergy symptoms and flare-ups.

In other words, cutting back on exposure may reduce our rhinitis severity because it can lighten the allergen load on our bodies. While we may be able to reduce exposure, avoiding allergens is quite difficult, and will not necessarily prevent or correct the underlying condition, as we'll elaborate on further.

Here are a few strategies we can use, when appropriate, to reduce many of the more common allergens:

> **Find out** precisely what we are allergic to. Consider the diagnostic section in the first chapter. Removing the wrong allergens can result in a lack of exposure, reducing our tolerance to the allergen, with the possibility of becoming sensitized to it after a re-exposure.

> **Clean the house:** Yes, it is not fun to clean the house. But it can be done weekly or semi-monthly, depending upon the house's use. Removing dust and microscopic debris will also remove the food for dust mites: skin flakes. We all slough off skin throughout the house, and this becomes our dust mites' favorite food.

> **Dusting** with a wet cloth and vacuuming with a HEPA (High-Efficiency Particular Arresting) filter are good strategies. The HEPA filter will keep some allergens and their sources in the bin and not back out through the blower. Cleaning the walls is often overlooked. Dust mites, mold and bacteria can all dwell on vertical surfaces just fine, thank you. To test a vacuum cleaner's integrity, we can turn off the lights and shine a flashlight into its exhaust. The particulates of a leaky vacuum will show up in the light.

> **Bedding can be washed** at least every two weeks in hot water. Observations have shown that wash water needs to be heated to 130 degrees F to kill dust mites.

> **Blinds** are better window coverings than curtains. Curtains can accumulate mold, dust mites and pollen. They are typically difficult to wash and dry, and for that reason, they rarely get washed in most households. Blinds are very easy

to clean even while still on the window. Removing them and hosing them down outside is probably a better strategy.

➤ **Household cleaners** can be natural. These include baking soda, vinegar, lemon and borax. These are all, to relative degrees, also antimicrobial.

➤ **Tubs and bathrooms** can be cleaned frequently, before mold forms. Mold grows in moist, dark places, so those areas of the bathroom can be cleaned more frequently than areas exposed to sunshine.

➤ **The best floors** are wood, stone or ceramic tiles. Vinyl flooring is better than carpet, but inferior to natural materials. Carpets and floor mats attract and house pollens, dust mites and insects. The floor can be periodically washed with vinegar and rubbing alcohol.

➤ **Carpets** can be regularly vacuumed. The application of tannic acid products can reduce dust mite populations. If dust mite allergies exist, having someone else do the vacuuming is not a bad idea.

➤ **Houseplants** are great for the house because they can give off significant oxygen. But beware that their soils can breed molds, and some may pollenate. Best if plants are kept where there is plenty of sunlight in contact with the soil.

➤ **Wearing a mask** during mowing is not a bad idea for those with grass pollen allergies. Or having someone else mow.

➤ **Fresh, natural air** is best assuming no pollen allergy. Windows are best left open in the right environment. Fresh air helps our airways purge allergens. Environments with smog and/or fireplace smoke can be blocked from entering the home to the degree possible, but be careful of the build-up of indoor pollutants. Most houses harbor worse air inside than outside. We might consider an environmental filter.

Creating an Allergy Safe Room

Anyone with active allergies can consider having a safe room. A safe room is a room in the house where we can go if we are feeling an episode coming on, or in the midst of one. The idea of a clean room is that it is clear of potential allergens and major toxins, while providing a calming, relaxing environment. Here are a few things that can be done to establish and maintain a safe room:

Floors: The safe room can have bare floors that are easily cleaned. Hard wood, stone or ceramic tiles are preferred. Vinyl flooring is next down the list. Carpets and floor mats can be removed. Any floor covering

can invite dust, dirt, mold, bacteria and dust mites. The floor can be periodically washed with vinegar and rubbing alcohol.

Walls: Cleaning the walls periodically is a good idea. Vinegar is a great
cleaner for walls because it can also eliminate mold spores. Just a quick
wipe is all that would be needed. Clearing the ceiling corners of cobwebs
might also be a good idea. These collect debris.

Furniture: Natural wood furniture is probably best for the clean
room. It can be simple and easy to dust. Fancy furniture with lots of
nooks and crannies will collect dust, mold and microorganisms. Sofas or
beds can be covered with an easily washable fabric. Plastic or vinyl covers
can be put on to mattresses or sofas for dust mite allergic-asthmatics, but
these can also outgas formaldehyde or plasticizers. Better to stick with
natural coverings if possible. Best to have a washable fabric and have
mattresses covered with linens.

Houseplants: Best to keep these out of the clean room, at least for
the hypersensitive.

Air: Fresh is best, unless outdoor air is smoggy, pollen-filled (for pollen-sensitive people) or otherwise toxic. The clean room should have
good windows with screens, preferably windows that let in sunlight
(sunlight will decrease the populations of molds and dust mites. A HEPA
(high-efficiency particle-arresting) air filter may be installed in the room,
especially during times where outdoor or indoor air is questionable.

Water: The clean room should be kept dry. Water will feed molds and
fungi. Look for leaks into the window sills. Humidifiers are not a good
idea in the clean room, because the moisture can breed molds.

Pets: Pets can be kept out of the clean room. They can track in a variety of microorganisms, dust, dirt, moisture, and their own allergens in
the form of dander.

Chemicals: The clean room can be clear of pesticides, fragrances, in-
cense, and other chemicals. If bugs are a problem, borax or traps in adjacent rooms could be considered.

Air Filtration Strategies

Reducing allergen and toxin load somewhat may be accomplished
with good filtration systems. Here are the main types:

Air purifiers: These can significantly remove allergens from the air,
as they draw air through a filter and then push the air out. Studies have
shown that air purifiers can significantly increase the quality of life among
the hypersensitive (Brodtkorb *et al.* 2010).

Electric ion generating machines generate negative ions. Ionizers
have been reputed to remove dust and mold spores. However, this has yet
to be proven. While dust and soot may be attracted to negative ions, they

are likely to remain airborne, or possibly end up on floors or furniture to be picked up again.

The amount of ions generated by these machines may also be of concern. While outdoor air may range from 500 to 5,000 negative ions per cubic centimeter, and indoor air may only have a couple hundred per cubic centimeter, negative ion generators can easily pump out from ten thousand to ten million negative ions per cubic centimeter. At these higher levels—especially over a million—negative ions can become irritating to mucous membranes. They can irritate the throat, the eyes, and the lungs. Quite simply, our bodies were not designed for this level of negative ions.

A Cochrane review (Blackhall *et al.* 2003) of six good quality studies concluded that ionizers exerted no significant effects upon lung function, symptoms or medication use among 106 asthmatics.

Ozone generators may be effective at removing bacteria, because bacteria require oxygen to live, and ozone depletes their oxygen levels. For this reason, a good ozone generator will often create a fresher smelling indoor environment. While ozone is not the same as smog, which has carbon or sulphur molecules connected to the molecules, ozone is an atmospheric response to smog, as ozone helps stabilize oxygen levels and clear out other molecules. Ozone has not been proven to remove dust.

At the same time, higher ozone levels may also result in lung irritation and allergic response. As mentioned earlier, the FDA limits ozone generating machines in medical devices (used in hospitals and clinics) to emit no more than 50 parts per billion. The bottom line with both ionizers and ozone generators is that the atmosphere contains a fragile balance of components: It is not a random mixture. The level of ozone present in outdoor pollution reflects the atmosphere's cleansing process. In other words, the decision to use these machines should be made carefully, and the composition of fresh air is likely healthier than any machine-driven composition.

High-Efficiency Particular Arresting (HEPA) filters: A HEPA filter is a better strategy for removing dust, dander and other particulates. HEPA filters are designed to pick up over 99.9% of particulates sized .3 microns and larger. HEPA filters can be installed onto air and heater air ducting systems to significantly remove dust, dander, and allergens.

Electrostatic air filters for forced air systems can be a good choice. These HEPA filters typically filter between ninety and a hundred percent of dander, mold, mites, dust, soot, and bacteria. Many of these filters come with the ability to clean and reuse, allowing us to clean them as often as needed—which should be at least monthly if use is constant.

Environmental filters are good alternatives, especially for cold urban environments. These draw in, filter and heat outdoor air. This maximizes circulation, ventilation and temperature control: The best of all worlds.

Pillowcase filters: This air filtration device is designed to filter the nighttime air through the pillowcase. One study (Stillerman *et al.* 2010) tested this with 35 adults who had allergic rhinoconjunctivitis and sensitivities to either dander or dust mites. The device was found to reduce 99.99% of allergen particulates greater than .3 microns within the patients' breathing zones. The patient group using the filtration device was found to have significantly fewer allergy symptoms and better quality of lie than the placebo group.

Do We Have to Know Our Allergens?

"Absolutely" is the typical response by an allergist or conventional health provider. But this also assumes that by reducing our exposure to the allergen, we can reduce our symptoms of hypersensitivity. However, this is not necessarily true. Hypersensitivity is not caused by allergen exposure. It is caused by an underlying condition.

For example, Spanish researchers (Torrent *et al.* 2006) collected dust samples of 1,474 homes of children that were three months old. They also tested blood levels of IgE in 1,019 of the children. The IgEs they tested for were for the allergens *Der p1* (dust mites) and *Fel d1* (cat dander). Although they confirmed the children's sensitivity to them, the researchers found no link between household levels of these allergens, and asthmatic or allergic symptoms. In other words, higher exposure did not predicate increases in allergy or asthma episodes.

This simply means that as the underlying condition continues, our hypersensitive condition will continue, and possibly migrate to other sensitivies. While we may not react to our local pollens now, we might in the future if we are allergic to other environmental allergens.

This doesn't mean that knowing our allergen doesn't have its place. Certainly it would be helpful as steps are taken to remove the causes of the underlying conditions.

Some research has shown reduced allergy incidence when allergens are avoided, such as found in research from the UK's St Mary's Hospital (Arshad *et al.* 2007). In this study of 120 children, those who had reduced allergen exposure using mattress covers, dust mite sprays (acaricide), and hydrolyzed anti-allergy formula had lower levels of allergy symptoms. However, in this study the results are confounded by the hydrolyzed milk, which in itself reduces milk allergies—known to predicate other allergies.

We actually do not need more research to confirm that exposure does not cause allergies. Besides the research showing that rural dwellers have fewer pollen allergies, we also know from research mentioned earlier that families with less income and from third-world countries have less allergy incidence. These cultures certainly have more exposure to allergens.

Besides, a lifetime of trying to avoid allergens is a complicated life indeed. It is one filled with worry and anxiety, not to mention lots of work.

Unless we want to wear a hazmat suit and breathing tank all day, it is nearly impossible for a person with allergies to completely and permanently avoid exposure to most allergens.

We might as well put all this effort into eliminating the underlying condition.

Chapter Four
The Real Culprits

So far, we have investigated the statistics of who gets allergic rhinitis, the mechanics of the condition, and its triggers and allergens. These are not the real culprits, however. Why? Because everyone is exposed to these triggers and allergens. Unless we live in a bubble, each one of us is bombarded with pollens, molds, dust mite endotoxins, animal dander and so many other potential allergens. Yet the large majority of us do not have allergic rhinitis.

What are the real culprits, then?

A Popular Suspect: The Hygiene Hypothesis

A variety of studies over the past two decades have arrived at the conclusion that greater exposure to siblings, other children, animals, soil, infective microorganisms and other potential allergy triggers during childhood dramatically decrease the incidence of allergies. Let's look at a few of these studies.

Researchers from University of Chile's School of Medicine (Vargas *et al.* 2008) analyzed common trigger exposure levels among 1,232 Chileans. They reviewed their early infections, siblings, bedroom sharing, daycare and animal contact during their first five years of life.

They found that having fewer allergies and asthma was associated with having more siblings, being in daycare and having an early respiratory infection. Some of these cut the risk in half or more. Having contact with dogs during the first year of life reduced the risk of rhinitis, by over half. On the other hand, contact with poultry or cats during the early years increased rhinitis risk by over 40%.

Researchers from the Austria's Salzberg Children's Hospital (Riedler *et al.* 2001) studied 2,618 children from rural locations in Austria, Germany, and Switzerland. They also tested 901 for IgE antibodies. They found that children who lived around farm animals and drank farm milk had a quarter of the incidence of hay fever compared to the other children.

In other words, exposures to allergens do not cause lasting hay fever or allergies. What may trigger initial sensitivity is altogether different from what causes ongoing allergic hyperresponsiveness. It is not as though a person gets exposed to high levels of a particular allergen or trigger, and this alone causes hay fever.

Researchers from Finland's University of Turku (Kalliomäki and Iso-lauri 2002) concluded after a review of multiple studies that the sterile birthing environments among Western hospitals have reduced exposure to early microbes. This, they hypothesized, is a key reason that sensitivity and atopic diseases such as eczema, allergic rhinitis and asthma are on the rise among these Western nations. This proposed effect has been called the *Hygiene Hypothesis of Asthma and Allergy.*

The Finnish researchers in this study supported this hypothesis with immunological data illustrating that the immune system responds to microbial antigens—both pathogenic and non-pathogenic ones—with the expression of cytokines that balance the T-helpers produced by the infants.

This said, there are also some studies that have shown that exposure to some allergens increases the risk of allergies for some. In other words, the incidence of allergies, hay fever and asthma is not related purely to exposure.

Rather, the hygiene hypothesis is applicable to allergies as it relates to a healthy flexing of the immune system through exposure to *natural* elements: Those from the soil, plants, forests, farms, pastures, oceans and other natural environments, in other words. This means that exposure to pollens, soil organisms, molds, microorganisms from raw milk and other natural environmental sources tend to boost the immune system, while exposures to synthetic toxins burden the immune system.

Why? Remember the MHC from the second chapter. It is all about developing tolerance.

For example, researchers from the University Children's Hospital in Munich (Ege *et al.* 2007) used the Prevention of Allergy Risk Factors for Sensitization in Children Related to Farming and Anthroposophic Lifestyle Study to assess allergies in rural schoolchildren. The study included 8,263 school-age rural children from five European countries. They found that raising pigs, consuming farm milk, being involved in haying, frequenting animal sheds and the use of silage all reduced the incidence of asthma and hay fever. They also related fewer asthmatic cases to levels of exposure to endotoxins and extracellular polysaccharides. Endotoxins and extracellular polysaccharides are both produced by bacteria.

This was also confirmed by Italian researchers (Chellini *et al.* 2005) in a large study of six- and seven-year-olds and adolescents (13- to 14-year-olds). Children living in the more populated southern regions had significantly higher levels of allergies and asthma than did children among the more rural northern region. The researchers attributed the trend to increased pollution, more junk foods and exercising less—all characteristics found among Italian metropolitan areas. They added that obesity is more prevalent in Southern Italy as well.

While farm children are exposed to more natural microbiological elements and natural waste products, they are exposed to less man-made toxins. Thus, we would conclude the hygiene hypothesis should probably be reworded to be the *"natural immunity hypothesis."*

In other words, during infancy—assuming a synthetic toxin overload does not exist—exposure to pathogens strengthens the immune system. On the other hand, an overload of synthetic toxins together with pathogens can overwhelm the immune system, producing immunosuppression and systemic inflammation.

In another study supporting this conclusion, medical researchers from Switzerland's University of Basel (Waser *et al.* 2007) tested 14,893 children between the ages of five and 13 from five different European countries. The subjects included 2,823 children from farms and 4,606 children attending Steiner Schools (known for their farm-based living and natural health philosophy). They found that children on the farms—particularly those who drank farm milk—had significantly fewer allergies and asthma. A major component, as we'll discuss, related to the increase in probiotics within raw farm milk.

Researchers from Switzerland's University of Basel (Braun-Fahrländer *et al.* 1999) also found that allergies among rural areas were lower than among urban populations. This study analyzed 1,620 children, and the blood samples from 404 adolescents (13-15 years old). Of the total, 307 children (19%) were from families that farmed for a living. After screening out the influences of residence, education, number of siblings, smoking among the parents, pet ownership, home humidity and heating fuel use and other factors, the researchers discovered that children of farmers had significantly less incidence of hay fever than those whose parents were not farmers. Children of full-time farmers had over 75% less incidence of allergic rhinitis, while children of part-time farmers had 50% less incidence of allergic rhinitis.

One common factor among these studies is contact with the soil and other sources of microorganisms. Children of farming parents would necessarily have more contact with the soil via the farming operations. Whether this indirectly comes through their parents' contact or through their own contact could not be determined. Most likely, both.

Institute of Environmental Medicine scientists (Alfvén *et al.* 2006) also studied other relationships between allergies, among the same group of 14,893 children. Again, they found that growing up on a farm significantly reduced the incidence of all allergies and asthma. In addition, children from anthroposophic families had less allergy and asthma incidence than did non-farming children.

The anthroposophic lifestyle was developed by Austrian Rudolf Steiner. Dr. Steiner taught that health is brought about through a natural balance of living with nature, using alternative medicine and eating wholesome, organic foods.

These results show that the farming lifestyle is consistent with beng infected. Scientists from Sweden's Institute of Environmental Medicine (Rosenlund *et al.* 2009) studied the same 14,893 children to assess the relationship between infections and allergies. In addition, 4,049 children were tested with blood samples for IgE sensitivities. They found that children who had previous measles infections or vaccinations were significantly less likely to have allergies later on.

All this science adds up to the same conclusion: The immune system is somewhat like a muscle: If it is not stressed, it will become weakened. We see this same tendency not only among muscles, but also among the joints and bones of the body: Those who exercise more and put regular weight-bearing stress on their joints and bones tend to have stronger joints and bones. Those who do not, have more brittle and weakened joints and bones.

This very same issue occurs with the immune system. As a healthy immune system becomes exposed to various challenges, it becomes stronger. This is also called *expression*. The immune system is given a chance to express its various abilities. This expression of the immune system gives it strength, as the expression produces tolerance.

Immunosuppression and Systemic Inflammation

However, should the stress put on the immune system be outside our genetically-recognized stressors, the immune system can easily become overburdened. Comparing to the analogy above illustrating that exercise strengthens muscles and joints; getting hit by a truck would not strengthen the muscles or joints. Getting hit by a truck would damage the muscles and break bones and joints. Why? Because the body was not genetically designed to be hit by a truck. Our bodies are simply not equipped to be hit by trucks.

We can compare the exposures to various industrial chemicals, food toxins and other pollutants to being hit by a truck: The immune system simply was not designed to deal with these sorts of challenges. While the body can, as we discussed in the second chapter, work to break down these abnormal toxins and rid the body of their parts, the body can easily become overwhelmed by doing so. The body is no way as efficient in this process as it is in removing natural exposures such as pollens, molds, insect endotoxins and so on.

Suppression is the opposite of expression. The immune system can be suppressed by two occurrences:

➢ The immune system is not stressed enough.

➢ The immune system is stressed too much

One might think that these two circumstances are mutually exclusive. But they aren't. In fact, in many people, especially in the modern age, they occur simultaneously. How so?

Remember the research showing how hay fever was initially found almost exclusively among the aristocratic classes. Now let's combine this information with the research showing that those with a naturally-stressed immune system have fewer allergies. Even today, as we look at the CDC information from the first chapter, we see that people in families with higher incomes have more allergies.

What is the common denominator? In earlier times, aristocratic and wealthy families were most known for their less contact with nature, and their increased cleanliness. They showered more than families with less income. They washed their hands more, and were found out of doors less frequently.

This is still common today, as wealthier families tend to have more indoor entertainment, and less contact with nature. Children from wealthier families have bigger and better toys, keeping them further away from outdoor sports. Wealthier families also tend to have less contact with the masses. In other words, they under-stress their immune systems.

But these wealthier groups also are known for something else: Their increased use of synthetics and rich processed food diets.

This of course, leads to the other side of the equation: the overstressing of the immune system, leading to systemic inflammation. Is there any evidence for this conclusion? Plenty.

The Evidence for Systemic Inflammation in Allergies

Researchers from University of Pennsylvania's School of Medicine (Brown-Whitehorn *et al.* 2010) found that allergic rhinitis—as well as asthma, atopic dermatitis and eosinophilic esophagitis—all shared the same signs of underlying systemic inflammation. These included Th2 inflammation at the disease site, increased TGF-beta expression and eosinophilic inflammation.

Allergy researchers from Turkey's Ege University School of Medicine (Onbasi *et al.* 2005) studied 38 patients with allergic rhinitis to grass pollen (in season) alongside 25 healthy subjects and 24 subjects with gastroesophageal reflux (GERD). They found that the allergic patients had the highest levels of eosinophil accumulation in the blood and tissues than the other groups—a sign of systemic inflammation.

This issue of a build-up of eosinophils is now identified as an emerging issue associated with the dramatic rise in allergies, asthma and other inflammatory conditions. Researchers from Australia's Royal Children's Hospital and the University of Melbourne (Heine *et al.* 2011) have been studying the relationships between eosinophilic esophagitis (EoE) and allergies and asthma—along with gastrointestinal conditions such as gastroesophageal reflux (GERD) and others.

As we discussed in Chapter Two, high levels of eosinophils is related to a systemic inflammatory response. The immune system is launching a large scale inflammatory attack on the region.

C-reactive protein also indicates a systemic inflammatory condition. Researchers from the Texas Tech University Health Sciences Center (Arif *et al.* 2007) studied the relationships between C-reactive protein (CRP) and asthma among 8,020 adults over the age of twenty, using the U.S. National Health and Nutrition Examination Survey. They found that those in the highest quarter of CRP levels had a 60% greater risk of current asthma than those with lower CRP levels. Those with the highest quartile of CRP levels had more than double the incidence of asthmatic wheezing, and more than triple the incidence of nighttime coughing.

A plethora of research has shown that higher eosinophils and C-reactive protein levels point to systemic inflammation occurring somewhere in the body. What causes inflammation? We'll investigate this thoroughly in this chapter.

Systemic inflammation indicates that the immune system is overburdened. The extent or combination of the elements mentioned simply overwhelms the immune system. Typically, the immune system can resolve most of these problems when it is presented with a small amount or a few of them at a time. But when an avalanche of them becomes too great, the immune system goes on alert, resulting in systemic inflammation.

Systemic inflammation is the immune system's version of all-out war. The immune system begins to launch the nukes. These can include fever, vomiting, diarrhea, swelling and pain—as we discussed in the second chapter.

Let's more specifically discuss lifestyle choices that produce or worsen systemic inflammation within the body, producing immunosuppression. In other words, these are *contributing causes*. This means that just one of these lifestyle choices may not in itself cause hypersensitivity. But any one of these in considerable amounts, or a combination thereof, can overwhelm the immune system—producing systemic inflammation.

Systemic Inflammation Factors

The following list summarizes conditions that collectively contribute to systemic inflammation, which in turn leads to hypersensitivity:

1) ***Toxemia:*** An overload of toxins that produce radicals.
2) ***Antioxidant enzyme deficiencies:*** An undersupply of antioxidizing enzymes that stabilize radicals, including glutathione peroxidase, glutathione reductase, catalase and superoxide dismutase.

3) ***Dietary antioxidant deficiencies:*** An undersupply of antioxidants from our foods to help stabilize radicals.

4) ***Barriers to detoxification:*** Lifestyle or physiological factors that block our body's ability to rid waste products and toxins.

5) ***Poor dietary choices:*** A poor diet burdens the body with toxins, unstable fatty acids, refined sugars and overly-processed foods.

6) ***Immunosuppression:*** A burdened or defective immune system.

7) ***Infections:*** In a burdened or defective immune system, infections with microorganisms become amplified, as the body easily reaches it critical mass of being able to manage multiple intruders. This amplification can result in not only a hypersensitive state: It can result in life-threatening illness.

The complete list of toxins that can accumulate in the body or otherwise overwhelm the body is gigantic. However, we can categorize them generally in one major respect: Most are synthetic chemicals, or other byproducts from our interference with nature's normal ecosystems. This means air pollutants, chemical toxins, fabricated materials like plastics, synthetic food additives and so on. Let's discuss a few of these here.

Lipid Peroxides

A critical component involving systemic inflammation is glutathione peroxidase—an enzyme produced in the liver. Glutathione peroxidase is the leading enzyme responsible for the breakdown and removal of lipid hydroperoxides. Lipid hydroperoxides are oxidized fats that damage cell membranes. As they do this, they create pores in the cell. The resulting damage eventually kills most cells. Lipid hydroperoxides are one of the most damaging molecules within the body. They are responsible for many deadly metabolic diseases, including heart disease, artery disease, Alzheimer's disease and many others.

When lipid hydroperoxides accumulate in the body, they can also damage the cells of the airways, causing irritation and inflammation. The damage from lipid hydroperoxides stimulates an inflammatory response. Researchers have called the initial signal from the cell that initiates this inflammatory response *lipid peroxidation/LOOH-mediated stress signaling.* In other words, the cells are stressed by lipid peroxidation, and this initiates a distress signal to the immune system.

This distress signal stimulates the contraction of the smooth bronchial muscles while stimulating leukotriene activity—which delivers cytotoxic (cell-destroying) T-cells and eosinophils into the region. This stimulates the production of more mucous, which drowns the cilia and restricts the clearing of mucous, resulting in the classic blocked nose of allergic rhinitis.

The production of more mucous is intended to clear out damaged cells and toxin parts. In other words, much of the increased mucous that drowns the cilia and blocks the nose is caused by the influx of dead cell matter from lipid hydroperoxide damage.

By virtue of removing lipid hydroperoxides, glutathione peroxidase—not to be confused with glutathione reductase—regulates pro-inflammatory arachidonic acid metabolism. In other words, glutathione regulates the release and populations of those pro-inflammatory mediators known for allergic episodes, the histamines. Histamine activity is directly associated with the damage created by lipid hydroperoxides. Thus, when lipid hydroperoxide levels are reduced by glutathione peroxidase, inflammatory histamine density is reduced.

Selenium is required for glutathione peroxidase production. Should the body be overloaded with lipid hydroperoxides, more glutathione is required to clear out the damage. As more glutathione is produced, more selenium is utilized, which runs down selenium levels.

This mechanism was illustrated by research from Britain's South Manchester University Hospital (Hassan 2008). The researchers studied 13 aspirin-induced asthmatics along with a matched (healthy) control group. They found that the asthmatics maintained higher levels of selenium in the bloodstream—especially among blood platelets. This high selenium content in the bloodstream correlated with higher glutathione peroxidase activity. The research illustrated how selenium is used up faster through this glutathione peroxidase process.

Lipid peroxidation means that the lipids that make up the cell membrane are being robbed of electrons. This 'robbing' results in an unstable cell membrane. Let's take a look at the process of lipid peroxidation.

The first step takes place with the entry of a reactive oxygen species into the proximity of the cell. Reactive oxygen species are elements that require an electron—such as hydrogen ($H+$)—in order to become stable.

Fatty acids that make up the membranes of cells are the likely candidates for peroxidation. Remember, the name "lipid" refers to a fatty acid. Fatty acids include saturated fats, polyunsaturates, monounsaturates, and so on (see fatty acid discussions later on).

Several types of lipids make up the cell membrane. Fatty acids will combine with other molecules to make phospholipids, cholesterols and glycolipids. Saturates and polyunsaturates are typical, but there are several species of polyunsaturates. These range from long chain versions to short versions. They also include the cis- configuration and the trans- configuration. Cell membranes that utilize predominantly cis- versions with long chains are the most durable. Those cell membranes with trans- configurations can be highly unstable, and irregularly porous. This is one reason why trans fats are not good. The other reason is that trans fats easily become peroxidized.

Cell membranes with more long chain fatty acids are more stable and are less subject to peroxidation. Shorter chains that provide more double bonds are less stable, because these are more easily broken. Also, mono-unsaturated fatty acids such as GLA are more stable.

Once the fatty acid is degraded by an oxygen species, it becomes a fatty acid radical. The fatty acid will usually become oxidized, making it a peroxyl-fatty acid radical. This radical will react with other fatty acids, forming a vicious cycle involving radicals called cyclic peroxides.

This is basically a chain reaction that, if it isn't stopped, results in the cell membrane becoming completely destroyed and dysfunctional. This forces the cell to signal to the immune system that it is under attack and about to become malignant. The T-cell immune response will often initiate the cell's self-destruct switch: TNF—tumor necrosis factor. Alternatively, the cell may be directly destroyed by cytotoxic T-cells. The combined process stimulates inflammation. As these cells are killed or self-destruct, they are purged from the system—provoking increased mucous formation.

While this peroxidation and cell destruction is taking place, the immune system is not simply standing by. The body enters the state of systemic inflammation. This results in the immune system launching an ongoing supply of eosinophils, neutrophils and mast cells, ready to release granulocytes like histamine when the body is exposed to any IgE trigger.

In other words, due to this ongoing peroxidation, the immune system is on a hair-trigger. Imagine a person at work who is stressed from being buried in work and a myriad of problems. You walk into their office and they immediately react: "And what do *you* want?" they ask, frantically.

If they were not overloaded with work, problems and deadlines, your coming into their office would probably not be met with such a frantic response. But since they were overloaded, they reacted (*hyper* reacted is a better word) more defensively than needed, *because they thought you were going to add to their workload.*

We will discuss strategies to secure better, more stable fatty acids in detail later. In the meantime, let's dig deeper into what causes the reactive oxidative species that produces lipid peroxidation.

Reactive Oxygen Species
Let's take a step back and analyze this situation a little deeper. The initiation process of the lipid peroxidation is started by a reactive oxygen species. What is this?

This is also often called a free radical. A free radical is an unstable molecule or ion that forms during a chemical reaction. In other words, the molecule or ion needs another electron, ion or molecule to stabilize it. Once it is stable, it is not reactive.

Thus, free radicals damage cells and the tissues by stealing their atomic elements.

Nature produces many, many free radicals. However, nature typically accompanies radicals with the molecules, atoms or ions that stabilize the radical. In the atmosphere, for example, radicals become stabilized by ozone and other elements. In plants, radicals become stabilized by anti-oxidants from nutrients derived from the sun, soil and oxygen. In the body, radicals are stabilized by antioxidizing enzymes, nutrients and other elements. These include glutathione peroxidase, as we discussed earlier.

Confirming this, the research from South Manchester University Hospital mentioned earlier concluded with a comment that the increased glutathione peroxidase activity related to radical oxidation: *administration of aspirin to these patients increases the generation of immediate oxygen products…*"

Another anti-oxidation process within the body utilizes the *superoxide dismutase* (SOD) enzyme. The SOD enzyme is typically available within the cytoplasm of most cells. Here SOD is complexed by either copper and zinc, or manganese—similar to the way selenium is complexed with the glutathione peroxidase enzyme. Several types of SOD enzymes reside within the body—some in the mitochondria and some in the intercellular tissue fluids. SOD neutralizes superoxides before they can damage the inside and outside of the cell—assuming the body is healthy, with sub-stantial amounts of SOD. The immune system produces superoxides as part of its strategy to attack microorganisms and toxins.

Another broad anti-oxidation process utilizes *catalase*. Here the body provides an enzyme bound by iron to neutralize peroxides to oxygen and water. It is a standard component of many metabolic reactions within the body.

Yet another enzyme utilized for radical reduction is *glutathione reductase*. This enzyme works with NADP in the cell to stabilize hydrogen peroxide oxidized radicals before they can damage the cell.

Notice that all of these antioxidizing enzymes require minerals. We have seen either selenium, copper, zinc, manganese or iron as necessary to keep these enzymes in good supply. Many other minerals and trace elements are used by other antioxidant and detoxifying enzyme processes. These minerals, and many of the enzymes themselves, are supplied by various foods and supplements, as we'll discuss further.

Another tool that the healthy body utilizes to stabilize radicals are the antioxidants supplied by plant foods. Plants produce antioxidants to protect their own cells from radical damage. Thus, their plant material contains a host of these oxidation stabilizers, which our bodies use to neutralize radicals.

Where do these oxidative radicals and lipid-peroxidizing elements come from? Primarily from two sources: the diet and exposure to toxins. We'll devote a chapter on diet to discuss this aspect in detail. For now, let's discuss the toxins we are exposed to that result in oxidative radicals, which in turn lead to immunosuppression.

The Link Between Synthetic Toxins and Allergies

Clinical research by Professor John G Ionescu, Ph.D. (2009) concluded that environmental pollution is clearly associated with the development of hypersensitivities. Dr. Ionescu's research indicated that environmental noxious agents, including many chemicals, contribute to the total immune burden, producing increased susceptibility for intolerances due to inflammation.

Environmental toxins are also sensitizing in themselves, producing new trigger allergens. Professor Ionescu draws this conclusion from studying more than 18,000 atopic patients:

> *"Beside classic allergic-triggering factors (allergen potency, intermittent exposure to different allergen concentrations, presence of microbial bodies dyand sensitizing phenols), the adjuvant role of environmental pollutants gains increasing importance in allergy induction."*

According to Dr. Ionescu, toxic inputs such as formaldehyde, smog, industrial waste, wood preservatives, microbial toxins, alcohol, pesticides, processed foods, nicotine, solvents and amalgam-heavy metals have been observed to be mediating toxins that produce the physical susceptibilities for allergic sensitization and subsequent inflammation.

This is also consistent with findings of other scientists—as discussed—that chemicals overload the immune system and cause inflammation.

Chemical toxins such as DDT, dioxin, formaldehyde, benzene, butane and chlorinated chemicals tend to accumulate within the body's tissues. This is because many of these are fat-soluble. In other words, they become lipid peroxides. Other compounds tend to clear the body faster because they are not fat soluble. (Non-fat soluble synthetics can also cause toxicity issues if they are regularly presented to the body.)

Research has indicated that these fat-soluble synthetic toxins predispose us to a body-wide status of systemic inflammation. This is because these synthetic toxins form radicals within the body that cannot be easily neutralized. Because synthetics or their presentation are new to nature, the body does not have the innate immune factors to easily neutralize them.

This is a gigantic subject, so here we will summarize the major categories and sources of toxic chemicals in our daily lives.

Consumer Toxins

In conjunction with a mandate to lower toxin levels among the state's residents, in 2010 the Minnesota Department of Health compiled and released a list of the most toxic chemicals used in consumer products, building materials, pesticides, hair dyes, detergents, aerosols, cosmetics, furniture polish, herbicides, paints, cleaning solutions and many other common products. The list also referenced research connecting the toxins to disease conditions.

The list contained 1,755 chemicals.

These all produce radicals. For each of these, the liver and immune system must launch a variety of macrophages, T-cells and B-cells to break them apart and escort them and the cells they damage out of the body. This means each toxin adds to the load the immune system must carry.

Illustrating this, researchers from Germany's National Research Center for Environment and Health (Kohlhammer *et al.* 2006) studied 2,606 adults, and found out that those who had frequented swimming pools as children had a 74% higher incidence of hay fever as adults. The researchers concluded that: *"Impaired integrity of the lung epithelial by exposure to chlorination by-products might facilitate a closer contact to allergens and therefore could result in higher rates of hay fever."*

We might compare this to moving dirt. A small handful of dirt can be carried around easily, and dispersed without much effort. However, a truckload of dirt is another matter completely. What can we do with a truckload of dirt? If we dumped a truckload of dirt on our lawn, we'd have a hill of dirt that would bury the access to our front door and annihilate our lawn and/or garden.

This is a useful comparison because while our bodies can handle a small amount of toxins quite easily, modern society is increasingly dumping toxic 'dirt' into our atmosphere, water and foods, effectively inundating our bodies 'by the truckload.'

With this increased burden, the research shows that the body's defenses are lowered. The mucosal membrane is weakened. This translates to an immune system that feels more threatened due to being compromised. This leads to an immune system on high alert and hypersensitive.

Plasticizers and Parabens

Today, plasticizers and parabens are common amongst many of our medications, toys, foods packaged in plastic, and other consumer items. Phthalates are also found in many household items. While phthalates have shorter half-lives than some toxins, they have been implicated in asthma and allergies, as well as cancers and other conditions. Many cosmetics and antiperspirants contain parabens. They are thus readily absorbed into the skin where they can provoke inflammatory responses (Crinnion 2010).

Heavy Metals

Heavy metals are elements that exist naturally in trace quantities within our soils, waters and foods. However, extraordinary levels of heavy metals such as cadmium, lead and mercury are produced by humanity's industrial complex in the manufacturing of various consumer items.

We can cite many studies that have associated heavy metal exposure to immunosuppression. Mercury is one of these.

For example, in multicenter research from the Department of Medicine from the Lavoro Medical Center in Bari, Italy (Soleo *et al.* 2002), researchers studied the effects of low levels of inorganic mercury exposure on 117 workers. They compared these with 172 general population subjects. They found no difference in the white blood cell count between the two groups. However, the worker group exposed to mercury had increased levels of CD4+ and CD8+ cytokines, and CD4+ levels were particularly high. These indicated a state of systemic inflammation. In addition, significantly lower levels of interleukin (IL-8) occurred among the exposed workers—indicating immunosuppression.

This research concluded that even low levels of environmental exposure to mercury and other heavy metals (beyond the trace levels normally found in nature) suppresses the immune system and stimulates inflammation. At toxic levels, they act like radicals within our bodies.

Pharmaceuticals

Practically every synthetic pharmaceutical can break down into free radicals and add to our body's total toxin burden. This is because the body must eventually break down any synthetic chemical in order to purge it from the body. The isolated or active chemical within the pharmaceutical may have its biological effect upon the body, but the chemicals in the medication must all be broken down at some point. The body rarely if ever utilizes these chemicals as nutrients, in other words. They are foreigners to the body, and easily become unstable.

If the body has enough available enzymes such as glutathione, it will readily break down these chemical molecules into neutralized forms that can be excreted in urine, sweat, exhalation or stool. Otherwise, many of these foreigners remain in the body, where their unstable molecular forms can harm cells and tissues.

Even if they are all broken down, this breakdown and disposal process requires work by the body's detoxification systems. This means that they burden or stress a system that must remove many other toxins within the body, including other environmental toxins, microorganisms and their endotoxins, inflammatory mediators, broken-down cells and other toxins the body must get rid of. As a result, the body becomes easily overwhelmed by other foreigners, such as pollens, molds and other allergens.

Illustrating this, researchers from Norway's Oslo University Hospital (Bakkeheim *et al.* 2011) studied 1,016 mothers and their children from birth until six months old, and then followed up with the children at 10 years old. They found that acetaminophen use by the mother during the first trimester significantly increased incidence of hay fever at age ten. Furthermore, girls given acetaminophen had more than double the asthma incidence at age ten.

Researchers from the Infants Hospital of Mexico Allergy Department (Del-Rio-Navarro *et al.* 2006). They recruited 5,006 six- and seven-year-old boys and girls, and 6,576 13- to 14-year-olds. They found that a history of taking antibiotics or acetaminophen during the first year of life increased the risk of contracting allergic rhinitis and atopic dermatitis among the six- and seven-year-olds—with a 50% increase in incidence.

Medical researchers from Norway's Haukeland University Hospital (Macsali *et al.* 2009) found, in a study of oral contraceptives and asthma among 5,791 women, that oral contraceptive use increased the incidence of asthma with hay fever by 48%, asthma alone by 42% and hay fever alone by 25%. They also found that oral contraceptives increased wheeze with shortness of breath. They concluded that: *"Women using oral contraceptive pills had more asthma. This was found only in normal weight and overweight women, indicating interplay between sex hormones and metabolic status in effect on the airways."*

A number of pharmaceuticals have been shown to trigger or worsen allergic hypersensitivity and asthma. These include:

➤ Acetaminophen
➤ Anti-arrhythmia drugs
➤ Anti-nausea drugs (e.g., dimenhydrinate)
➤ Anti-Parkinson's drugs
➤ Anti-psychotic drugs (e.g., phenothiazines and lithium)
➤ Anti-viral drugs (e.g., cidofovir, protease inhibitors)
➤ Aspirin
➤ Barbiturates
➤ Benzodiazepines, anti-anxiety drugs
➤ Beta-blockers
➤ Blood pressure medications (e.g., guanethidine)
➤ Cephalosporin, sulfonamide antibiotics
➤ Cholinesterase inhibitors
➤ Ibuprofen

➤ Selective Serotonin Reuptake Inhibitors (SSRIs) and Antide-pressants (e.g., fluoxetine, fluvoxamine, paroxetine)
➤ Sleeping drugs (e.g., diphenhydramine)
(Mindell and Hopkins 1998)

Even some of the more common over the counter pharmaceuticals can cause havoc. Consider the overuse of aspirin, which can cause salicylate sensitivity and even aspirin-allergic asthma. There are also many other medications that contain salicylates, such as cough syrups, antihistamines and other medications. Salicylate sensitivity has been known to cause bronchial congestion, wheezing, hives, GI pain, upset stomach, indigestion, rhinitis and other symptoms.

Over time, the isolated salicylates in aspirin can damage the mucosal membrane in the stomach and intestines, producing sensitivity (Goldstein *et al.* 2008). For this reason, stomach bleeding can result from the overuse of aspirin and other salicylate medications.

We should note that herbs and other plants also contain salicylates. However, in whole foods and plants, the salicylates are typically buffered by other natural compounds. For this reason, plants are not known to cause salicylate sensitivity. However, once a person becomes allergic or sensitive to salicylates from aspirin or other medications, they may also become sensitive to a variety of salicylates, including those in other medications as well as salicylates in some foods and herbs.

We should add that naturally formed salicylates are extremely healthy constituents in plants. They balance the immune system and slow inflammation. For this reason, salicylates have also been shown to reduce cardiovascular disease and even reduce some cancers (Din *et al.* 2010). Many of these properties stem from the fact that salicylate constituents are produced to help plants themselves defend against disease.

Furthermore, salicylate-containing herbs such as peppermint, meadowsweet and willow contain a number of natural constituents that buffer and balance the effects of their salicins, while achieving similar anti-inflammatory effects as salicylate pharmaceuticals (Schmid *et al.* 2001). Thus, salicylates should be considered the innocent bystanders. The real culprit is the overuse of the isolated and synthetic pharmaceutical versions of these natural plant compounds.

The Tryptophan Defect

As another example of the potential for pharmaceuticals to stimulate systemic inflammation, many children with asthma and allergies have illustrated a defect in the availability of tryptophan. Tryptophan is an amino acid critical for a number of processes in the body. If tryptophan is not properly metabolized, it can remain in the body at unhealthy high levels. This can be evidenced by extraordinary high levels of xanthurenic and knurenic acid in the urine.

One of the problems with high levels of tryptophan is that tryptophan is the precursor of serotonin. Thus, high tryptophan levels produce high levels of serotonin. And high serotonin levels can cause over-contraction among the smooth muscles of the airways—producing wheezing.

Another link between tryptophan and airway hypersensitivity is the indoleamine dioxygenase enzyme, or IDO. IDO regulates eosinophil inflammation, and tryptophan reduces IDO availability. This means that increased tryptophan presence in the blood has the effect of leaving eosinophils unregulated—which are directly involved in asthma and allergic episodes.

Researchers from Innsbruck Medical University (Kositz *et al.* 2008) analyzed the blood of 44 allergic patients along with 38 healthy persons. They found that tryptophan levels were significantly higher among the allergic subjects. They concluded that: *"Higher tryptophan levels may result from lower indoleamine 2,3-dioxygenase activity in atopics."*

Researchers from the Mahidol University Medical School in Bangkok (Maneechotesuwan *et al.* 2008) studied 34 asthmatic patients who were being treated with beta-agonist medications. They found that all the patients had low levels of IDO activity and knurenine levels that would indicate high tryptophan levels.

There is also reason to believe that oral steroids may increase the loss of vitamin B6 levels (Holt 1998). Vitamin B6 (pyridoxine) is required to metabolize and reduce tryptophan levels. Vitamin B6 also happens to diminish the effectiveness of steroid medications, because it inhibits steroid update into the nucleus and DNA (Gropper *et al.* 2008).

This scenario also (ironically) implicates certain pharmaceuticals used for asthma symptoms, including steroids and theophylline medications. While they can temporarily decrease asthma symptoms, they can also reduce levels of vitamin B6, which in turn increases tryptophan availability. This effectively produces continuous inflammation associated with high eosinophil levels by virtue of decreased levels of the IDO enzyme.

This effect was confirmed by researchers (Sur *et al.* 1993) studying 31 asthmatic patients. They found that the medication theophylline significantly reduced pyridoxine (vitamin B6) levels within the patients.

Another study (Collipp *et al.* 1975) found that asthmatic symptoms were significantly improved, together with a reduction of asthma medications, after B6 supplementation. This study followed 76 asthmatic children who were given 200 milligrams per day of vitamin B6 for five months.

While these specific pharmaceuticals may be of concern, any synthe-sized chemical has the potential to increase the body's total toxic burden, imbalance nutrient levels, and raise the risk of systemic inflammation.

Air pollutants

A number of studies have shown that pollen allergies increase during periods and regions with heavy air pollution.

This was shown by researchers from Sweden's University (Böttcher *et al.* 2006) tested 30 Estonian and 76 Swedish infants and found that living in a polluted industrial area during the first two years of life substantially increased incidence of asthma and allergies.

According to a 2007 *American Lung Association State of the Air* report, 46% or about 136 million Americans live within a county having *"unhealth-ful"* levels of either ozone or particle-based outdoor pollution. Over 38 million Americans live in a county with *"unhealthful"* levels of both ozone and particle pollution. A third of Americans live in *"unhealthful"* ozone level counties.

Interestingly, this is substantially better than a 2006 report indicating that almost half of Americans live in ozone-rich areas. It is unlikely that the source of ozone pollution—carbon emissions—went down this much in a year. Most likely—just as the ozone hole has been fluctuating with atmospheric rhythms—there are complicated relationships between weather systems, temperature, pressure and so on.

Meanwhile, more than ninety-three million Americans—about one in three—live in areas seasonally high in short-term particle pollution and about one in five Americans lives in an area of high year-round particle pollution. Unlike the fluctuating ozone levels, the number of high particle pollution areas has steadily increased over the past few years.

Clean air contains about 78% nitrogen, 21% oxygen, .9% argon, .03% carbon dioxide and a host of other trace elements. Depending upon the location and source, outdoor air pollution can contain carbon monoxide, nitrogen dioxide, sulphur dioxide, excess carbon dioxide, ammonia, vari-ous particulates, chlorofluorocarbons (CFCs), radon daughters, and a variety of toxic metals and volatile organic compounds (VOCs).

These can also be found in the home or on the job. Coal miners, for example, are exposed to coal dust and soot, together with exhaust, with minimal ventilation. Agricultural workers, landscapers and horticulture workers are exposed to chemical pesticides and herbicides. Teachers and healthcare workers are exposed to the contaminants that occupy their respective buildings and ventilation systems.

Exposure to specific toxins requires extensive ventilation and filtra-tion systems. Whether these come in the form of protective breathing gear or building HVAC systems, the toxin exposures within a workplace must be minimized. Reducing exposure is, in fact, one of the driving purposes of the U.S. Occupational Safety and Health Administration (OSHA). Toxin exposure at the workplace has reached such significant levels that OSHA has put in place many regulations, such as Material Safety Data Sheets (MSDS), in efforts to protect workers from the effects of workplace toxins.

Why such an effort to protect workers from toxins? Today there are in the neighborhood of 100,000 different synthetic chemicals available in the marketplace. The chemical industry has produced many workplace chemicals for industrial uses over the past century, and many of these chemicals have been subsequently found to be carcinogenic or otherwise toxic. Keeping track of the effects and safeguards of each of these chemical toxins is a dizzying affair. Yet it is theoretically the responsibility of any business to make efforts to protect its workers from these toxins. We'll discuss this further later on.

Volatile organic compounds (VOCs) also burden the immune system with toxicity. Exposure to aromatic compounds increases the incidence of allergies and asthma. These include aromatic compounds such as trichloroethene, toluene and benzene. These can be found in many paints, glues, solvents, rubbers and many other workplace materials. Industries that use aromatic hydrocarbon solvents must provide significant ventilation and protection to avoid poisoning their workers.

There are several types of air pollution. The first is *air particle* pollution—when particulate size ranges from .1 micron to 10 microns. This type of pollution is from soot, typical of automobile exhaust, industrial smoke stack exhaust, fireplace smoke, and smoke from forest fires, barbeques and other combustion. Soot is also called *black carbon* pollution, because the excess carbon burn off from burning fossil fuels is the primary component.

Noxious gases are another type of pollution category. These include gasses such as carbon monoxide, chlorine gas, nitrogen oxide, sulphur dioxide and various other chemical gases and vapors. CFCs are a type of noxious gas.

While these two pollution types are distinct, they are often tough to differentiate. Many pollutants are actually vaporized liquids. Molecules become suspended in vapor, appearing like gases or liquid vapors. They are airborne elements derived from synthetic solid and liquid compounds.

There are a number of pollutants pervading building ventilation systems and indoor facilities. To this we can add outdoor pollution entering the house. Examples of indoor pollutants include formaldehyde emitted by foam, treated wood plastics, and chlorine gas emitted in indoor swimming pools.

Let's review each of these forms of air pollution in more detail.

Ozone

Smog is primarily made up of ozone. There are two forms of ozone: The ozone that naturally makes up part of the stratosphere, often referred to as the ozone hole; and the ozone within the lower atmosphere, or troposphere. This latter ozone is called tropospheric ozone or ozone pollution. This form of O_3 gas is caused not by a nature's interaction between radiation and the atmosphere, but through the reaction between fuel vapors from automobiles and sunlight. For this reason, smog levels tend to peak during hot weather.

Smog levels are also higher in warmer regions like Southern California and urban areas in the southern U.S., such as Atlanta. Other cities also experience greater smog levels during the summer months. Wherever higher concentrations of vehicles combine with warm sunshine, smog levels go up. The 'perfect storm' of almost constant sunshine, warm weather, and vehicle concentration makes Southern California one of the worst smog and ozone regions in the United States.

Ozone will oxidize on a cellular and internal tissue level when taken into the body. These tissues will be damaged in almost the same way other oxidized radicals damage tissues. Ozone is readily absorbed through the alveoli as a gas. From there it can enter the bloodstream and damage artery walls and tissues. Ozone is also a major lung tissue irritant, causing inflammation and epithelial cell damage. This can result in decreased lung capacity and/or decreased lung growth development among children.

Ozone is directly linked to the incidence and worsening of allergies, asthma, bronchitis, and COPD. Recent research indicates that this mechanism is the oxidation of lung surface lipids that line the cells of the lung. These oxidized lipids stimulate inflammation as the body seeks to mitigate ozone's damaging effects. The oxidation stimulates scavenger macrophages, which bind to the oxidized lipids in an effort to reverse the damage (Postlethwait 2007).

This means that ozone will release unpaired oxygen radicals, which can interfere with biomolecular bonds within the body. While oxidation is a natural part of our metabolism, too much oxidization—especially when an abundance of radicals are released—can damage tissues, blood vessels and organ systems.

Ozone has some redeeming qualities as well. Generated ozone gas is used in a number of positive ways. Ozone therapy is gaining recognition among the alternative medical community. Ozone is used in hot tubs as a purification measure. It is also used as an industrial cleaning and sanitizing substance. Ozone is part of our natural mix of gases in our air as well. Typical levels are between 25 and 75 parts per billion.

However, dangerous ozone levels occur with higher levels of carbon monoxide levels, sulphur dioxide, and other pollutants. Like the canary in the coalmine, high ozone levels provide a good indicator of unhealthy air. When combined with other pollutants, ozone has a worsening detrimental effect upon the body.

The EPA's Air quality index rates 85 parts per billion of ozone as unhealthy for sensitive people, and over 105 ppb as unhealthy for anyone. As ozone levels rise, it can irritate the lungs and throat, increasing the potential for inflammatory throat and lung infections. As a result, indoor ozone generating machines—which have become popular over the last decade—are discouraged by both the EPA and the FDA if they emit levels higher than 50 parts per billion.

Ironically, higher ozone levels in the air reflect its cleansing action upon other pollutants. Ozone is part of the atmosphere's normalizing systems. The very same cleaning and antibacterial effect we have begun to utilize are part of the earth's detoxification mechanisms to clean and break down particulate pollution. This doesn't mean it is healthy to breathe in ozone at these levels, however.

Particulates

Particulate pollution can trigger allergies, asthma and produce severe toxicity. PM(10-2.5) refers to a particle size from 2.5 micron to 10 micron, and PM(2.5) refers to particle sizes below 2.5 micron. 2.5 micron or less is a *fine particulate*, while less than .1 micron is *ultra-fine*. Ultra-fine particles may also be considered noxious gas pollutants, because their molecular size is small enough to pass through the alveoli into the bloodstream.

Particles above 10 micron in size are usually trapped by the cilia and mucous membranes in the nose, throat, or mouth. As mentioned earlier, in healthy people, these are usually disposed through the movement of mucous or broken down by immune cells.

Fine particulates are small enough to escape this labyrinth and get into our lungs, but they are usually too large to get directly into the bloodstream—again assuming mucous membranes. These particles can become lodged in the tissues of the airways and slowly break down. As they break down, their radicals become absorbed and dumped into the bloodstream. This accumulation of toxins can quickly overburden the liver and bloodstream, producing an inflammatory airway response. In other words, the pollution of the air quickly becomes the pollution of our bloodstream and liver—producing systemic inflammation.

The chemical makeup of these toxins depends upon the source of the pollution. Particle pollution caused by automobile exhaust will have various fluorocarbons and nitrate particles, while coal fired power plants will emit large numbers of sulphur dioxide molecules.

Course particulate pollutants are typically caused by mining, construction, or demolition. Building demolition can rain fumes of various dangerous substances a mile or more from the demolition site.

The most blatant illustration of the demolition effect is the World Trade Center bombing of 2001. The collapse of the towers caused such a toxic fume that there are still thousands of people suffering from a slow poisoning of the lungs. Dangerous chemicals like asbestos, formaldehyde and many others were breathed by thousands of people.

This effect was not limited to rescuers and those who escaped from the twin towers. Many others who happened to be in the vicinity are now suffering. One of the more prevalent diseases has been *sarcoidosis*—a life-threatening inflammation of the lungs. As toxin radicals build up and damage the airway tissues, scar tissue forms—making allergic rhinitis seem like a walk in the park.

This scar tissue affects the elasticity and efficiency of the lungs, causing life-threatening lung collapse. A recent study released by nine doctors (Izbicki *et al.* 2007) who researched the delayed health effects at Ground Zero reported that firefighters and rescue workers were diagnosed with sarcoidosis at a rate of five times the incidence rate prior to 9/11.

An epidemic of allergies and asthma was also an unfortunate result of the Trade Center bombing. While we know asbestos is toxic to the airways, it is still a popular building material. Many structural components of new buildings use asbestos as an ingredient. Because it is a cheap fire retardant material, buildings still go up using it. Asbestos has been linked to thyroid cancer and lung cancer in many studies, which caused a number of high profile lawsuits and residential building restrictions.

Another inflammation trigger released when buildings collapse or are demolished is benzene. Benzene has been identified as a carcinogen, and certain types of leukemia are associated with benzene exposure. Other toxins thought to be released by building collapse include mercury, lead, cadmium, dioxin, polycyclic aromatic hydrocarbons (PAHs) and polychlorinated biphenyls (PCBs). Many of these components are still used to build buildings. All of them were used in buildings a few decades ago, when many of our current skyscrapers were built.

Besides the more publicized cases of cancer and sarcoidosis, ailments associated with the WTC bombing include allergies, reactive-airways syndrome, asthma, chronic throat irritation, gastroesophageal reflux disease (GERD—also referred to as heartburn) and persistent sinusitis. Other cases thought to be associated with the WTC have included miner's lung and thyroid cancer. While many thought these disorders were temporary, new diagnoses have continually increased. This is because toxins can build up and reside in lung tissue cells, affecting future lung capacity for many years to come. Studies on firefighters involved in the rescue report an average loss of 300 milliliters of lung capacity (Senior 2003).

Exposure to these sorts of particulates may not be symptomatic for years after the exposure. This was certainly the case with those exposed to Agent Orange in Vietnam. Cases of prostate cancer, skin cancer, and chronic lymphocytic leukemia did not appear in some veterans for decades later (Beaulieu and Fessele 2003).

Particulate pollution or soot is the most dangerous form of outdoor pollution. Auto exhaust, aerosols, and chemicals from power plants and wood burning are the major sources. While the particles themselves are too small to be seen by the naked eye, they can be seen as a whole in the form of a haze in the sunlight. An avalanche of these foreigners can overwhelm an already over-taxed or suppressed immune system. Furthermore, they can corrupt the mucosal membranes with radicals, serving to weaken the very protective layer that keeps nature's intruders like pollens away from the epithelial tissues.

Fragrances

The volatile scents and fragrances used in deodorizers, decorations, soaps, and furniture can trigger allergies, along with being downright toxic. While a fragrance might smell like flowers or delicious foods, the typical commercial fragrance contains at least ninety-five percent synthetic chemicals. A single perfume may contain more than 500 different chemicals. Benzene derivatives, aldehydes, toluene, and petroleum-derived chemicals are just a few synthetics used in commercial fragrances. Toluene alone, for example, has been linked to allergies among previously healthy people.

Does this mean we can become allergic to these volatiles? It is possible, but unlikely. More likely, the chemicals simply corrupt our immune systems and mucosal membranes with radicals, making us more sensitive to other allergens such as pollens and molds.

For this reason, we should carefully consider any product containing an ingredient called "fragrances." This includes laundry detergents, dishwashing and other soaps, shampoos and other types of hair products, disinfectants, shaving creams, fabric softeners, fragrant candles, air fresheners, and of course perfumes and colognes. Discernment also should also be given to the word "unscented," as this still may have some of the same synthetics, used instead as fragrance masking elements.

In one study (Anderson and Anderson 1997), mice were cruelly submitted to breathing with a commercial air freshener for one hour at different concentrations. A number of concentrations, including levels typically used by humans in everyday use, caused sensory and pulmonary irritation, decreased breathing velocity, and functional behavior abnormalities.

Another study, performed by the same researchers (Anderson and Anderson 1998) and published a year later, revealed that mice who were cruelly subjected to five commercial colognes or toilet water for an hour suffered various combinations of negative effects, including sensory irritation, pulmonary irritation, decreased airflow expiration, and neurotoxicity.

We might also add that many plants also produce volatile organic compounds. These include fragrances from flowers, trees and other plants. While these volatiles are common in nature, an overstressed immune system could conceivably react with rhinitis symptoms.

Household Air Pollutannts

The modern home typically contains many airborne toxins, which can overload the body with radicals.

The same researchers mentioned above (Anderson and Anderson 2000) found that pulmonary irritation and decreased lung capacity results from the use of synthetic mattress pads. They identified respiratory irritants such as styrene, isopropylbenzene and limonene among polyurethane mattresses. When subjecting organic cotton mattresses to the same test, the results were quite the opposite. Increased respiratory rates and tidal breathing volumes were observed with organic fiber mattresses. The authors noted in each of the above studies that any of these toxin sources could be at least a contributing factor in the rampant rise of allergies among developed countries.

Fabric softener emission is also a dangerous source of air toxicity. Several known irritants and toxins are typically found in fabric softeners, including styrene, isopropylbenzene, thymol, trimethylbenzene and phenols. In yet another study, Anderson and Anderson cruelly subjected mice to five commercial fabric softener emissions for 90 minutes using laundry dryers. The results clearly illustrated that fabric softeners significantly irritate airways. These negative health effects were also seen resulting from emissions of clothing driers containing fabric softener pads.

The researchers (Anderson and Anderson 1999) also found that pulmonary toxicity resulted from commercial diapers, adding that a number of chemicals found in diapers were known to be pulmonary and sensory irritants. They form radicals, in other words.

Another potential indoor radical source is the propellant. Propellants are used in sprays and pump bottles to disperse fluids. While chlorofluorocarbons (CFCs) have been practically eliminated from aerosols, today's aerosols and pump sprays often involve the use of toxic volatile organic compounds (VOCs). Noxious propellants such as isobutane, butane and propane will typically linger in the air for several minutes after spraying. They can also form radicals and trigger rhinitis.

Smoking

Tobacco smoke also produces a hazardous form of indoor pollution. The American Cancer Society estimated in 2004 that 160,000 Americans die each year from lung cancer caused by smoking. Lung cancer maintains between an eleven and fifteen percent chance of survival beyond five years. It should be noted that the highest rates of global lung cancer occur for both men and women in North America and Europe (Field *et al.* 2006). These are also countries where indoor smoking is more prevalent.

Cigarettes release a variety of toxins, which include carbon monoxide, nicotine, aldehydes, ketones and other radical-forming agents—many of which are also carcinogens. These can easily burden the immune system with radical overload. This is especially true when they pervade the environment of a child, or the bloodstream of the mother.

Recent research has indicated that not only is second-hand smoke dangerous to non-smokers, but it has more than twice the amount of tar, nicotine and other radical-forming agents than the smoker inhales. While the smoker will inhale the smoke through the filtering mechanism provided by the packed tobacco inside the cigarette paper—and many cigarettes also have additional filters to capture toxins—the second-hand smoker will breathe all the smoke. Second-hand smoke contains five times the amount of carbon monoxide—the lethal gas that de-oxygenates the blood—than the smoker inhales.

Second-hand smoke also contains ammonia and cadmium. Its nitrogen dioxide levels are fifty times higher than levels considered harmful, and the concentration of hydrogen cyanide approaches toxic levels. Constant exposure to second-hand smoke increases the risk of lung disease by 25%, and increases the risk of heart disease by 10%. Second-hand smoke exposure has also been irrefutably linked to emphysema, chronic bronchitis, asthma, rhinitis and other conditions. Third-hand smoke can also trigger sensitivities.

First-, second- and third-hand smoke poisoning is a significant cause for immunosuppression and systemic inflammation. The Centers for Disease Control's National Health and Nutrition Examination Survey from 1999-2008 (CDC 2010) revealed that between 2007 and 2008, about 88 million American nonsmokers over the age of three were consistently exposed to secondhand smoke. The good news is that the detectible blood nicotine levels among nonsmokers have declined from 52% between 1999 and 2000 to 40% between 2007 and 2008. Still, 40% is simply not acceptable. It should be noted that rates were the highest among children living in households below federal poverty levels.

Researchers from the Respiratory Diseases Department of France's Hospital of Haut-Lévèque in Bordeaux (Raherison *et al.* 2008) studied 7,798 children among six cities in France. This focused on asthma and hay fever among families who smoked. They found that about 20% of all the children were exposed to tobacco via their mother's smoking. Furthermore, they found that children born of mothers who smoked during pregnancy had significantly greater incidence.

Researchers from Austria's Innsbruck Medical University (Horak *et al.* 2007) studied second-hand smoking amongst 1,737 preschool children. They found that nearly 46% of the participating children were exposed to second-hand smoke in the home. Children in poorer homes had greater exposure levels. The researchers found that tobacco smoke exposure during pregnancy increased the incidence of hay fever.

Asbestos

Asbestos exposure has become less likely since the Environmental Protection Agency passed the Asbestos Ban and Phase Out Rule as part of the Toxic Substances Control Act in 1989—which was for the most part overturned in 1991 by the U.S. Fifth Circuit Court of Appeals. What remain are various specific bans such as those from the Clean Air Act and the remnants of the Toxic Substances Control Act, including some continued restrictions supported by Congressional rulings.

The CAA has stimulated various bans since 1973. The bottom line is that although paper- and cardboard-based asbestos has been banned along with certain spray-on versions, many products still contain asbestos. These include cement sheets, clothing, pipe wrap, roofing felt, floor tiles, shingles, millboard, cement pipe, and various automotive parts.

Beyond the banned items, there is no ban preventing manufacturers from using asbestos. The important thing to remember is that the EPA does not monitor manufacturers for their ingredients. In general, asbestos inclusion into today's building materials should be considered a given.

And of course, asbestos is a significant source of radicals in the body.

Formaldehyde

Formaldehyde falls in the same category. Today so many building materials and furniture are built using formaldehyde. These include pressed wood, draperies, glues, resins, shelving, flooring, and so many other materials. The greatest source of formaldehyde appears to be those materials made using *urea-formaldehyde* resins. These include particleboard, plywood paneling, and medium density fiberboard.

Among these, medium density fiberboard—used to make drawers, cabinets and furniture tops—appears to contain the highest resin-to-wood ratio. Another sort of resin called *phenol-formaldehyde* or PF resin. PF resin apparently emits substantially less formaldehyde than the UF resins. The PF resin is easily differentiated from UF resin by its darker, red or black color. The incidental *off-gassing* of formaldehyde into the indoor environment from these resins results from sun, heat, sanding and demolition. As the formaldehyde slowly off gasses, it becomes a constant inflammation and hypersensitivity trigger as it makes contact with the body's tissues.

But these are not the only sources of formaldehyde. The *Final Report on Carcinogens* by the National Toxicology Program included this statement about formaldehyde:

"Occupational exposure to formaldehyde is highly variable and can occur in numerous industries, including the manufacture of formaldehyde and formaldehyde-based resins, wood-composite and furniture production, plastics production, histology and pathology, embalming and biology laboratories, foundries, fiberglass production, construction, agriculture, and firefighting, among others. In fact, because formaldehyde is ubiquitous, it has been suggested that occupational exposure to formaldehyde occurs in all work places. Formaldehyde is also ubiquitous in the environment and has been detected in indoor and outdoor air; in treated drinking water, bottled drinking water, surface water, and groundwater; on land and in the soil; and in numerous types of food. The primary source of exposure is from inhalation of formaldehyde gas in indoor settings (both residential and occupational); however, formaldehyde also may adsorb to respirable particles, providing a source of additional exposure. Major sources of formaldehyde exposure for the general public have included combustion sources (both indoor and outdoor sources including industrial and automobile emissions, home cooking and heating, and cigarette smoke), off-gassing from numerous construction and home furnishing products, and off-gassing from numerous consumer goods. Ingestion of food and water can also be a significant source of exposure to formaldehyde."

Other Building Materials

There are many other toxins—including many yet to be discovered—in our building materials. Certainly, from the above information, we can safely say that any kind of building or decomposition of a modern building will likely impart various hazardous chemicals, most likely including asbestos and formaldehyde.

This means that the air during any kind of sanding, crushing, fire or demolition should be treated with extreme caution. Using a particle or gas mask is more than a good idea under these circumstances, though it should be noted that most particle masks do not form a tight enough bond with the face to filter much at all. Best is to use a gas filter or a mask with a rubber barrier that fits tightly onto the face.

With regard to off-gassing, prior to bringing in any type of new furniture or wood into the house, it is best to off-gas the product by setting it in the sunshine for a couple of days or at least for a full day. As the sun's radiation connects with the material, many of its radical-forming agents are disassociated and released. Not such a good thing for the environment, but at least they will disburse outside of our immediate breathing environment. Off-gassing can help us avoid more than potent hypersensitivity triggers: We can also reduce the body's free radical burden.

Fresh paint can also set off a hypersensitivity episode. This is because paint typically contains VOCs. These can also irritate the airways and produce radicals in the body.

Carbon Monoxide

Carbon monoxide is a substantial indoor air toxin and radical-forming agent. Carbon monoxide is released by burning gas, kerosene, or wood. It can thus arise from the use of wood stoves, fireplaces, gas stoves, generators, automobiles, kitchen stoves, and furnaces. Low concentrations of carbon monoxide in the indoor environment might cause fatigue and even chest pain.

Higher concentrations may result in headaches, confusion, dizziness, nausea, vision impairment and fever. This is due to carboxyhemoglobin formation in the bloodstream, which takes place when carbon monoxide attaches to hemoglobin instead of oxygen. This will in effect starve the body of oxygen, and higher concentrations can easily lead to death.

Acceptable carbon monoxide levels in households are about .5 to 5 parts per million. Levels near a gas stove might be 5 to 15 ppm. An improperly vented or leaking stove might cause 30 ppm or more near the stove, which becomes hazardous. The U.S. National Ambient Air Quality Standard for maximum carbon monoxide levels outside is 35 ppm for one hour and 9 ppm for eight hours. Standards for indoor carbon monoxide have not been determined. Even a pilot (a stove can be used without a pilot) can trigger hypersensitivity.

Making sure that every appliance is vented properly is task number one in avoiding carbon monoxide poisoning. The appliance should also be checked for leaks, and those leaks should be sealed prior to use. Central heating systems should be inspected for leaks as well. Idling the car in the garage is hazardous. Open fireplaces should be avoided indoors, and wood stove doors should be kept closed. We shouldn't solely rely upon the draft up the fireplace chimney for the escape of carbon monoxide.

Nitrogen Oxide

Nitrogen oxide is a gas byproduct of most engines and practically any gas-run appliance. Gas stoves, water heaters, wood stoves, gas heaters and cars are probably the biggest emitters in the home. Homes without these appliances will have very low levels of NO_2 compared to outside. Homes with these appliances may have double the levels. Nitrogen oxide at these levels can imbalance the body, forming radicals in the tissues.

Researchers from Birmingham Heartlands Hospital (Tunnicliffe *et al.* 1994) tested one hour exposure to nitrogen dioxide on ten mild asthmatics with dust mite allergies. Forced expiratory volume (FEV1) levels were tested with non-NO_2 air, air with 100 parts per billion of NO_2, and air containing 400 ppb of nitrogen dioxide. FEV1 levels were 27% lower between the non-NO_2 air and the 400 ppb of NO_2 air. The average FEV1 among the allergic-asthmatics was nearly three times lower in the 400 ppb NO_2 air than in the clear air. The 100 ppb NO_2 air content did not seem to make a significant difference in FEV1, however. This gives us a yardstick for determining unhealthy NO_2 levels.

Radon

Radon is another indoor pollutant worth consideration as a contributor to the body's immune burden. It is estimated that almost 12% of American cancer deaths from lung cancer (about 19,000 deaths a year) result from radon exposure (Field *et al.* 2006). Radon is caused by exposure to disturbed soils and rocks. Increased radon exposure occurs when a house is not properly ventilated, especially in cold weather. Cold outside weather combined with an unventilated warm indoor environment creates an energy vacuum, drawing radon into the house and keeping it there. Houses without adequate coverage over ground soils (such as in an open basement or crawl space) may have greater radon exposure.

Transportation Air

Many other indoor pollutants exist, depending upon the structure and condition of the environment. For example, automobiles, trains, planes, or buses can provide a whole range of radical-forming agents, from carbon monoxide to lead, formaldehyde and plasticizers—which can off-gas (also called *outgassing*), especially when the weather gets warmer.

This is especially the case for new cars. That 'new car smell' is the toxic off-gassing of a mixture of plasticizers, formaldehyde and other synthetics. In the case of older cars, air vents may be clogged with a number of molds, dust and bacteria, which may spray out whenever the "air" is turned on.

It might help to periodically clean out the filters of any car—especially older ones. In the case of a newer car, we might also consider leaving the windows cracked while parking in sunny locations between drives for a few weeks, to let the various materials outgas.

Sick Buildings

Over the last thirty years, researchers have become increasingly aware that certain buildings, especially older ones with older ventilation systems, can make people sick. This effect is often termed *sick building syndrome*, or SBS. The major symptoms reported in SBS include chronic fatigue, brain fog, headaches, allergies, nausea, chronic sore throat, bronchial conges-tion, and higher allergy incidence. There is thus little doubt sick buildings can increase inflammatory events and allergic rhinitis.

SBS is indicated when multiple workers or inhabitants of a building complain of one or more of these symptoms soon after beginning to work or live in the building. Sometimes, however, SBS can develop over time, or directly after or during an extreme change in the weather. A hu-mid summer or heavy rainfall period, for example, may stimulate a growth in mold in the ventilation system. After a smoggy summer in a city or during a fire season, the ventilation system may become clogged with soot. Workers or occupants of the building need to speak up and request from management that filters and vents be periodically cleaned and flushed. The upholstery, walls and other parts of workplaces should also be cleaned periodically.

All of these sources of pollutants are toxins. Once within the body they produce unstable oxidative radicals, which damage cells and tissues. An overload of these toxins produces immunosuppression and systemic inflammation.

The Lessons of Immunotherapy

Nothing illustrates immunosuppression and tolerance in allergies bet-ter than immunotherapy. Why? Because during immunotherapy, we are exposed to very small amounts of an allergen, with gradual increases over time. With these gradual increases, the immune system begins to develop a tolerance to the allergen. The result is a decrease in hypersensitivity reac-tions. After we review the science, we'll discuss what mechanisms are at play with regard to allergic rhinitis.

There are several types of immunotherapy. The types used for aller-gies include *sublingual immunotherapy* (SLIT), *specific oral tolerance induction* (SOTI), *nasal immunotherapy* and *subcutaneous immunotherapy*.

Sublingual immunotherapy places precisely-dosed tablets or drops containing extracts of the trigger under the tongue. Immunotherapy medical suppliers have created various tablets and drops of specific aller-gens/triggers. These allow the dose to be measurable. They also allow for minute doses. Specially-trained health professions typically administer this form of immunotherapy.

Specific oral tolerance induction is typically utilized for food-triggered allergies. Here small amounts of the allergen are eaten daily or periodically under supervision, beginning with miniscule doses. The doses are then increased gradually, thereby increasing the immune system's tolerance to that food.

Nasal immunotherapy has also been used with success, although it has proved primarily beneficial for rhinitis symptoms.

Subcutaneous immunotherapy inserts a small amount of the trigger under the skin. This is usually done with a needle by shallow injection, performed by an experienced health professional. Some allergists—especially those from Europe—have been trained in these techniques.

As we will see from the research, immunotherapy is becoming a frequent treatment among Asian and European doctors for allergy and asthma sufferers—and with great success. As of 2003, over a third of allergies were treated with immunotherapy in Europe (Canonica *et al.* 2003). Today that rate is significantly higher.

The impact of immunotherapy can be significant on someone with allergic hypersensitivity. Let's look at some studies that show how immunotherapy has successfully helped people with various types of allergies:

Researchers from the Respiratory Disease Center in Italy's Papardo Hospital (D'Anneo *et al.* 2010) conducted a sublingual immunotherapy (SLIT) study using 30 adult patients allergic to dust mites with either asthma or rhinitis. They gave the patients a four-day dosing build-up phase of doubling dose, followed by maintenance dosing for the next year—using a commercial immunotherapy formulation called Allergoid.

Using skin prick tests and global symptoms scores, they found that the SLIT group became significantly more tolerant to dust mites at the end of the twelve months, while the control group showed no changes. There were no severe adverse events during the SLIT treatment. The researchers concluded: *"Even with this short four-day up-dosing, the Allergoid SLIT proves to be safe. In addition, it is already effective in patients allergic to HDM after 12 months..."*

Researchers from China's Xinjiang Medical University (Ma and Muzhapaer 2010) gave 32 children with dust mite-allergic asthma sublingual immunotherapy and conventional treatment or just conventional asthma treatment for one year. After the year, the immunotherapy group required less medication to control their asthma than the control group. Symptom scores also significantly decreased among the immunotherapy group and forced expiratory flow increased from 25% to 75% among the immunotherapy group. Specific IgE levels were lower among the immunotherapy group as well. The immunotherapy resulted in no severe adverse effects.

Researchers from Turkey's Ministry of Health and Ankara Diskapi Children's Diseases Training and Research Hospital, Ankara (Reha and Ebru 2007) studied 107 patients who either had sensitivities to dust mites or pollen with either immunotherapy or typical pharmaceuticals. After follow-ups for four years, 81% of the dust mite group and 77% of the pollen group no longer had these sensitizations among the immunotherapy group; compared with 39% of the control group.

Researchers from Germany's Frankfurt University (Zielen *et al.* 2010) gave subcutaneous immunotherapy (SCIT) to 65 asthmatic children sensitive to dust mites. Children treated with house dust mite SCIT together with their medication were able to cut their asthma control medication doses by more than half during the first two years of treatment. The SCIT group significantly improved in peak expiratory flow tests compared to the control group as well.

A newer version of immunotherapy is the mite vaccine. Here is a small amount of the mite allergen is injected into the patient one or multiple times. In a test by Thailand researchers (Visitsunthorn *et al.* 2010), it was found that the Siriraj Mite Allergen Vaccine given to 17 people resulted in no systemic or significant local reactions. Thus this new treatment method—like subcutaneous immunotherapy—appears to be safe.

Researchers from Sweden's Sahlgrenska University Hospital (Höiby *et al.* 2010) gave subcutaneous immunotherapy (SCIT) to 61 patients with birch pollen allergies. They utilized a polymerized birch pollen extract developed specifically for immunotherapy. The therapy consisted of injections of increasingly weekly doses for four weeks, followed by maintenance doses every six weeks for 18 months. The researchers then measured the results during the 2006 birch pollen season. They found that the SCIT-treated patients had significantly fewer symptoms and more tolerance to birch pollen.

The need for medications was also less for the SCIT group. The SCIT group showed significantly increased levels of specific IgG1 and IgG4 immunoglobulins and lower counts of IL-4- and IL-13-producing PBMC—illustrating increased tolerance and lower levels of inflammation. Across all the injections, there were only 29 patients that suffered (mild) reactions, and 17 of those were in the placebo group. None of the reactions required treatment.

Specific immunotherapy has been established for pollen-food sensitivities in many studies. Swiss researchers (Bucher *et al.* 2004) used specific immunotherapy for 27 birch pollen-allergic subjects that either had allergies to apple or hazelnut. Fifteen of the 27 volunteers were given immunotherapy and the others were controls. They were given increasing doses of one gram to 128 grams of either fresh apples or ground hazelnuts over a year's time. After the year, 87% of the immunotherapy group (13) had increased tolerance of apple or hazelnuts with no adverse symptoms. The average amount of increase in the allergen food was about 20 grams—ranging from 12 grams to 32 grams.

Researchers from the Division of Allergy and Immunology of the National Jewish Health association (Katial *et al.* 2010) studied oral tolerance using a protocol they described as aspirin desensitization. They gave 21 adults with aspirin-triggered asthma a desensitization dose of aspirin for two days, followed by 650 mg of aspirin twice daily (classified as high-dose) for six months. After the six months, levels of inflammatory mediators IL-4 and matrix metalloproteinase 9 (MMP-9) fell off significantly compared to the beginning of the treatment. The patients were significantly desensitized to aspirin.

Food allergy immunotherapy has also proved successful, and it is now a standard practice among European doctors. The author's book on food allergies has additional information on food allergy immunotherapy, but here are a few studies illustrating the successes of immunotherapy:

Researchers from France's University Hospital of Nancy (Morisset *et al.* 2007) tested SOTI with 60 milk allergy children, aged between 13 months and 6.5 years old; and 90 egg allergy children, ages 12 months to eight years old. They were randomized, and given either allergen elimination diets or gradual SOTI desensitization by feeding small amounts of the allergen. After six months, skin prick testing and IgE testing revealed that sensitivities continued in only 11% of the milk SOTI group, and 30% of the egg SOTI group. This means the success rates were 89% and 70%, respectively.

Allergy researchers from the University of Rome (Meglio *et al.* 2004) gradually desensitized (SOTI) 21 milk allergy children within six months by feeding increasing amounts of milk daily, with a goal of 200 ml per day of eventual tolerance. Within the six months, 71% of the children (15 of 21) accomplished the 200 mL daily intake. Of the rest, three (14%) were able to tolerate 40-80 ml per day, and only three of the 21 children (14%) failed the SOTI treatment completely. This rendered a total success rate of 86%.

Researches from Italy's University of Trieste (Longo *et al.* 2008) found that even children with extreme allergic responses to milk could significantly benefit from oral immunotherapy protocol. They divided 60 severely milk-allergic children five years old or higher into two groups. The first group of 30 was given immediate oral immunotherapy of gradually increasing amounts of milk for one year. The other group remained on a milk elimination diet throughout the year. After the year, 11 become completely tolerant to milk while 16 of the children became partially tolerant. That means that out of the 30 *severely allergic* children, 90% (27 out of 30) became tolerant to milk to one degree or another.

Many more studies have confirmed the same findings: That 80-90% of allergies can be reversed through the use of immunotherapy.

Transylvania University researchers (Agache and Ciobanu 2010) found in their study of 33 asthmatic children and 82 asthmatic adults that asthma was more frequent and severe among those who did not utilize allergen-specific immunotherapy for their hay fever allergies, which, in most cases, preceded their asthma diagnosis.

The newest form of allergy immunotherapy is the Ultra Rush method. This increases the rate of introduction and increase of the allergen, often producing results within a week or two. The risk of this therapy is increased by virtue of pushing the immune system. Therefore, ultra-rush immunotherapy must be conducted in a clinical setting monitored by people skilled in anaphylaxis.

This was illustrated by research from the Allergy Unit at the University Hospital Germans Trias i Pujol in Badalona, Spain (Roger *et al.* 2011). Here Ultra Rush technique outcomes were surveyed for reactions. Out of 218 patients, 32 adverse reactions were reported among 27 of the patients. All the reactions were considered "mild or moderate," with no serious or life-threatening reactions.

Nature also conducts immunotherapy. Researchers from Turkey's Hacettepe University School of Medicine (Celikel *et al.* 2006) studied 444 beekeepers with a history of receiving bee stings. More than half of the beekeepers were stung more than 100 times in the previous year, and yet only 29 of the beekeepers sustained systemic reactions—6.5% of the 444. The researchers commented: *"The incidence of systemic reactions in Turkish beekeepers is low, which might be due to the protective effect of a high frequency of bee stings."*

The beekeepers received immunotherapy, in other words. By being stung repeatedly, they began to tolerate the bee sting venom.

What is the mechanism that causes the immune system to become tolerant, and why does this tolerance begin with small increments of the allergen?

Mechanisms of Immunotherapy: Building Tolerance

Let's consider this carefully. When a weakened immune system is exposed to a large amount of the allergen, it reacts with a hyperinflammatory event. But when the immune system is exposed to very small amounts of the same allergen in increasingly larger doses, it learns to tolerate the allergen.

It is not as though the immune system simply "gets used to" the allergen. It is not like learning to tolerate a bad boss at work. The immune system is re-learning to handle the foreigner as it should.

This again is the concept of burden. When the immune system is overloaded with a foreigner, it will respond in a systemic fashion. If it is exposed to a small amount, then localized factors such as IgA, probiotics,

T-cells and B-cells work locally to rid the area of the potential threat. This of course, is how a healthy body will eliminate the foreigner.

This localized elimination process in turn communicates to the immune system that this foreigner can easily be gotten rid of using less extraordinary means. As the immune cells communicate the successful elimination of small quantities of the foreigner, the immune system learns to handle more.

Again building immunity is similar to building muscle strength. We could compare this with weight-lifting:

If we put 250 lbs of barbell weights on top of the chest of a 180-lb person, they would likely collapse and maybe even break a few ribs from the weight.

But if we took the same person, and put them on a weight-lifting program for a year, we could probably easily get them to a point where they would easily lift the 250 lbs off their chest.

Such a training schedule would equate to immunotherapy.

In this weight-lifting program, we'd probably start them on lifting 50 lbs, then 100 lbs, then 150 lbs, then 200 lbs, then eventually the 250 lbs. Gradually, as we added weight to their lifting, we would be increasing their strength to a point where they could lift the whole weight load.

As we review the other contributing culprits of allergic rhinitis, we'll be circling back to this concept of building immunity. Later we'll also discuss "training" methods to increase our immunity.

Defective Mucous Membranes

As we illustrated with the University of Melbourne research on eosinophilic esophagitis, many allergy sufferers also deal from gastroesophageal reflux (GERD). This and other research points to the fact that the association between allergies and GERD is not merely a coincidence: The two conditions are somehow connected. How and why are they connected? Let's review the science on their relationship, and then answer this question:

Researchers from Lebanon's Balamand University (Waked and Salameh 2008) studied 5,522 children from 22 schools for incidence of asthma, allergic rhinitis and atopic eczema alongside gastroesophageal reflux among other associations. They found that GERD was significantly associated with asthma, allergic rhinitis and atopic eczema.

Scientists from Australia's Griffith University Medical School (Sugnanam *et al.* 2007) studied eosinophilic esophagitis along with gastroesophageal reflux and allergies among 45 children and 33 other patients. They found that allergies were significantly associated with eosinophilic esophagitis. The children showed more allergies to foods, while the adults had more allergic rhinitis. Airborne allergies and allergic rhinitis, they found, appears to increase with age, following four years old. In addition, nearly a quarter of the EE/allergy patients had a history of having anaphylaxis.

Medical researchers from Munich University (Müller *et al.* 2007) studied randomly-selected 117 eosinophilic esophagitis patients, consisting of 9 children and 108 adults (72% were male). They found that 82% of the adults' symptoms appeared mostly between the age of 21 and 30 years old. GERD symptoms were found among 70% and 47%, while allergies were found among 49% of the EE patients.

In a study we discussed earlier, University of Vermont researchers (Dixon *et al.* 2006) found that asthmatics with gastroesophageal reflux disease (GERD) symptoms had twice the occurrence of either sinusitis or rhinitis.

Background on GERD

Before we can better understand the relationship between allergies, eosinophilic esophagitis and GERD, we should review the science on GERD itself.

Studies have shown that GERD incidence is higher among more developed countries—and significantly greater in those countries whose populations eat primarily a 'western' diet.

This is illustrated dramatically by comparing GERD rates between China and the U.S.

Researchers from the University of Hong Kong (Wong *et al.* 2003) conducted a study of GERD among Chinese populations. In total, 2,209 adult volunteers participated in the study. The research discovered that 2.5% of the population experienced some heartburn weekly, 9% experienced heartburn monthly, and nearly 30% experienced some heartburn at least once in the past year.

In comparison, about a third of the U.S. population experiences heartburn at least monthly, and about 10% experience heartburn daily (Friedman *et al.* 2008). About 18-20% of Americans experience heartburn weekly (Locke *et al.* 1997).

In other words, Americans experience heartburn about 7.6 times more frequently than do the Chinese (18-20% versus 2.5%). That means that Americans have 760% more weekly heartburn than the Chinese. Furthermore, slightly more Americans experience daily heartburn than the number of Chinese who experience heartburn monthly. This could be translated to Americans having over thirty times more severe heartburn. However it is calculated, Americans have dramatically more GERD than the Chinese.

In addition to diet, we can also include air pollution and stress as possible GERD factors. However, we should note that cities in China are significantly more crowded, with more pollutants—especially in the way of soot and heavy metals—than U.S. cities. So the difference relates to other key lifestyle differences—the prominent of which are diet and stress.

The assumption has been that asthma- and allergy-related GERD is associated with stomach acid leaking into the esophagus and bronchial passages, where it theoretically irritates the airways. Unfortunately, this theory has not panned out well in the research:

Researchers from Brazil's University of São Paulo Medical School (Araujo *et al.* 2008) studied the relationship between acid infusion and GERD-associated asthma. They monitored the esophageal pH and bronchial responsiveness among 20 GERD-asthma patients. They found that acid-infusion did not increase bronchial hyperresponsiveness among the GERD-related asthmatics. They concluded: *"These findings strongly question the significance of acid infusion as a model to study the pathogenesis of GERD-induced asthma."*

Researchers from Norway's Østfold County Hospital (Størdal *et al.* 2005) studied 38 children who presented with asthma and gastroesophageal reflux. They were given acid suppression medication omeprazole or placebo for 12 weeks, while undergoing monitoring for esophageal pH control.

Repeated pH monitoring confirmed that the acid suppression medication indeed inhibited acid secretion in the children. However, the total symptom scores were not significantly different between the omeprazole group and the placebo group. Lung function and asthma medication use were also comparable between the two groups. The researchers concluded: *"Omeprazole treatment did not improve asthma symptoms or lung function in children with asthma and GERD."*

This and other research confirms that the leaking of acids into the esophagus is not the primary cause for GERD-related asthma.

The Mucosal Conclusion

The mechanism that binds these conditions—GERD, eosinophilic esophagitis, asthma and allergic rhinitis—is the health of the mucosal membranes that line the airways, the nasal region, the esophagus, and the stomach.

This is also illustrated by research from the University of Helsinki (Renkonen *et al.* 2010) that found birch pollen allergen readily transported through the epithelium of allergic patients, but not non-allergic subjects. Healthy people did not have this transport mechanism defect.

Furthermore, medical researchers from the University of Helsinki (Toppila-Salmi *et al.* 2011) found that among those allergic to birch pollen, the birch pollen protein allergen was "rapidly and actively" transported through the mucous membrane and the airway epithelium. Healthy patients, on the other hand, had a "strong epithelial response" when challenged by the birch allergen.

This means that the mucous membranes and epithelial layer of skin in the nasal cavities of allergic people readily lets allergens cross the skin into the tissues and bloodstream—sparking an allergic IgE response—while non-allergic people actively fight off the allergen before it intrudes into the tissues and bloodstream. Non-allergic people have stronger IgA, immune cell and probiotic systems within the mucosal membranes. The Helsinki researchers confirmed this as they concluded:

"Epithelium has emerged as an active and complex organ with mechanical, biochemical and immunological functions. The increasing awareness that epithelium interacts actively with allergens might provide new targets for the prevention and management of allergy."

Researchers from the China-Japan Union Hospital and Jilin University (Zhu *et al.* 2009) found that patients with allergic rhinitis had a greater expression of thymic stromal lymphopoietin (TSLP) among the epithelium of the nasal and other airway regions. They harvested samples from 22 allergic patients and 11 healthy control patients.

TSLP is a signalling protein that is associated with increased T-cell activity. TSLP stimulates a pathway that increases the binding of allergens. In other words, TSLP is part of the immune system's process for a hyper-response when the IgA system within the airway mucosal membranes and epithelia has been weakened.

GERD takes place because there are two conditions within the stomach. The first is the thinning of the mucosal membrane that lines the stomach. This membrane protects the stomach from the acids presented by the gastric cells and acidic foods. The gastric acids, meant to destroy microorganisms in our foods and help break down the nutrients, do not irritate the stomach of healthy persons. A healthy person produces sufficient alkaline mucous in the stomach to protect the cells from the acid.

A situation that also occurs in some GERD patients is the weakening of the sphincter muscle at the entry of the stomach from the esophagus. This muscle controls the valve that keeps stomach acids and foods from backing up into the esophagus. Most medical experts propose that this is the result of overeating and/or going to bed after a big meal.

The problem with this theory is that many people who overeat and go to bed full do not experience heartburn. Surely, these people also experience a backup of food and acids from the stomach, yet they do not ex-

161

perience heartburn. Holiday meals are a good example. After a gigantic holiday meal, people will roll around for the next few hours with their esophagi crammed with food, as it is gradually admitted into the stomach.

Only a small percentage of these people who regularly overeat will experience GERD. Therefore, we can conclude that overeating and the subsequent sphincter weakening is also not the sole cause of GERD.

We also know that for many, GERD follows the use of certain medications. These include, beta-blockers, NSAIDs, COX inhibitors, sedatives, antidepressants, calcium channel blockers, progestin and others.

What is the connection? Now we have more associations to consider: asthma, GERD, certain medication use, and heartburn from stomach acids and foods.

Again, there can only be one issue that truly links all of these: The health of the mucosal membranes. The stomach, esophagus and the airways are each coated with protective mucosal membranes.

The stomach is coated with a protective gastric mucosal membrane. The esophagus and airways are also coated with protective mucosal membranes. Special mucosal glands within the cell matrix of all three epithelial regions secrete a combination of protective mucopolysaccharides, glycoproteins and ionic fluids. These are further complexed by probiotics and immune cells, which protect their epithelial cells from infection and toxins. Should the mucosal membranes weaken, food and acids can impact the epithelial cells, much the way pollen can impact the epithelial tissues of our nasal cavities.

The Causes of Corrupted Mucosal Membranes

Many things can corrupt the mucosal membranes:

Certain medications, such as the ones mentioned above, will interrupt the cyclooxygenase enzyme pathway. One of the cyclooxygenase enzyme pathways stimulates the secretion of mucosal glands throughout the body. In addition, nutrient deficiencies, dehydration, toxin overload and/or stress can change the content and the volume of these all-important mucosal secretions: Again not just in the stomach, but among all mucosal secretions. This is why the same acid-blocker and anti-inflammatory medications that halt mucosal secretions can also cause dry mouth.

Now should the mucosal secretions be halted from nutrient deficiencies, dehydration, nervousness, toxin overload and/or stress, the mucosal glands will not produce enough of the protective coating over those epithelial regions. This leaves the epithelia cells in these regions exposed to stomach acids in the case of GERD, and toxins or other allergy triggers in the case of allergic rhinitis.

This is the reason why GERD often accompanies allergies, asthma, and eosinophilic esophagitis: These factors corrupt the body's ability to produce and maintain healthy mucosal membranes. This in turn opens these tissues up to damage from allergens and toxins—which in turn produces inflammation as the immune system responds to radicals.

Weakened Probiotic Colonies

Can defective probiotic deficiencies directly cause allergic rhinitis? Let's look at the evidence.

Most people think of the intestines when they hear the word probiotics. Yes, it is true that the intestines host the majority of the body's probiotic bacteria. However, nearly all of the body's mucosal membranes house probiotics. Our probiotics are therefore at home within our oral cavity, sinus cavity, larynx, pharynx, esophagus and airways. They line these regions and guard their territories (also part of our body) with tenacity. They attack and take apart invading viruses, bacteria, fungi and a variety of toxins. As we've discussed earlier, they also alert our immune system of pending invasions.

Our intestinal bacterial are critical to the health of the sinuses, nasal region, eyes and airways. Consider, for example, a Swiss study, which showed how a probiotic yogurt affected the nasal tissues:

Scientists from the Swiss National Accident Insurance Institute (Glück and Gebbers 2003) gave 209 human volunteers either a conventional yogurt or a combination of *Lactobacillus* GG (ATCC 53103), *Bifidobacterium* sp. B420, *Lactobacillus acidophilus* 145, and *Streptococcus thermophilus* every day for 3 weeks. Nasal microbial flora was measured at the beginning, at day 21 and at day 28. Significant pathogenic bacteria were found in most of the volunteers' nasal cavities at the beginning of the study. The consumption of the probiotic-enhanced milk led to a 19% reduction of pathogenic bacteria in the nasal cavity. The researchers concluded that, *"The results indicate a linkage of the lymphoid tissue between the gut and the upper respiratory tract."*

This is only the tip of the iceberg. Let's review more of the research.

Probiotics, Pollen Allergies and Allergic Rhinitis

Probiotic mechanisms have been increasingly connected to inflammatory and allergic responses. They play a critical role in maintaining the mucosal membranes. This relates directly to respiratory allergic responses.

Researchers from Finland's National Public Health Institute (Piirainen *et al.* 2008) found that *Lactobacillus rhamnosus* GG fed to pollen-allergic persons for 5-½ months resulted in lower levels of pollen-specific IgE, higher levels of IgG and higher levels of IgA in the saliva. This is consistent with lower sensitivity, greater immunity, and a greater tolerance for pollens.

Japanese scientists (Xiao *et al.* 2006) gave 44 patients with Japanese cedar pollen allergies *Bifidobacterium longum* BB536 for 13 weeks. The probiotic group had significantly decreased symptoms of rhinorrhea (runny nose) and nasal blockage versus the placebo group. The probiotic group also had decreased activity among plasma T-helper type 2 (Th2) cells and reduced symptoms of Japanese cedar pollen allergies. The researchers concluded that the results: *"suggest the efficacy of BB536 in relieving JCPsis symptoms, probably through the modulation of Th2-skewed immune response."*

Researchers from Japan's Kansai Medical University Kouri Hospital (Hattori *et al.* 2003) gave 15 children with atopic dermatitis either *Bifidobacterium breve* M-16V or a placebo. After one month, the probiotic group had a significant improvement of allergic symptoms.

Japanese scientists (Ishida *et al.* 2005) gave a drink with *Lactobacillus acidophilus* strain L-92 or a placebo to 49 patients with perennial allergic rhinitis for eight weeks. The probiotic group showed significant improvement in runny nose and watery eyes symptoms, along with decreased nasal mucosa swelling and redness compared to the placebo group. These results were also duplicated in a follow-up study of 23 allergy sufferers by some of the same researchers.

Scientists from Britain's Institute of Food Research (Ivory *et al.* 2008) gave *Lactobacillus casei* Shirota (LcS) to 10 patients with seasonal allergic rhinitis. The researchers compared immune status with daily ingestion of a milk drink with or without live *Lactobacillus casei* over a period of five months. Blood samples were tested for plasma IgE and grass pollen-specific IgG by an enzyme immunoassay.

Patients treated with the *Lactobacillus casei* milk showed significantly reduced levels of antigen-induced IL-5, IL-6 and IFN-gamma production compared with the placebo group. Levels of specific IgG also increased, while pro-inflammatory IgE decreased in the probiotic group. The researchers concluded that: *"These data show that probiotic supplementation modulates immune responses in allergic rhinitis and may have the potential to alleviate the severity of symptoms."*

Japanese researchers (Odamaki *et al.* 2007) gave yogurt with *Bifidobacterium longum* BB536 or plain yogurt to 40 patients with Japanese cedar pollinosis for 14 weeks. *Bacteroides fragilis* significantly changed with pollen dispersion. The ratio of *B. fragilis* to bifidobacteria also increased significantly during pollen season among the placebo group but not in the *B. longum* group. Peripheral blood mononuclear cells from the patients indicated that *B. fragilis* microorganisms induced significantly more Th2 cell cytokines such as interleukin-6, and fewer Th1 cell cytokines such as IL-12 and interferon. The researchers concluded that: *"These results suggest a relationship between fluctuation in intestinal microbiota and pollinosis allergy. Fur-*

thermore, intake of BB536 yogurt appears to exert positive influences on the formation of anti-allergic microbiota."

Researchers from the Department of Otolaryngology and Sensory Organ Surgery at Osaka University School of Medicine in Japan (Tamura *et al.* 2007) studied allergic response in chronic rhinitis patients. For eight weeks, patients were given either a placebo or *Lactobacillus casei* strain Shirota. Those with moderate-to-severe nasal symptom scores at the beginning of the study and given probiotics experienced significantly reduced nasal symptoms.

Research confirms this relationship. For example, researchers from Finland's University of Turku (Kalliomäki *et al.* 2001) gave the probiotic *Lactobacillus GG* or placebo to mothers of children with a high risk of allergies during pregnancy; and to their infants for six months. They found the incidence of allergies among the children given probiotics was half the incidence of the placebo group.

Allergy researchers from Helsinki University (Kuitunen *et al.* 2009) gave a probiotic blend of two lactobacilli, bifidobacteria, propionibacteria and prebiotics, or a placebo to mothers of 1,223 infants with a high risk of allergies during the last month of pregnancy term. Then they gave their infants the dose from birth until six months of age. They evaluated the children at five years of age for allergies. Of the 1,018 infants who completed the dosing, 891 were evaluated after five years. Among the Cesarean-birth children, allergy incidence was significantly lower in the probiotic group compared to the placebo group (24% versus 40%).

Japanese researchers (Kubota *et al.* 2010) analyzed the intestinal bifidobacteria from 29 patients who were allergic to Japanese cedar pollinosis (JCPsis). They found that those patients with more than three bifidobacteria species had significantly lower levels of allergen-specific IgEs in their blood—resulting in less severity. Those patients with less than three species had greater allergy severity and more IgEs in the blood.

A year earlier, some of the same researchers (Kubota *et al.* 2009) found that intestinal probiotics respond to allergen reception. They found that cedar pollen-allergic patients responded differently to supplemented probiotics than did the healthy subjects. This illustrated that the probiotics specifically responded to their allergic responses.

Researchers from Japan's Chiba University School of Medicine (Yonekura *et al.* 2009) gave *Lactobacillus paracasei* strain KW3110 or a placebo for three months to 126 patients who had allergies to cedar. They began the treatment one month prior to cedar pollen season. The probiotic group had a significant reduction of rhinitis symptoms. They also had significantly reduced eosinophil cationic protein (ECP) counts in the bloodstream and had higher quality of life scores.

Finnish researchers (Ouwehand *et al.* 2009) studied 47 children with birch pollen allergies. They gave the children either a combination of Lactobacillus acidophilus NCFM and Bifidobacterium lactis Bl-04 or a placebo for four months. They began the treatment before the birch pollen season. They took nasal swabs and analyzed for inflammatory eosinophils, as well as IgA and probiotics in the feces. As the pollen season progressed, the probiotic group had significantly fewer symptoms of rhinitis—by up to a third less for blocked nose. Also, the probiotic group also had nearly 40% lower levels of eosinophils among their nasal tissues.

University of Helsinki researchers (Viljanen *et al.* 2005) treated 230 milk-allergic infants *Lactobacillus* GG, four probiotic strains, or a placebo for four weeks. Among IgE-sensitized allergic children, the LGG provoked a reduction in symptoms while the placebo group did not.

Allergy Hospital researchers from Helsinki University (Kuitunen *et al.* 2009) gave a probiotic blend of two lactobacilli, bifidobacteria, propionibacteria and prebiotics, or a placebo to mothers of 1,223 infants with a high risk of allergies during the last month of pregnancy term. Then they gave their infants the dose from birth until six months of age. They evaluated the children at five years of age for allergies. Of the 1,018 infants who completed the dosing, 891 were evaluated after five years. Allergies among the cesarean-birth children—which have higher rates of allergies—were nearly half in the probiotic group compared to the placebo group (24.3% versus 40.5%).

University of Milan researchers (Arslanoglu *et al.* 2008) found that a mixture of prebiotics galactooligosaccharides (GOS) and fructooligosaccharides (FOS) reduces allergy incidence. A mix of these or a placebo was given with formula for the first six months after birth to 134 infants. The incidence of allergic symptoms in the prebiotic group was half of what was found among the placebo group. The researchers concluded that: *"The observed dual protection lasting beyond the intervention period suggests that an immune modulating effect through the intestinal flora modification may be the principal mechanism of action."*

Scientists from Britain's Institute of Food Research (Ivory *et al.* 2008) gave *Lactobacillus casei* Shirota (LcS) to 10 patients with seasonal allergic rhinitis. The researchers compared immune status with daily ingestion of a milk drink with or without live *Lactobacillus casei* over a period of five months. Blood samples were tested for plasma IgE and grass pollen-specific IgG by an enzyme immunoassay. Patients treated with the *Lactobacillus casei* milk showed significantly reduced levels of antigen-induced IL-5, IL-6 and IFN-gamma production compared with the placebo group. Levels of specific IgG also increased and IgE decreased in the probiotic group. The researchers concluded that: *"These data show that probiotic supple-*

mentation modulates immune responses in allergic rhinitis and may have the potential to alleviate the severity of symptoms."

Probiotics and Immunosuppression

As we've discussed, allergies are directly related to an overloaded and burdened immune system. This is also called systemic inflammation and immunosuppression. Probiotics are nature's smart army corps of engineers. They will help rebuild cellular functions, immune cell function, and help stimulate better immune system responses. Rebuilding our immune system is the absolute requirement for anyone seeking to reverse the effects of diseases related to systemic inflammation and immunosuppression—such as allergic rhinitis.

Hundreds of studies have illustrated probiotics' direct affect upon immunosuppression. Here we will show a tiny sampling.

A review from the Wright State University Boonshoft School of Medicine (Michail *et al.* 2009) found that probiotics showed a rebalancing of the Th2/Th1 balance—increasing the anti-inflammatory Th1 side and decreasing the inflammatory Th2 side. They commented: "Probiotics have been shown to modulate the immune system back to a Th1 response. Several in vitro studies suggest a role for probiotics in treating allergic disorders."

Researchers from the University of Arkansas' Medical School (Wheeler *et al.* 1997) studied 15 asthmatic adults in two one-month crossover periods with placebo or yogurt containing *L. acidophilus*. The probiotic consumption increased immune system interferon gamma and decreased eosinophils—both markers for systemic and airway inflammation.

Japanese scientists (Hirose *et al.* 2006) gave *Lactobacillus plantarum* strain L-137 or placebo to 60 healthy men and women, average age 56, for twelve weeks. The probiotic group had increased Con A-induced proliferation (acquired immunity), increases in IL-4 production by CD4+ T-cells, and a more balanced (anti-inflammatory) Th1:Th2 ratios.

Researchers from Britain's Scarborough Hospital (McNaught *et al.* 2005) gave a placebo or *Lactobacillus plantarum* 299v to 103 critically ill patients along with conventional therapy. On day 15, the probiotic group had significantly lower serum (anti-inflammatory) IL-6 levels compared to the control group.

Researchers from the Department of Immunology at Japan's Juntendo University School of Medicine (Takeda *et al.* 2006) gave a placebo or *Lactobacillus casei* Shirota to 9 healthy middle-aged adults and 10 elderly adults daily for three weeks. After three weeks of supplementation, *L. casei* significantly increased natural killer cell activity (stimulated immunity) among the volunteers, especially among those who had low NK-cell activity before probiotic supplementation.

Researchers from the University of Vienna (Meyer *et al.* 2007) gave healthy women yogurt with *Lactobacillus bulgaricus* and *Streptococcus thermophilus*, with or without *Lactobacillus casei*. After two weeks, both yogurt groups had significantly increased blood levels of tumor necrosis factor-alpha (TNF-a)—by 24% in the regular yogurt group and by 63% in the *L. casei* yogurt group. They also observed significantly higher levels of cytokines interleukin (IL)-1beta (by 40%) and interferon gamma (by 108%). In addition, IL-10 decreased during *L. casei*-enhanced yogurt treatment, but then significantly increased after the yogurt treatment was stopped (by 129%). These are all signs of strengthened immunity.

Researchers from Finland's University of Turku (Ouwehand *et al.* 2008) gave a placebo, *Bifidobacterium longum*, or *Bifidobacterium lactis* Bb-12 to 55 institutionalized elderly subjects for 6 months. The probiotic groups showed modulated pro-inflammatory cytokine TNF-alpha and cytokine IL-10 levels compared with the placebo group.

Scientists from Spain's University of Navarra (Parra *et al.* 2004) investigated the effects of fermented milk with *Lactobacillus casei* DN114001 on 45 healthy volunteers aged 51-58. The probiotic group showed increased oxidative burst capacity among monocytes, and increased NK-cell tumor suppression activity. The researchers concluded that *L. casei* can have *"a positive effect in modulating the innate immune defense in healthy-middle-age people."*

Researchers from Tokyo's Juntendo University School of Medicine (Fujii *et al.* 2006) gave 19 preterm infants a placebo or *Bifidobacterium breve* supplementation for three weeks after birth. Anti-inflammatory serum TGF-beta1 levels in the probiotic group were elevated on day 14 and remained elevated through day 28. Messenger RNA expression was enhanced in the probiotic group on day 28 compared with the placebo group. The researchers concluded: *"These results demonstrated that the administration of B. breve to preterm infants can up-regulate TGF-beta1 signaling and may possibly be beneficial in attenuating inflammatory and allergic reactions in these infants."*

Scientists from the Department of Oral Microbiology at Japan's Asahi University School of Dentistry (Ogawa *et al.* 2006) found that *Lactobacillus casei* supplementation significantly decreased cedar pollen-specific IgEs, thymus, chemokines, eosinophils, and interferon-gamma levels compared to the placebo group—all signs of strengthened immunity.

Dr. Oner Ozdemir, M.D. at the SEMA Research and Training Hospital in Turkey, characterizes the issue with an understanding of immune and probiotic mechanisms:

> *"Development of the child's immune system tends to be directed toward a T-helper 2 (Th2) phenotype in infants. To prevent development of childhood allergic/atopic diseases, immature Th2-*

dominant neonatal responses must undergo environment-driven maturation via microbial contact in the early postnatal period. Lactic acid bacteria and bifidobacteria are found more commonly in the composition of the intestinal flora of nonallergic children. Epidemiological data also showed that atopic children have a different intestinal flora from healthy children. Probiotics are ingested with live health-promoting microbes that can modify intestinal microbial populations in a way that benefits the host; and enhanced presence of probiotic bacteria in the intestinal microbiota is found to correlate with protection against atopy."

What Causes Probiotic Deficiencies?

The central causes are toxins, stress and the overuse of antibiotics and other sanitation strategies. Some of the same things associated with allergies, in other words. The use of antibiotics has soared over the past few decades—suspiciously over the same period that allergy rates have also soared. Today, over 3,000,000 pounds of pure antibiotics are taken by humans annually in the United States. This is complemented by the approximately 25,000,000 pounds of antibiotics given to animals each year.

Meanwhile, many of these antibiotics are given erroneously or are ineffectual. The Centers for Disease Control states that, *"Almost half of patients with upper respiratory tract infections in the U.S. still receive antibiotics from their doctor."* The CDC further explains that, *"90% of upper respiratory infections, including children's ear infections, are viral, and antibiotics don't treat viral infection. More than 40% of about 50 million prescriptions for antibiotics each year in physicians' offices were inappropriate."*

Indeed, the growing use of antibiotics has also created a Pandora 's Box of *superbugs*. As bacteria are repeatedly hit with the same antibiotic, they learn to adapt. Just as any living organism does (yes, bacteria are alive), bacteria learn to counter and resist repeatedly utilized antibiotics. As a result, many bacteria today are resistant to a variety of antibiotics. This is because bacteria tend to adjust to their surroundings. If they are attacked enough times with a certain challenge, they are likely to figure out how to avoid it and thrive in spite of it.

This has been the case for a number of other new antibiotic-resistant strains of bacteria. They have simply evolved to become stronger and more able to counteract those antibiotic medications.

This phenomenon has created *multi-drug resistant organisms*. Some of the more dangerous MDROs include species of *Enterococcus, Staphylococcus, Salmonella, Campylobacter, Escherichia coli,* and others. Superbugs such as MRSA are only the tip of the bacterial iceberg.

Another growing infectious bacterium is *Clostridium difficile*. This bacterium will infect the intestines of people of any age. Among children, this is one of the world's biggest killers—causing acute, watery diarrhea. It is also a growing infection among adults. Every year, *C. difficile* infects tens of thousands of people in the U.S. according to the Mayo Clinic. Worse, *C. difficile* are increasingly becoming resistant to antibiotics, and infections from clostridia are growing in incidence each year.

Researchers from the Norwegian University of Science and Technology (Mai *et al.* 2010) found that early antibiotic use increased the likelihood of allergies at age eight. Over 3,300 children were studied for antibiotic use and respiratory conditions at the ages of two months, one year, four years and eight years. Of all groups, 43% of the children received antibiotics. A third of the children had a respiratory infection, including pneumonia, bronchitis or otitis. The researchers found that those who used antibiotics during their first year of life had increased rates of wheeze and eczema by age eight.

Childhood Allergies and Probiotics

Probiotics are critical during the first few weeks of life, and a deficiency during that period can result in allergies because the immune system is not ready to 'stand up on its own.' Consider some of the science supporting this:

Research from Sweden's Linköping University (Böttcher *et al.* 2008) gave *Lactobacillus reuteri* or a placebo to 99 pregnant women from gestational week 36 until infant delivery. The babies were followed for two years after birth, and analyzed for eczema, allergen sensitization and immunity markers. Probiotic supplementation lowered TGF-beta2 levels in mother's milk and babies' feces, and slightly increased IL-10 levels in mothers' colostrum. Lower levels of TGF-beta2 are associated with lower sensitization and lower risk of IgE-associated eczema.

German researchers (Grönlund *et al.* 2007) tested 61 infants and mother pairs for allergic status and bifidobacteria levels from 30-35 weeks of gestation and from one-month old. Every mother's breast milk contained some type of bifidobacteria, with *Bifidobacterium longum* found most frequently. However, only the infants of allergic, atopic mothers had colonization with *B. adolescentis*. Allergic mothers also had significantly less bifidobacteria in their breast-milk than non-allergic mothers.

Researchers from Tokyo's Juntendo University School of Medicine (Fujii *et al.* 2006) gave 19 preterm infants placebo or *Bifidobacterium breve* supplementation for three weeks after birth. Anti-inflammatory serum TGF-beta1 levels in the probiotic group were elevated on day 14 and remained elevated through day 28. Messenger RNA expression was enhanced for the probiotic group on day 28 compared with the placebo group. The researchers concluded that: *"These results demonstrated that the administration of B. breve to preterm infants can up-regulate TGF-beta1 signaling and may possibly be beneficial in attenuating inflammatory and allergic reactions in these infants."*

In a study from the University of Western Australia School of Pediatrics (Taylor *et al.* 2006), 178 children born of mothers with allergies were given either *Lactobacillus acidophilus* or a placebo for the first six months of life. Those given the probiotics showed reduced levels of IL-5 and TGF-beta in response to polyclonal stimulation (typical for allergic responses), and significantly lower IL-10 responses to vaccines as compared with the placebo group. These results illustrated that the probiotics had increased allergen resistance among the probiotic group of children.

Medical researchers from the University of Siena (Aldinucci *et al.* 2002) gave 450 grams per day of either probiotic yogurt or partially skimmed milk to 20 infants for four months. Thirteen infants had rhinitis and seven were healthy. Symptoms and mucosal health were significantly better among the yogurt group.

Probiotics and the Hygiene Hypothesis

The reality is that the body naturally houses many infectious bacteria, including *E. coli* and *Clostridium difficile*. However, probiotic colonies typically keep their populations minimized and under control. When probiotic populations are deficient, these bacteria can grow out of control and stimulate systemic inflammation. This means that they hygiene hypothesis must take into account the ability of probiotic colonies to control other infective microorganisms.

This control and balance is illustrated by *H. pylori* infections. Researchers from the New York University's School of Medicine (Chen and Blaser 2008) studied the colonization of *Helicobacter pylori* within the digestive tract and childhood asthma. Using a cross-sectional analysis of NHANES 1999-2000 data on 7,412 persons, they found that the incidence of allergic rhinitis is significantly lower among those with childhood *H. pylori* infections.

Those children who contracted *H. pylori* were also about 40% less likely to have asthma before the age of five. The risk of current asthma among the children was even lower, at nearly 60% lower incidence. Research over the next year by these scientists concluded similar findings.

The implications of this are quite complicated. When we review the worldwide populations of asthma and *H. pylori*, we find that populations with higher infection rates of *H. pylori* also have significantly fewer cases of asthma among children.

An interesting association becomes evident with respect to worldwide rates of GERD and ulcers. For people living in developed (first world) countries, especially in the U.S., ulcer rates are quite high (some 70%-90%) among those who have *H. pylori* infections. The rate is high enough to conclude—as many physicians have—that ulcers are caused by *H. pylori* infections.

The interesting caveat to consider, however, is that third-world and developing countries have some of the world's *lowest* rates of ulcers (and allergies), yet these countries also have massive *H. pylori* infection rates. While western countries might have *H. pylori* infections in 10-20% of the population, third world countries see upwards of 75% of their children hosting a *H. pylori* infections—with seemingly no ill effects.

The research correlating *H. pylori* with reduced risk of allergy is not simply a matter of a single microorganism. Rather, the digestive tract is chock full of so many species of microorganisms. By focusing on just this one microorganism, many health professionals are missing the bigger picture: The balance between the hundreds of different species living in our digestive tracts.

As we'll discuss further, the western diet discourages probiotic colonization in the digestive tract. In a healthy digestive tract—as exhibited among third world countries—legions of probiotic cultures keep *H. pylori* populations—and many other microorganisms—in check. *H. pylori* may populate, but they are controlled by beneficial species of probiotics.

This realization is now becoming obvious by a few astute scientists: *"This bacterium has been the dominant organism in our stomach for tens of thousands of years, and it can't disappear from us without consequences,"* said New York University School of Medicine's Dr. Blaser, the leading researcher of the NHANES 2008 study. *"This is probably the first time in human history that we have children who are growing up without Helicobacter guiding their immune responses. By the repeated courses of antibiotics given to children, we are changing human microecology and we don't know what we are doing."*

Anti-Allergic Probiotic Strategies

The key to the equation is our probiotic colonies. Let's jump to the practical side, and discuss methods to increase our probiotic populations:

Fermented Foods

Probiotics supplemented by eating fermented foods or supplements give us temporary residents. They will typically endure for a couple of weeks before they leave. However, this period allows them to provide numerous benefits. They also help set up an environment conducive to the regrowth of our resident populations. We can also keep replenishing their populations through regular eating of fermented foods, as our ancestors have done for thousands of years.

Illustrating the ability of probiotic foods to reduce hyperreactivity, researchers from the Department of Food Science and Human Nutrition at the University of Illinois (Frias *et al.* 2008) studied the hypersensitivity response (or, as the researchers termed it, *"immunoreactivity"*) of soybeans in the cracked bean form and in the flour state before and after fermentation with probiotics. They fermented some of the cracked beans and flour with *Aspergillus oryzae*, *Rhizopus oryzae*, *Lactobacillus plantarum*, and *Bacillus subtilis*. These culturing bacteria are commonly used to make various probiotic fermented foods such as tempeh and sauerkraut.

The researchers used ELISA tests and the Western blot test to quantify IgE immunoglobulin response within human plasma. They found that the fermented soy dramatically decreased reactivity to the soybeans and flours. Soy flour fermented with *L. plantarum* exhibited the highest reduction, with 96-99% less immunoreactivity. *R. oryzae* and *A. oryzae* reduced immunoreactivity by 66% and 68% respectively. *B. subtilis* resulted in 81% to 86% reductions in immunoreactivity.

In addition to these results, a positive side effect of the fermentation was the improvement of the protein quality of the soy products. After fermentation with *R. oryzae*, for example, levels of the amino acids alanine and threonine were increased, making the soy products more nutritious.

This and other research illustrates what healthy colonies of probiotics can do to lower the body's hypersensitivity response. This keeps us healthy, which also keeps them healthy.

Traditional yogurt is produced using *L. bulgaricus* and *S. thermophilus*. Commercial preparations sometimes include *L. acidophilus* in addition, but the use of *L. acidophilus* in the starter will rarely result in the final product containing *L. acidophilus*. This is because *L. bulgaricus* is a hardy organism, and it will easily overtake *L. acidophilus* within a culture. Note also that commercial yogurt preparations pasteurized after culturing will contain few or no living probiotics in the final product. Some manufacturers culture the milk after pasteurization. This can result in a healthy probiotic culture.

Here are a few other fermented foods/beverages available:
- Kefir
- Kimchi
- Miso
- Shoyu
- Tempeh
- Lassi
- Sauerkraut
- Raw milk
- Kombucha

Assuming they are traditionally cultured and not pasteurized after culturing, each of these will provide healthy probiotics. More information on these probiotic foods may be found in the author's book, *Probiotics— Protection Against Infection.*

Many health experts agree that commercial milks, cheeses and butters are not suggested for those with hypersensitivity. However, milk can be considered when it is either cultured with probiotics (such as yogurt and kefir), or consumed in a naturally raw state. Raw, probiotic-rich milk contains a host of vitamins, proteins, nucleotides, minerals, probiotics, immunoglobulins and healthy fatty acids. Raw milk also helps support the intestinal barrier.

Raw whole milk can be a substantial food for children, and pregnant or lactating mothers, assuming:

> ➤ The cows have been primarily grass-fed. When cows eat grass, they have stronger immune systems, stronger probiotic colonies, and milk that is more nutritious.

> ➤ The cows receive no synthetic or genetically modified growth hormones. Growth hormones injected into cows have been shown to produce higher levels of IGF-1 in the milk and human body after drinking milk from growth hormones-injected cows. The American Public Health Association stated the following in a 2009 Policy Release after a review of the research: *"Elevated IGF-1 levels in human blood are associated with higher rates of colon, breast, and prostate cancers."* Growth hormones also speed puberty, as evidenced by research from the University of Cincinnati's College of Medicine (Biro *et al.* 2010) that examined 1,239 girls from 6-8 years old. They found that girls in this age group are reaching puberty at double the rate they did just ten years ago.

> ➤ The cows receive little or no antibiotics. These antibiotics will travel through the milk into the body. Here they can weaken our immune systems and set up a greater susceptibility of antibiotic-resistant microorganisms.

> ➤ The milk (from grass-fed cows) is not pasteurized. Pasteurization kills all the beneficial microorganisms cows provide that promote healthy probiotics in our bodies.

> ➤ The dairy is certified by the state and is regularly tested for microorganisms.

Note that lactose-intolerant persons should do fine with fresh raw milk from an organic dairy. Many raw milk drinkers are lactose-intolerant.

How does this work? The probiotics in the cow have large colonies of lactobacilli. These species derive energy from breaking down lactose, and they produce lactase.

Probiotic Supplementation Strategies

After reviewing hundreds of human clinical studies—some quoted in this book and many more discussed and referenced in the author's two books about probiotics: *Probiotics—Protection Against Infection* and *Oral Probiotics*—below are the probiotic species shown in research to have the most usefulness in reducing systemic inflammation and allergic hyperreactivity. Please refer to these books for scientific references and a thorough description of each:

Intestinal Probiotics
Lactobacillus acidophilus
Lactobacillus helveticus
Lactobacillus casei
Lactobacillus rhamnosus
Lactobacillus reuteri
Lactobacillus bulgaricus
Bifidobacterium bifidum
Bifidobacterium infantis
Bifidobacterium longum
Bifidobacterium animalis/B. lactis
Bifidobacterium breve
Streptococcus thermophilus
Saccharomyces boulardii

Oral Probiotics (nasal, sinus, oral, airways)
Lactobacillus salivarius
Lactobacillus rhamnosus
Lactobacillus plantarum
Lactobacillus reuteri
Streptococcus salivarius

Supplement Format

The main consideration in probiotic supplementation is consuming *live* organisms. These are typically described as "CFU," which stands for *colony forming units*. In other words, live probiotics will produce new colonies once inside the intestines. Heat-killed ones are not as beneficial, although they can also stimulate the immune system. So the key is keeping the probiotics alive while in the capsule and supplement bottle, until we are ready to consume them. Here are a few considerations about probiotic supplements:

Capsules: Vegetable capsules contain less moisture than gelatin or enteric-coated capsules. Even a little moisture in the capsule can increase the possibility of waking up the probiotics while in the bottle. Once woken up, they can starve and die. Enteric coating can minimally protect the probiotics within the stomach, assuming they have survived in the bottle. Some manufactures use oils to help protect the probiotics in the stomach. In all cases, encapsulated freeze-dried probiotics should be refrigerated (no matter what the label says) at all times during shipping, at the store, and at home. Dark containers also better protect the probiotics from light exposure, which can kill them.

Powders of freeze-dried probiotics are subject to deterioration due to increased exposure to oxygen and light. Powders should be refrigerated in dark containers and sealed tightly to be kept viable. They should also be consumed with liquids or food, preferably dairy or fermented dairy. Powders can also be used as starters for homemade yogurt and kefir.

Caplets/Tablets: Some tablet/caplets have special coatings that provide viability through to the intestines without refrigeration. If not, those tablets would likely be in the same category as encapsulated products, requiring refrigeration.

Shells/Beads: These can provide longer shelf viability without refrigeration and better survive the stomach. However, because of the size of the shell, these typically come with less CFU quantity, increasing the cost per therapeutic dose. Another drawback may be that the intestines must dissolve this thick shell. An easy test is to check our stool to be sure that the beads or shells aren't coming out the other end whole.

Lozenges: These are the best way to supplement oral probiotics. A correctly formulated chewable or lozenge can inoculate the mouth, nose and throat with beneficial bacteria to compete with and fight off pathogenic bacteria as they enter or reside in our mouth, nose, throat and airways of the lungs.

We listed on the previous page those probiotics that thrive among healthy mucous membranes of the airways, sinuses and oral cavity. As we discussed in the research, several of these, notably *L. reuteri*, have been shown to increase airway health and decrease lung infections.

However, most of the probiotics in a lozenge will not likely survive the stomach acids and penetrate the intestines. So lozenges are best utilized for the oral region and airways rather than for intestinal probiotic supplementation.

The research illustrates that lozenges provide an excellent way to help prevent new infections and sore throats during increased exposures. The lozenge or chewable format allows the probiotics to colonize around our gums and throat. From there they can easily translocate to the nasal cavities and airways to arm our mucosal membranes.

Liquid Supplements: There are several probiotic supplements in small liquid form. One brand has a long tradition and a hardy, well-researched strain. A liquid probiotic should be in a light-sealed, refrigerated container. It should also contain some dairy or other probiotic-friendly substrate, giving the probiotics some food while awaiting delivery to the intestines.

Probiotic Hydrotherapy: This method of supplementation is a great way to implant live colonies of probiotics into the lower colon. Colon hydrotherapy (or colonic) is one of the healthiest things we can do for preventative and therapeutic health in general. Colon hydrotherapy is performed by a certified colon hydrotherapist who uses specialized (and sanitary) equipment to flush out the colon with water. This colon flushing usually takes about 30 minutes. Once the process is complete, the hydrotherapist can "insert" a blend of probiotics into the tube and "pump" the probiotics directly into our colon. Colon hydrotherapy is a wonderful treatment recommended for most anyone, especially those with disorders related to systemic inflammation and allergic hypersensitivity.

Colonic treatments are relatively inexpensive when compared to their benefit. Two to three colonics a year are often recommended for ultimate colon health. Those with sensitive or irritable bowels should consult with their health professional before submitting to a colonic, however.

Probiotic Dosage: A good dosage for taking oral intestinal probiotics for prevention and maintenance can be ten to fifteen billion CFU (*colony forming units*) per day. Total intake during an illness or therapeutic period, however, will often double or triple that dosage. Much of the research shown in this text utilized 20 billion to 40 billion CFU per day, about a third of that dose for children and a quarter of that dose for infants. (*B. infantis* is often the supplement of choice for babies at far smaller doses.)

Supplemental oral probiotic dosages can be far less (100 million to two billion), especially when the formula contains the hardy *L. reuteri*.

People who must take antibiotics for life-threatening reasons can alternate doses of probiotics between their antibiotic dosing. The probiotic dose can be at least two hours before or after the antibiotic dose. (Always consult with the prescribing doctor.)

Remember that these dosages depend upon delivery to the intestines. Therefore, a product that passes into the stomach with little protection would likely not deliver many colonies to the intestines. Such a supplement would likely require higher dosage to achieve the desired effects.

Increased Intestinal Permeability

This discussion of probiotics and allergies opens up what many consider the unthinkable: Allergies are associated with the health of the intestines and most notably, the barrier that separates the contents of the intestines from the bloodstream.

Let's examine the science closely.

The consensus of the research is that the gastrointestinal tract, from the mouth to the anus, is the primary defense mechanism against antigens as they enter the body. The mucous membrane integrity, the probiotic system, digestive enzymes, and the various immune cells and their mediators work together to orchestrate a "total blockade" structure using the mucosal membranes. However, should these barriers be weakened or become imbalanced, hypersensitivity can result due to increased exposure of the epithelial layers.

When it comes to the intestinal barrier, weaknesses can be influenced by a number of factors, including toxins, diet, and other environmental factors (Chahine and Bahna 2010).

In other words, poor dietary choices, toxin exposures and environmental forces related to lifestyle and living conditions can damage the integrity of mucosal membranes—not just in the esophagus, airways and stomach: A weakened intestinal mucosal membrane exposes intestinal cells to digestive acids, undigested foods, microorganisms, undigested food macromolecules, and toxins.

These contribute to overloading the immune system, producing systemic inflammation and hypersensitivity.

As discussed in Chapter Two, the intestines also have a microscopic barrier structure. The tiny spaces between the intestinal epithelial cells—composed of villi and microvilli—are sealed from the general intestinal contents with what are called tight junctions. Should the tight junctions become irritated by acids, toxins or pathogens (such as microorganisms) they will open up: Their barrier or seal will be broken.

When tight junctions are unnaturally open, the wrong molecules can cross the epithelium through a transcellular pathway. Researchers have found more than 50-odd protein species among the tight junction. Should any of these proteins fail due to exposure to toxins in the form of radicals, the barrier can break down, allowing intestinal contents access to the bloodstream. Once these intestinal macromolecules access the body's internal tissues and fluids, they can stimulate a hyper-immune response: a systemic inflammatory response (Yu 2009).

As we'll find, many researchers are seeing the connection between intestinal permeability and allergic conditions. For example, Louisiana State University researchers (Chahine and Bahna 2010) found that the intestinal wall uses specific immunologic factors to defend the body against antigens. Their research showed that a defective lining leads to allergic responses and hypersensitivity reactions. They named the cause of these inflammatory responses *"defects in the gut barrier."*

The Intestinal Permeability Index

How do scientists and physicians test for increased intestinal permeability? Intestinal permeability is typically measured by giving the patient indigestible substances with different molecular sizes. Urine samples then show relative levels of these, illustrating degrees of intestinal permeability. For example, alcohol-sugar combinations such as lactulose and mannitol are often used. These indicate intestinal permeability because of their different molecular sizes. A few (typically 5-6) hours after ingestion, the patient's urine is tested to measure the quantities of these two molecules in the urine.

Because lactulose is a larger molecule than mannitol, greater permeability will be indicated by high lactulose levels in the urine relative to mannitol levels. Intestines with normal permeability will have little lactulose absorption.

These relative levels create a ratio between lactulose and mannitol, which scientists call the L/M ratio. This L/M ratio is used to quantify intestinal permeability. When the lactulose-to-mannitol ratio is higher, more permeability exists. When it is lower, less (more normal) intestinal permeability exists. Higher levels are compared using what many researchers call the *Intestinal Permeability Index.*

Other large molecule substances are also sometimes used to detect intestinal permeability using the same protocol of measuring recovery in the urine over a period of time. These other substances include polyethylene glycols of various molecular weights, horseradish peroxidase, EDTA (ethylenediaminetetraacetic acid), CrEDTA, rhamnose, lactulose, and cellobiose. Because these substances are not readily metabolized in the intestine or blood, and have large molecular sizes, they can also give accurate readings on the relative intestinal permeability. Let's see how researchers have used the Intestinal Permeability Index to discover how allergic rhinitis and other allergies are linked to intestinal permeability:

Medical researchers from Kuwait University (Hijazi *et al.* 2004) studied 32 asthmatic children together with 32 matched healthy children. They conducted a lactulose/mannitol test to determine intestinal permeability among both groups. They found that the asthmatic group exhibited more than three times the levels of intestinal permeability than did the control group. They also eliminated other possible relationships, such as eczema and inhaled steroid use.

179

Researchers from Sweden's University Hospital in Uppsala (Knutson *et al.* 1996) studied 12 patients with allergic asthma who were sensitive to birch pollen—along with 12 healthy controls. They found that exposure to the birch pollen allergen increased the intestinal permeability of the allergic group, but not the healthy group. They concluded: *"This would suggest less organ specificity and more general allergic recognition shared by several immunocompetent tissues in the body, probably mediated by circulating IgE antibodies."*

Intestinal Permeability and Childhood Allergies

As we discussed previously, research has confirmed that many children develop allergic rhinitis a few years after having milk allergies as younger children. Early food allergies, as we've discussed, are also associated with allergic rhinitis later on. The research confirms intestinal permeability and milk allergies.

Researchers from the Department of Pediatrics of the Cochin St Vincent de Paul Hospital in Paris (Kalach *et al.* 2001) studied intestinal permeability and cow's milk allergy among children as they aged. The research included 200 children who exhibited symptoms of cow's milk allergies. Of this 200, 95 were determined as allergic using challenge testing. This left 105 children as control subjects. The researchers measured intestinal permeability using the L/M ratio. They found that the L/M ratio was significantly greater among the milk-allergic children. Abnormal intestinal permeability levels were present among 80% of the milk-allergic children who had digestive symptoms, and 40% of children who exhibited anaphylactic symptoms. Furthermore, L/M ratios improved among older children who became more tolerant to milk.

Medical researchers from Italy's University of Naples (Troncone *et al.* 1994) tested intestinal permeability among 32 children aged from three months old to 84 months old. They utilized a ratio related to L/M called the cellobiose/mannitol (C/M) ratio. Of those who had allergy symptoms after a challenge with milk, 90% had significantly increased C/M ratios, indicating increased intestinal permeability.

Researchers from France's St. Vincent de Paul Hospital (Dupont *et al.* 1989) measured intestinal permeability using mannitol and lactulose among 12 milk-allergic children; 28 children with atopic dermatitis; and 39 healthy children. L/M ratios indicated that intestinal permeability in the milk-allergic group was three times higher than the healthy group when they drank milk.

Another study from the Paris' Cochin St Vincent de Paul Hospital (Kalach *et al.* 2001) studied 64 children with milk allergy symptoms, and found that higher intestinal permeability levels were also associated with anemia.

French INSERM researchers from the Hospital Saint-Lazare (Heyman *et al.* 1988) studied intestinal permeability with milk allergy among infants. They tested 33 children ages one month to 24 months, which included 18 healthy infants and 15 with milk allergies, using the protein marker horseradish peroxidase together with jejunal biopsies. No absorption permeability was seen in the control children over two months of age, illustrating that *"gut closure probably occurred earlier in life."* However, milk allergy children had about eight times the permeability levels than the healthy children.

The diet of the mother is an important issue, as we've discussed. French doctors (de Boissieu *et al.* 1994) reported a one-month-old breast-fed boy who had regurgitation, diarrhea, feeding difficulties, and malaise—typical of breast milk sensitivities. They conducted intestinal permeability tests on the mother and her baby. The physicians concluded that the mother's breast milk had induced intestinal permeability in the baby.

The child's symptoms continued without improvement after the mother eliminated dairy products from her own diet. Then the mother withdrew egg and pork from her diet. The withdrawal of egg and pork resulted in an almost immediate disappearance of allergy symptoms in the child.

The doctors tested the child again for intestinal permeability after provocation with mother's milk (the same test done previously). Intestinal permeability levels were now normal in the child. The doctors concluded that sensitivities can be transferred from mother to baby through breast milk.

Increased Intestinal Permeability and Systemic Inflammation

Once permeability is increased in the intestinal tract, it is likely that the immune system is greatly burdened by the many strange and different molecular structures now gaining entry into internal tissues and bloodstream. What is known is that once permeability is increased, a self-perpetuating cycle of increased permeability and immune hypersensitivity produces more intestinal dysfunction and inflammation (Heyman 2005).

Researchers from Ontario's McMaster University (Berin *et al.* 1999) studied the role of cytokines in intestinal permeability. They found that interleukin-4 (IL-4) increased intestinal permeability and increased horseradish peroxidase (HRP) transport through intestinal walls. They found that IL-4 was inhibited by the soy nutrient genistein, and anti-IL-4 antibodies also reduced the HRP transport. The researchers concluded that: *"We speculate that enhanced production of IL-4 in allergic conditions may be a predisposing factor to inflammation by allowing uptake of luminal antigens that gain access to the mucosal immune system."*

181

Research has indicated that CD23 encourages the transport of intestinal IgE and allergens across intestinal epithelium. This opens a gateway for antigen-bound IgE to move across (transcytose) the intestinal cells. This sets up the immune response of histamine and inflammatory conditions related to intestinal permeability (Yu 2009).

Researchers from the University of Cincinnati College of Medicine (Groschwitz *et al.* 2009) determined that mast cells are critical to the regulation of the intestinal barrier function. The type and condition of the mast cells seems to affect the epithelial migration through intestinal cells.

Researchers from the Cincinnati Children's Hospital Medical Center (Forbes *et al.* 2008) found that interleukin-9 appears to help stimulate, along with mast cells, increased intestinal permeability. The researchers found that this *"IL-9- and mast cell-mediated intestinal permeability"* activated conditions for hypersensitivity.

French INSERM researchers (Desjeux and Heyman 1994) concluded that increased protein permeability in milk allergies follows what they called *abnormal immunological response.* This abnormal immune response, they observed, leads to general mucosal and systemic inflammation.

What Causes Increased Intestinal Permeability?

The causative forces of increased permeability are not very different from the other associations with allergies: an overload of toxins, pharmaceuticals, probiotic deficiencies, nutrient deficiencies, breast milk deficiencies, metabolic stress and others have been identified as potential causes of increased intestinal permeability.

For example, the Desjeux and Heyman INSERM research mentioned above based their conclusions on the observation that the pro-inflammatory protein beta-lactoglobulin stimulated lymphocytes that released increased levels of cytokines tumor necrosis factor-alpha (TNF alpha) and gamma interferon. The cytokines stimulated an inflammatory response that in turn disturbed the intestinal cell wall barrier.

In other words, radical formation from toxins, unhealthy foods or other stressors disrupts the intestinal mucous membrane. This irritates the intestinal barrier, producing inflammation within the intestinal wall. This in turn opens gaps in the intestinal barrier.

Medical researchers from the University Hospital in Groningen, The Netherlands (van Elburg *et al.* 1992) point out that the intestinal immunity mechanisms, which include IgA immunoglobulin and cell-mediated immune factors—and the brush barrier in general—do not completely mature until after about two years of age. Until this time, the barrier is extra sensitive to toxins and/or poor dietary choices.

Researchers from the Medical University of South Carolina (Walle and Walle 1999) found that mutagens formed when frying meat are implicated in producing intestinal permeability. These mutagens, such as phenylimidazo-pyridine, were studied for their possible transport across human Caco-2 intestinal cells. The absorption was characterized as *"extensive and linear."*

Equilibrium exchange tests showed that the mutagens form substrates with intestinal transporters. This indicates the connection between diet and allergies—specifically heavy red meat diets.

Medical researchers from Finland's University of Helsinki (Kuitunen *et al.* 1994) studied permeability using beta-lactoglobulin with 20 infants through eight months old. One week after they weaned from breast milk, bovine beta-lactoglobulin levels were found in the bloodstream among 38% of the infants. After two weeks, 21% retained beta-lactoglobulin in the bloodstream.

Research from Germany's Otto-von-Guericke University (Schönfeld 2004) found that dietary phytanic acid increases intestinal permeability through a function of ionic exchange and disruption of mitochondrial membranes. Damage to mitochondria may also explain the production of the inflammatory cytokine IL-4 within intestinal cells. We'll discuss the sources of phytanic acid later.

After extensive research, medical scientists from the Department of Internal Medicine at France's University Hospital (Moneret-Vautrin and Morisset 2005) found that the risk factors for severe anaphylaxis include agents that produce increased intestinal permeability—which include alcohol, aspirin, beta-blockers and angiotensin-converting enzyme (ACE) inhibitors.

Researchers from Rush University's Division of Gastroenterology and Nutrition and the Rush-Presbyterian-St. Luke's Medical Center in Chicago (DeMeo *et al.* 2002) has proposed that the gastrointestinal tract maintains one of the body's biggest areas offering exposure to the outside environment. This is because everything we eat ends up facing the intestinal walls.

The Rush University researchers illustrated in their research that disruptions to the gut barrier follow inputs including nonsteroidal anti-inflammatory drugs, free radical peroxidation, adenosine triphosphate depletion (metabolic stress) and damage to the epithelial cell cytoskeletons that regulate tight junctions. They also pointed out evidence that associates gut barrier damage to immune dysfunction and sepsis—infection from microorganisms. This of course also alludes to the defenses provided by our probiotic microorganisms, which keep populations of infective microorganisms minimized—as we discussed in the probiotic section.

Medical researchers from the University of Southampton School of Medicine (Macdonald and Monteleone 2005) have suggested that this epidemic of intestinal permeability among industrialized nations has been creating genetic mutations that produce greater levels of permeability among successive generations. This of course provides the link between greater susceptibility for asthma and allergies among those with parents having these conditions.

Thus, we can conclude that intestinal permeability is not simply a creative explanation for allergic hypersensitivities made without substantiation. It is a scientifically proven fact.

Probiotics and Intestinal Permeability

Our probiotics line the mucosal membranes that line our digestive tract. Here they police the intestinal cells and excrete acids that help manage the pH of the mucosal membrane. Should probiotic colonies be damaged by toxins, infection, antibiotics or poor dietary choices, their symbiotic relationship with our intestines can come to an end or become severely limited. This effectively alters the mucosal membrane and leaves the intestinal cells more exposed to food particles and toxins.

Should our probiotic colonies become scarce and our mucosal membranes are altered, larger peptides, toxins and even invading microorganisms are allowed to have contact with the cells of the intestines. This irritates the intestinal cells, producing an inflammatory immune response. This inflammatory immune response in turn hurts the ability of the intestinal brush barrier to keep larger food proteins and toxins from invading our tissues and bloodstream.

As we described in Chapter Two, the intestinal brush barrier includes the mucosal layer of enzymes, probiotics and ionic fluid. This forms a protective surface medium over the intestinal epithelium. It also provides an active nutrient transport mechanism. It contains glycoproteins and other ionic transporters, which attach to nutrient molecules, carrying them across intestinal membranes. However, this mucosal membrane is supported and stabilized by the grooves between the intestinal microvilli. Should the probiotics become damaged, the entire mucosal brush barrier begins to break down—allowing toxins access to our tissues and bloodstream.

The health of our probiotics and the health of the brush barrier can be threatened by similar factors. Alcohol is one of the most irritating substances to our probiotics and the mucosal brush barrier in general (Bongaerts and Severijnen 2005).

Research has also revealed a link between intestinal permeability and liver damage (Bode and Bode 2003). Alcohol consumption has also been associated with intestinal permeability (Ferrier *et al.* 2006).

In addition, many pharmaceutical drugs, notably NSAIDs, have been identified as damaging to probiotics and the mucosal brush barrier integrity. Foods with high arachidonic fatty acid content (such red meats); low-fiber, high-glucose foods; and high nitrite-forming foods have been shown to inhibit probiotic growth. Toxic substances such as plasticizers, pesticides, herbicides, chlorinated water and food dyes are also implicated in the loss of probiotics. Chemicals that increase PGE-2 response also negatively affect permeability (Martin-Venegas *et al.* 2006).

In addition, the overuse of antibiotics can cause a die-off of our resident probiotic colonies. When intestinal probiotic colonies are reduced, pathogenic bacteria and yeasts can outgrow the remaining probiotic colonies. Pathogenic bacteria growth invades the brush barrier, introducing an influx of endotoxins (the waste matter of these microorganisms) into the bloodstream, together with some of the microorganisms themselves.

Inflammatory responses resulting from increased intestinal permeability have now been linked to sinusitis, allergies, psoriasis, asthma, arthritis and other inflammatory conditions.

Let's look at some of the research directly linking intestinal permeability to the health of our probiotics:

Researchers from Greece's Alexandra Regional General Hospital (Stratiki *et al.* 2007) gave 41 preterm infants of 27-36 weeks gestation a formula supplemented with *Bifidobacterium lactis* or a placebo. After seven days, bifidobacteria counts were significantly higher and head growth was greater. After 30 days, the lactulose/mannitol ratio (marker for intestinal permeability) was significantly lower in the probiotic group as compared to the placebo group. The researchers concluded that, *"bifidobacteria supplemented infant formula decreases intestinal permeability of preterm infants and leads to increased head growth."*

German scientists (Rosenfeldt *et al.* 2004) gave *Lactobacillus rhamnosus* 19070-2 and *L. reuteri* DSM 12246 or a placebo to 41 children. After six weeks of treatment, the frequency of GI symptoms were significantly lower (10% versus 39%) among the probiotic group as compared to the placebo group. In addition, the lactulose-to-mannitol ratio was lower in the probiotic group, indicating to the researchers that, *"probiotic supplementation may stabilize the intestinal barrier function and decrease gastrointestinal symptoms in children with atopic dermatitis."*

Researchers from the People's Hospital and the Jiao Tong University in Shangha (Qin *et al.* 2008) gave *Lactobacillus plantarum* or placebo to 76 patients with acute pancreatitis. Intestinal permeability was determined using the lactulose/rhamnose ratio. Organ failure, septic complications and death were also monitored. After seven days of treatment, microbial infections averaged 38.9% in the probiotic group and 73.7% in the placebo group. Furthermore, only 30.6% of the probiotic group colonized potentially pathogenic organisms, as compared to 50% of patients in the control group. The probiotic group also had significantly better clinical outcomes compared to the control group. The researchers concluded that: *"Lactobacillus plantarum can attenuate disease severity, improve the intestinal permeability and clinical outcomes."*

The microbiology researchers from the Radboud University Nijmegen Medical Centre in The Netherlands (Bongaerts and Severijnen 2005) concluded their research on the link between intestinal permeability and allergies with the following statement:

> *"Adequate probiotics can (i) prevent the increased characteristic intestinal permeability of children with atopic eczema and food allergy, (ii) can thus prevent the uptake of allergens, and (iii) finally can prevent the expression of the atopic constitution. The use of adequate probiotic lactobacilli, i.e., homolactic and/ or facultatively heterolactic l-lactic acid-producing lactobacilli, reduces the intestinal amounts of the bacterial, toxic metabolites, d-lactic acid and ethanol by fermentative production of merely the non-toxic l-lactic acid from glucose. Thus, it is thought that beneficial probiotic microorganisms promote gut barrier function and both undo and prevent unfavorable intestinal micro-ecological alterations in allergic individuals."*

Other Factors that Contribute to Allergies

Breastfeeding

Research is increasingly illustrating that breastfeeding is critical to the strength of baby's immune system. This of course directly relates to the risk of allergies and asthma. A wealth of breastfeeding research has found that babies breastfed from healthy mothers have a lower incidence of many diseases, higher rates of growth, and stronger immune systems. Breast milk contains a healthy blend of proteins, fatty acids, vitamins, nucleotides and colostrum—an immunity boosting substance made up of immunoglobulins and probiotics. Breast milk also contains the prebiotics galactooligosaccharides (scGOS) and fructooligosaccharides (FOS).

Researchers from the University of Puerto Rico School of Medicine (González *et al.* 2010) studied 175 children and their mothers. Exclusive breastfeeding resulted in significantly lower rates of allergies among the children.

Researchers from University of Cincinnati's Department of Internal Medicine (Codispoti *et al.* 2010) studied 361 children, 116 with allergic rhinitis. They found that longer breastfeeding among African American children decreased the rates of allergies by 20%. They also found that children with multiple siblings in the home had a 60% reduced incidence of allergies.

Breast milk is critical because newborns have under-developed mucosal membranes and their immune systems are still developing. For this reason, it is a sensitive time for the mucosal membrane-lined airways. Breast milk has been shown to stimulate greater levels of IgA within the mucosal membranes (Brandtzaeg 2010).

Illustrating the effect of a lack of breastfeeding on mucosal membrane health, researchers from Italy's Siena University (Garzi et al. 2002) found that infants given formula instead of breast milk had significantly greater incidence of gastroesophageal reflux (GERD) and milk allergies.

Scientists from the Center for Infant Nutrition at the University of Milan (Arslanoglu et al. 2008) found that the galactooligosaccharides (GOS) and fructooligosaccharides (FOS) (present in healthy breast milk) can reduce the incidence of atopic dermatitis (AD) and various infections through six months of age. A group of 134 non-breastfed infants was given either a prebiotic-supplemented formula or formula without prebiotics. Follow-ups continued until age two. Rates of asthma, atopic dermatitis and allergic urticaria were significantly higher among the infants given the placebo formula.

The bottom line: Exclusive breastfeeding through about the first four months reduces the risk of allergies, because our immune systems become better prepared to tolerate allergens and fight off toxins.

C-Sections

According to recent information published by the National Center for Health Statistics, almost a third of all births in the United States are by Cesarean section. Cesarean sections have increased by some 50% in the United States between 1996 and 2008—from a little over 20% to 32%. While many believe that C-section bears little risk to the child, this is contradicted by the research.

In fact, C-section directly increases the risk of allergic hypersensitivity. Researchers from The Netherlands' National Institute for Public Health and the Environment (Roduit et al. 2009) studied the allergic status of 2,917 children with respect to whether they were born with a Cesarean section. They tested 1,454 of the children for IgE antibodies for inhalants and food allergens at age eight. They found conclusively that babies born with Cesarean section had significantly greater incidence of allergies.

C-sections also produce more milk allergies among children. Researchers from Finland's National Institute for Health and Welfare (Metsälä et al. 2010) studied all children born in Finland between 1996 and 2004 that were diagnosed with cow's milk allergies. In all, 16,237 allergic children were found. Children born by Cesarean section had 18% greater incidence of milk allergies.

C-sections produce more allergies of other types among children. Researchers from Germany's National Research Centre for Environment and Health and the Institute of Epidemiology (Laubereau *et al.* 2004) studied 865 healthy infants with allergic parents. They tested the babies at one, four, eight and twelve months old. They found that babies (147) born with Cesarean section had over double the incidence of allergic sensitivities than their peers (also with allergic parents) without C-section birth.

The mechanism relates to the fact that the vagina is colonized with billions of probiotic bacteria that inoculate baby with natural probiotics—an integral aspect of the immune system. The C-section deprives the child of these important probiotics during a critical moment of life.

Cesarean sections are often the result of induced birthing. Doctors now induce childbirth more often, and routinely. Induction leads to a greater risk of Cesarean sections. C-sections also increase the likelihood of the mother requiring pain medication during childbirth (Caughey *et al.* 2006), which can decrease important mucous secretions.

Dehydration

The fact that dehydration (lack of sufficient fluid intake) can contribute to allergies and hay fever has been confirmed by research. For example, after a significant review of multiple studies, the conclusion of scientists from Germany's Research Institute of Child Nutrition (Manz 2007) concluded that asthma and allergies are associated with dehydration.

The mucosal membranes of the airways and nasal cavities are made primarily of water. In a dehydrated state, our mucosal membranes thin and change pH. It is for these reasons that other research has found that many ulcerated conditions can be cured simply by drinking adequate water (Batmanghelidj 1997).

Water is directly involved in inflammatory metabolism. Research has revealed that increased levels of inflammatory mediators such as histamine are released during periods of dehydration in order to help balance fluid levels within the bloodstream, tissues, kidneys and other organs.

Our airways need to stay moist. Inadequate water intake will dehydrate the airways. This produces irritation and hypersensitivity. Research by Dr. Batmanghelidj (1987; 1990) led to the realization that the blood becomes more concentrated during dehydration. As this concentrated blood enters the capillaries of the respiratory system, histamine is released in an attempt to balance the blood dilution levels. This stimulates a tightening of the smooth muscles, causing constricted airways.

The immune system is also irrevocably aligned with the body's water availability. The immune system utilizes water to produce lymph fluid. Lymph fluid circulates immune cells throughout the body, enabling them to find intruders among the tissues. The lymph is also used to escort toxins out of the body.

Intracellular and intercellular fluids are necessary for the removal of nearly all toxins—and pretty much every metabolic function of every cell, every organ and every tissue system.

Water also increases the availability of oxygen to cells. Water balances the level of free radicals. Water flushes and replenishes the digestive tract. Thus, water is necessary for the proper digestion of food, as well as nutrition utilization. The gastric cells of the stomach and the intestinal wall cells require water for proper digestive function. The health of every cell depends upon water.

There is certainly good science supporting dehydration as a contributing cause for allergic hypersensitivity. Drinking ½ ounce of water per day for every pound of body weight is a good rule of thumb.

Sun Exposure/Vitamin D

Multiple studies have found that allergies and asthma are significantly greater among regions further from the equator and those with less sunlight exposure. In both Europe and the U.S.—with the exception of urban areas with greater air pollution—those living in Southern regions have shown significantly lower incidence of asthma and allergies along with fewer hospital visits.

Researchers from National Jewish Health (Searing and Leung 2010) reviewed the role of vitamin D with allergies. They found that there was significant evidence that vitamin D played an important role in allergies, and its deficiency is associated with greater incidence of allergic reactions.

Remember that the sun is our best source for vitamin D. Researchers from the Massachusetts General Hospital in Cambridge (Camargo *et al.* 2011) tested the cord blood of 922 newborn babies for vitamin D levels. They found that infants who developed a history of wheezing at 15 months and a diagnosis of asthma by five years old were more likely to have suffered deficiencies in vitamin D. Incidence also increased with lower vitamin D levels.

Researchers from the Children's Hospital Boston (Rudders *et al.* 2010) studied anaphylaxis emergency room visits throughout the United States. They found that those living in Southern regions had significantly lower incidence of anaphylaxis and far fewer hospital visits. The Northeast region had 5.5 visits per thousand, while the South had 4.9 visits per thousand. The researchers concluded that: *"These observational data are consistent with the hypothesis that vitamin D may play an etiologic role in anaphylaxis."*

Food allergies also appear to be related to the sun. In a study from Australia's Monash Medical School (Woods *et al.* 2001) food allergy rates were higher among Northern European countries than among Southern European countries.

Researchers from Finland's University of Helsinki (Erkkola *et al.* 2009) studied the relationship between supplemental vitamin D during pregnancy and the occurrence of asthma and allergic rhinitis in the child. Their study followed 1,669 mothers and children for five years.

They determined that the average vitamin D intake of the whole group was 5.1 micrograms from food and 1.4 micrograms from supplements. They found that increased vitamin D intake from foods significantly reduced the incidence of allergic rhinitis among the children.

Researchers have found that vitamin D levels are generally lower amongst minorities. This relates to the fact that darker skin pigmentation contains more melanin. Because melanin blocks UV from the sun, higher skin melanin levels require more sun for vitamin D production than lighter skin colors.

Vitamin D induces cathelicidin production (Grant 2008). Cathelicidins are proteins found within the lysosomes of macrophages and polymorphonuclear cells (PMNs). These immune cells are intensely antiviral and antibacterial in nature. They are also stimulated and regulated by vitamin D within the body.

Illustrating the effects of ultraviolet radiation on the health of the sinuses, a new treatment has emerged called *intranasal phototherapy*. This has been used effectively as a treatment for allergic rhinitis. The therapy irradiates nasal and sinus tissues with a low-dose combination of UVA and UVB light.

In a study from Hungary's University of Szeged (Garaczi *et al.* 2011), intranasal phototherapy or the medication fexofenadine HCl was given to 31 patients with seasonal allergic rhinitis for two weeks. The intranasal phototherapy group was given three treatments per week. At the end of the two weeks, the intranasal phototherapy group had significantly fewer symptoms, including less nasal obstruction, less nasal and palate itching and fewer other rhinitis symptoms. The fexofenadine group showed no significant change in comparison.

In another study on phototherapy, this one conducted by researchers from the UK's University of Worcester (Emberlin and Lewis 2009), 101 hay fever sufferers were given either intranasal phototherapy or a placebo treatment three times a day for two weeks. Just as in the Hungary research, after the two weeks, the phototherapy group had a significant reduction in hay fever symptoms. Symptom scores for sneezing, runny nose, watery eyes and itchy mouth were all significantly lower among the phototherapy group.

190

It is not difficult to extrapolate from this research that sunshine helps prevent allergies. This conclusion is also confirmed by research we discussed earlier, that regions with sunnier climates tend to have fewer allergies among their populations.

Additional effects and mechanisms of sunlight and vitamin D are discussed in the author's book, *Healthy Sun*.

Lack of Exercise

A plethora of research has shown that sedentary lifestyles dramatically increase the risk of allergies—and allergies are highest among those who do not exercise regularly.

Let's look at some of the research supporting these conclusions:

Researchers from Germany's National Research Center for Environment and Health (Kohlhammer *et al.* 2006) followed 2,429 children between 1992 and 2005. They closely reviewed their rates of allergies and the level of sports activities. After adjusting for other potential factors, they found that inactive children had double the incidence of hay fever compared to the active children.

Medical researchers from Portugal's University of Porto (Moreira *et al.* 2008) conducted a three-month physical training program on allergic asthmatic children. The exercise training program was found to significantly reduce allergic and mite-specific IgE levels.

Sleep

Sleep is super critical to immune function. For this reason, researchers and physicians find that allergic rhinitis is often accompanied by daytime sleepiness (Mansfield and Posey 2007).

Researchers from the Mannheim University Hospital (Stuck *et al.* 2004) tested 25 patients with allergic rhinitis alongside 25 healthy people. They conducted sleep studies (polysomnography) on both groups, together with extensive questionnaires. They found that poor sleep quality and more daytime sleepiness were associated directly with allergy severity: The poorer the sleep quality, the more severe the allergies. They also found that the healthy subjects slept better than the allergic rhinitis patients.

The connection here is that our immune system becomes extremely active when we sleep. Probiotics engage in high gear, and our various immune cells activate at higher levels. For this reason, our rate of detoxification increases during sleep. This might be compared to a clean-down of a food factory. The clean-down rarely occurs during production, because the clean-down process would interfere in the production process. Instead, the company waits until the night-shift, when the production lines are down for the night. Then they can clean everything.

In the same way, our immune systems switch into high gear when our body's normal metabolic processes are slowed. This occurs during sleep.

With insufficient sleep, there is insufficient detoxification. More radicals are left in the system, and the body must then work harder during normal metabolic activity (waking period) to try to detox. This relates directly to systemic inflammation. The body must work on a body-wide basis to defend itself against foreigners it would normally block with IgA and probiotics at the mucosal membrane.

This was illustrated by researchers from Chicago's Rush University Medical Center (Ranjbaran *et al.* 2007), who studied sleep abnormalities and their association with *"chronic inflammatory conditions (CIC) such as asthma, RA, SLE and IBD."* They found that changes in the *"sleep-wake cycle"* stimulate an increased systemic inflammation response. Their research showed that slow wave (deep) sleep reduces inflammation and strengthens immunity.

They also found that sleep disturbances can cause greater levels of inflammatory pain and fatigue, while reducing quality of life. This scenario is often seen amongst those with allergies. The researchers commented that the underlying mechanism causing a lack of sleep to spurn systemic inflammation relates to the *"dysregulation of the immune system."*

Asthma and sleep are related as well. Researchers from the Department of Medical Sciences of Sweden's Uppsala University (Leander *et al.* 2009) followed 290 subjects. They found that those who developed asthma had a greater incidence of sleep disturbances (30% versus 10%), depression (40% versus 20%) and difficulty relaxing (40% versus 13%) compared to those who were asthma-free.

Those who contracted asthma also had significantly lower levels of energy, appetite and sleep than those without asthma. Asthma sufferers also had less patience, less memory, lower fitness levels and less appreciation than those without asthma.

Furthermore, depression and anxiety have been specifically linked to a lack of REM-stage sleep. Refer to the author's book *Natural Sleep: Solutions for Insomnia* for more information on REM-sleep and the immune system; and strategies that facilitate deep sleep.

Anxiety and Stress

Stress and anxiety deplete the immune system because they increase the body's metabolic load. While we are stressed, our body's metabolism focuses on the stressor. This pulls the body's metabolism away from the processes related to the immune system and detoxification. Because the body has a fairly constant exposure to toxins, and some pathogens (such as bacteria and viruses) will grow in the absence of the immune system, the body's toxin load will increase during stress and anxiety.

Our ancestors became anxious and stressed over physical issues like being chased by tigers or enemies. Thus, our body is tuned to respond to anxiety by sending blood, nutrients and energy to our muscles, eyes, lungs and other facilities to help us get away or face the challenge. These functions all divert blood, nutrients and energy away from our immune system functions, our digestive systems and our mucosal membranes.

Anxiety and stress specifically inhibit the submucosal glands and thus the health and ionic balance of the mucosal linings. Let's think about this carefully: This means that when we are anxious, our mucosal membranes become weaker and maintain less immunity. This allows environmental elements like pollens and molds more immediate access to our nasal tissues. Instead of being blocked by our mucosal membranes, gathered up and broken down by IgAs, probiotics and immune cells, those pollens, molds, dust mite endotoxins and/or other potential allergens gain access to our tissues.

In this condition, the body's immune system must resort to a hyper-reactive, systemic immune response. The IgEs, B-cells and various inflammatory factors must face down the intruders in an all-out war of hypersensitivity.

This scenario is not speculative. It is backed up by plenty of research. For example, Department of Otolaryngology researchers from Beijing's Chaoyang Hospital (Lv et al. 2010) studied 337 adults with seasonal allergic rhinitis during allergy season. Using the internationally-recognized Symptom Checklist 90 (SCL-90) scoring system, they found that the allergic patients had significantly greater levels of depression, anxiety and hostility. They also found that those with a history allergic rhinitis or allergic eczema were more likely to have a history of anxiety, depression, compulsion and hostility.

This relationship between allergic rhinitis and anxiety, depression and stress has been confirmed by a plethora of other studies, including: Xi et al. 2009; Jernelöv et al. 2009; Kiecolt-Glaser et al. 2009; Postolache et al. 2007; and Ke et al. 2010.

Similar Underlying Issues among Other Rhinitis

NARES

A condition that is typically considered non-allergic, yet still includes hyper-inflammation and the invasion of eosinophils in the nasal region is called nonallergic rhinitis with eosinophilia (NARES). This condition has all the symptoms of allergic rhinitis, but in many cases does not maintain a basophil response, as does allergic rhinitis.

While no IgE-specific allergen is found in most cases of NARES, research illustrates that NARES maintains precisely similar immune system defects among the mucosal linings. It is also characterized by systemic inflammation. While there seems to be no smoking gun, NARES actually indicates there is no need for a smoking gun. The defective immune system apparent in NARES can still erupt in rhinitis symptoms, despite the lack of allergic response.

And like allergic rhinitis and so many other hyper-inflammatory conditions, NARES can still be triggered by environmental assaults such as chemicals, smoke, smog and others. NARES can also be triggered by dust mite endotoxins and pollen, though there does not appear to be a clear IgE response.

Nasal Polyps

Nasal polyps may form in the nasal region, where they can also produce nose block, runny nose and watery eyes. Nasal polyps are also symptomatic of a hyper-inflammatory state, however. Here, the immune system has stimulated vascular permeability to the degree that the tissues begin to expand out of control. Sometimes this can follow hay fever season, and sometimes it can seem isolated. Regardless of when polyps appear, they are still inflammatory responses.

Some confuse nasal polyps with cancer. They are not a sign of cancer. Polyps can actually occur almost anywhere in the body, although they are more prevalent among epithelial regions that have mucous membranes. Polyps can also appear in the colon, intestines, ear canal and throat.

Some research has indicated that polyps may be a response to increased levels of specific IgEs to bacteria superantigens (Pant *et al.* 2009). Here again, the immune system has elevated its threat level, but possibly to infective agents like bacteria and viruses.

Health professionals typically treat polyps with corticosteroids. This slows the hyper-inflammatory response—another indication that polyps are an inflammatory condition like allergic rhinitis.

Vasomotor Rhinitis

Vasomotor rhinitis is another hyper-reactive inflammatory condition that occurs in the nasal region. It typically causes nose blockage and runny nose, but not usually watery or itchy eyes—these two symptoms are typical of allergies. Vasomotor rhinitis is considered a nonallergic form of rhinitis, although, like NARES, it is still often triggered by pollutants, chemicals, dust and even pollen.

Vasomotor rhinitis is differentiated from NARES in that it does not typically involve eosinophils. This simply means that the immune system is responding with hyper-inflammation without the immunosuppressive state of eosinophilia. This is likely because the immune system is responding specifically to a certain type of toxin overload—either a different toxin or a different type of immune response, or both.

Vasomotor rhinitis is often considered an autonomic nerve response. Many doctors believe that the nerves lying close to the nasal area have become ultra-sensitive for some reason, causing them to react more deeply than normal.

However, we know from our discussion of the nasal epithelia that the mucosal membranes should be providing protection to the nasal epithelia. Therefore, vasomotor rhinitis is another result of defects among the nasal mucosal membranes—allowing rhinitis triggers to gain contact with the epithelia.

This gives rise to the reality that vasomotor rhinitis is a hypersensitive inflammatory response to toxins or pollutants. This may also relate to poor dietary habits, as we'll discuss in the next chapter.

We must remember that rhinitis—regardless whether it is allergic or nonallergic—is not a disease. Rather, it is a symptom of systemic inflammation throughout the body, combined with defects among the mucosal membranes of the nasal region and upper airways.

Sinusitis and Rhinosinusitis

As we mentioned briefly earlier, sinusitis is typically the result of an infection within the sinus cavities. Like the nasal membranes and the rest of the airways, the sinuses are lined with a mucous membrane that contains a variety of immune cells, probiotics, and IgA. These are typically strong enough to thwart the growth of any invading organism, be it viral, bacterial or fungal.

However, a weakening of the body's mucosal membranes, as we've discussed at length, will give pathogens an environment that allows them to grow and prosper. For bacteria, this means colonization. For viruses, this means a infection of epithelial cells. For fungi, this means a growth of spores and cultures that can spread to different areas.

These three infective microorganisms often arrive by way of air droplets; or for fungi, mold spores. Once they arrive in our nasal cavities, defective mucosal membranes allow them to set up shop in the dark, protected recesses of our sinus cavities. Here they can spread out into the nasal cavities—giving them more opportunity to translocate to other sinus regions.

As these colonies expand out from the sinuses, they can invade our lung tissues. This is often the predicament found in pneumonia, COPD and other infective lung disorders.

Antibiotics are often the treatment of choice by conventional doctors for sinusitis. While antibiotics might work for a bacterial infection of the sinuses temporarily, it will do little for a fungal or viral infection of the sinuses.

In addition, antibiotics can set up an environment for future invasions. This is because our probiotic defense team—which breaks down infective microorganisms before they can grow—can be seriously harmed by antibiotics.

Should this happen, we provide further access to microorganisms to enter our tissues and bloodstream: Our mucosal membranes are not adequately providing a barrier, in other words. They are not replete with immune cells, probiotics and IgA, along with ionic fluids that break these foreigners down before they have a chance to set up shop and/or make contact with our tissues and bloodstream.

Furthermore, once these infective organisms set up shop, they can also burden the immune system, provoking the state of systemic inflammation that facilitates the hypersensitive allergic condition.

Chapter Five

Anti-Allergy Nutrition Strategies

An exhausted immune system will inevitably react differently than a strong immune system to a perceived foreigner. Our diets directly affect our immune system strength and the health of our airways. Let's look at the research supporting these conclusions. Some of these studies point at systemic inflammation, and others focus upon asthma. Still, most of their conclusions are supported by studies specific to allergies. Furthermore, as we've discussed, there is about a 70% association between allergies and asthma.

Medical researchers from Greece's Department of Social Medicine and the University of Crete (Chatzi *et al.* 2007) studied 460 children and their mothers on Menorca—a Mediterranean island. They found that children of mothers eating primarily a Mediterranean diet (a predominantly plant-based diet) produced significantly lower rates of allergic rhinitis and asthma among the children. The researchers concluded: *"The results of this study suggest a beneficial effect of commonly consumed fruits, vegetables and nuts, and of a high adherence to a traditional Mediterranean diet during childhood on symptoms of asthma and rhinitis. Diet may explain the relative lack of allergic symptoms in this population."*

They found that mothers with a high Mediterranean Diet Score during pregnancy reduced the incidence of persistent wheeze among their children by 78%. Their children also had 70% lower incidence of allergic wheezing; and a 45% reduction in allergies among their children at age six (after removing other possible variables).

Another extensive predictive study was the International Study of Asthma and Allergies in Childhood (ISAAC). The study was conducted among eight Pacific countries, which included Samoa, Fiji, Tokelau, French Polynesia and New Caledonia. The research found that the major predicating factors in current asthma wheeze were regular margarine consumption, electric cooking, and maternal smoking. They found that the risk factors for increased rhinoconjunctivitis included the regular consumption of meat products, butter, margarine and nuts; along with regular television viewing, acetaminophen use and second-hand smoke. Allergic eczema was also associated with regular meat consumption, pasta consumption and butter consumption; along with regular television viewing, acetaminophen use and second hand smoke. The researchers concluded that: *"Regular meat and margarine consumption, paracetamol [acetaminophen] use, electric cooking and passive smoking are risk factors for symptoms of asthma, rhinoconjunctivitis and eczema in the Pacific."*

Medical researchers from Britain's University of Nottingham (McKeever *et al.* 2010) researched the relationship between diet and respiratory symptoms, including forced expiratory volumes. Their data was derived from 12,648 adults from the Monitoring Project on Risk Factors and Chronic Diseases in The Netherlands. They found that diets with higher intakes of meat and potatoes, and lower levels of soy and cereals, was linked to reduced lung function and lower expiratory levels (FEV1) levels. They also found that the heavy meat-and-potatoes diet produced higher levels of chronic obstructive pulmonary disease. They also found that a "cosmopolitan diet" with heavier intakes of fish and chicken (both of which are commonly fried) produced higher levels of wheeze and asthma.

Research from the University of Athens (Bacopoulou et al. 2009). Here 2,133 children at ages seven and eighteen were studied. The daily consumption of fruit and vegetables significantly reduced the risk of asthma symptoms through age 18.

Researchers from the Johns Hopkins School of Medicine (Matsui and Matsui 2009) studied 8,083 people over two years old using data from the National Health and Nutrition Examination Survey (2005-2006). They found that among patients diagnosed by a doctor as having asthma and/or wheeze in the last year, higher blood levels of folate was linked to lower total IgE levels—a sign of reduced allergy and hypersensitivity (atopy). They also found a dose-dependent relationship between higher folate levels and doctor-diagnosed wheeze and/or asthma.

Good sources of folate include lettuce, spinach, lentils, beans, asparagus and other plant-based foods.

Researchers from Mexico's Institute of National Public Health (Romieu et al. 2009) followed 158 asthmatic children and 50 healthy children from Mexico City for 22 weeks. Diet, lung function testing and sinus mucous analysis was done every two weeks. Diets with greater amounts of fruits and vegetables resulted in lower levels of pro-inflammatory IL-8 cytokines. A diet that most closely trended towards the Mediterranean Diet Index resulted in better lung function tests. Children with the higher Mediterranean Diet Index scores also scored the highest in forced expiratory volume (FEV1) testing. The researchers concluded: *"Our results suggest that fruit and vegetable intake and close adherence to the Mediterranean diet have a beneficial effect on inflammatory response and lung function in asthmatic children living in Mexico City."*

Another study by researchers from the University of Crete's Faculty of Medicine (Chatzi et al. 2007) surveyed the parents of 690 children ages seven through 18 years old in the rural areas of Crete. The children were also tested with skin prick tests for 10 common allergens. This research found that consuming a Mediterranean diet reduced the risk of allergic rhinitis by over 65%. The risk of skin allergies and respiratory conditions (such as wheezing) was also reduced, but by smaller amounts. They also found that greater consumption of nuts among the children cut wheezing rates in half, while consuming margarine more than doubled the incidence of both wheezing and allergic rhinitis.

Nutrition researchers from Italy's D'Annunzio University (Riccioni *et al.* 2007) also studied the relationships between nutrition and bronchial asthma. They found significant evidence that inflammatory activity associated with the asthmatic hyperresponse relates directly to the production of reactive oxygen species. Furthermore, they determined that the damage done by these free radicals produces *"specific inflammatory abnormalities"* within the airways of asthmatics.

A related study by these researchers (Riccioni *et al.* 2007) tested 96 people—which included 40 asthmatics and 56 healthy control subjects—for blood levels of vitamin A and lycopene. They found that lycopene and vitamin A levels were significantly lower among the asthmatic patients versus the healthy controls. They concluded that: *"Dietary supplementation or adequate intake of lycopene and vitamin A rich foods may be beneficial in asthmatic subjects."*

As part of the International Study on Allergies and Asthma in Childhood (ISAAC), a contingent of researchers from around the world (Nagel *et al.* 2010) convened to analyze studies on asthma and diet conducted between 1995 and 2005 among 29 research facilities in 20 different countries. In all, the dietary habits of 50,004 children ages eight through twelve years old were analyzed.

This study revealed that those with diets containing large fruit portions had significantly lower rates of allergies and asthma. This link occurred among both affluent and non-affluent countries. Fish consumption in affluent countries (where vegetable intake is less) and green vegetable consumption among non-affluent countries were also associated with reduced asthma. In general, the consumption of fruit, vegetables and fish was linked with less lifetime asthma incidence among the entire population. Frequent consumption of beef burgers, on the other hand, was linked with greater incidence of lifetime asthma.

Researchers from Spain's University of Murcia (Garcia-Marcos *et al.* 2007) examined the effects of diet on asthma in 106 six and seven year-old children. Utilizing a Mediterranean diet score along with a survey of symptoms, they found that eating a predominantly Mediterranean diet decreased severe allergies and asthma symptoms among the girls. Diets high in cereal grains produced 46% lower incidence of severe asthma. Frequent fruit eating decreased rhinoconjunctivitis incidence by 24%. In contrast, diets higher in fast foods produced 64% greater incidence of severe asthma and allergies.

Meanwhile, research from the National Center for Chronic Disease and Prevention (Cory *et al.* 2010) indicated that only 11-30% of adult Americans eat the recommended amounts of fruits and vegetables—some of the lowest levels in the world.

Nutrition scientists from Korea's Kyung Hee University (Oh *et al.* 2010) studied the relationship between allergies, asthma and antioxidants. They found by testing 180 allergic and 242 non-allergic Korean children that higher serum levels of beta-carotene, dietary vitamin E, iron and folic acid were associated with lower incidence of atopic reactions among the children. These antioxidant nutrients are derived primarily from plant-based foods.

Many other studies have shown these associations between diet and allergies. Researchers from the Allergy and Respiratory Research Group Centre for Population Health Sciences at the University of Edinburgh's Medical School (Nurmatov *et al.* 2010) analyzed 62 international asthma and allergy studies for control protocols and study design. They found that 17 of 22 well-designed studies that compared dietary fruit and vege-table intake with asthma and allergies showed that higher fruit and vege-tables in the diet lowered asthma and allergy incidence.

Their analyses found that asthmatic children had significantly lower levels of vitamin A; and that greater levels of vitamin D, vitamin E and zinc was *"protective for the development of wheezing outcomes."*

The researchers concluded that adequate intake of antioxidant vita-mins including vitamins A, C, and E were critical to reducing free radicals and inflammatory abnormalities. They also determined that antioxidants are able to reduce damage from incoming bacteria, viruses, toxins and xenobiotics (pollutants to the body). The researchers referenced a number of other studies that successfully associated oxidative stress with bronchial inflammation and subsequent hypersensitivities.

Researchers from Italy's University G. D'Annunzio Chieti (Riccioni and D'Orazio 2005) discovered in their research that persistent asthma is linked to an increase in reactive oxygen species. Their research also found that antioxidant nutrients such as selenium, zinc and other antioxidant vitamins have the potential to help reduce asthma symptoms and severity.

Consuming a predominantly plant-based diet (such as the Mediterra-nean diet), has clear results: It is linked with reduced allergy and asthma incidence and a reduction of systemic inflammation.

This also means that diets weighted too far towards animal-based foods—especially red meats—increase the likelihood of allergies and asthma, whether among mothers and their infants, adults in general, or children growing up.

These associations also confirm the well-researched relationship between a diet rich in antioxidants (plant-foods have more antioxidants) and strengthened immunity in general.

Problems with Red Meat

What is it about meats—particularly red meats—that is so bad? How do diets heavy in red meats contribute to increased levels of systemic inflammation and allergic hyperreactivity? Here is an abbreviated list of issues:

> *Fatty acid imbalances:* Red meats provide increased levels of saturated fats, which lead to greater levels of LDL cholesterol. LDL, remember, is more susceptible to lipid peroxidation.

> *Arachidonic acid overload:* Red meats and oily fish provide higher levels of arachidonic acid. Increased arachidonic acid levels in the body push the immune system towards inflammation.

> *Nitrites:* Red meats have greater levels of nitrites. This is especially true for processed and fried meats. As nitrites enter the body, they produce reactive nitrogen species. These damage cells and cell membranes, producing inflammatory peroxidation.

> *Dysbiosis:* Animal foods facilitate the growth of colonies of pathogenic microorganisms in the intestines. These produce endotoxins that damage cell membranes and tissues, stimulating inflammation, again through peroxidation.

> *Beta-glucuronidase:* Omnivore diets result in higher levels of beta-glucuronidase and other mutagenic enzymes. These enzymes directly damage cells and increase systemic inflammation.

> *Toxemia:* Animal foods typically contain a greater number of toxins compared to plant foods. This is because animals are *bioaccumulators:* They accumulate toxins. Many toxic chemicals are fat-soluble: The toxins thus accumulate among fat cells. Animals also produce and circulate various waste products, and their waste production increases during slaughter. Plant-based foods, by contrast, provide various antioxidants.

> *Protein metabolic stress:* Animal proteins require significant effort by the body to break them down into useable amino acid and smaller peptide form. The body utilizes single amino acids and small amino acid chains (peptides). Animal

proteins contain hundreds, even thousands of amino acids in a single molecule. This requires significantly more energy and enzyme production to break down and process these complex proteins.

> ***Acidic plasma:*** The excess proteins in animal foods produce greater levels of acids in the bloodstream and tissues, which can lead to toxemia. Remember, amino acids are acidic.

Let's review some of the science supporting these points:

Nitrites

Researchers from the Harvard School of Public Health (Varraso *et al.* 2007) studied the effects of nitrites in the diet and lung health. They analyzed 111 diagnosed cases of COPD between 1986 and 1998 among 42,915 men who participated in the Health Professionals Follow-up Study. The average consumption of high-nitrite meats (processed meats, bacon, hot dogs) was calculated from surveys conducted in 1986, 1990, and 1994. They found that consuming these meats at least once a day increased the incidence of COPD by more than 2-½ times over those who rarely ate high-nitrite meats.

These same Harvard researchers used a similar analysis of 42,917 men, but with more dietary parameters. This research found that the *"western diet"* consisting of refined grains, sugary foods, cured and red meats, and fried foods, increased COPD incidence by more than four times. Meanwhile, a *"prudent"* diet, rich in fruits, vegetables and fish, halved COPD incidence.

The same researchers from the Harvard School of Public Health studied lung function, COPD and diet among 72,043 women between 1984 and 2000 in the Nurses' Health Study. Diets that had more fruit, vegetables, fish and whole-grain products reduced the incidence of COPD by 25%. Meanwhile, a diet heavy in refined grains, cured and red meats, desserts and French fries increased the incidence of COPD by 31%.

Pathogenic Enzymes

In the early 1980s, Dr. Barry Goldin, a professor at the Tufts University School of Medicine, led a series of studies that found that certain diets promoted a group of cancer-causing enzymes. These included beta-glucuronidase, nitroreductase, azoreductase, and steroid 7-alpha-dehydroxylase. The enzymes were linked with cancer in previous studies. (Cancer is caused by the same types of cell damage that also stimulates systemic inflammation.)

A number of studies on vegetarians found lower levels of these mutagenic enzymes, while those eating animal-based diets had greater levels. Apparently, these cancer-related enzymes originate from a group of pathogenic bacteria that tend to occupy the intestines of those with diets rich in animal-based foods. It was discovered that the cancer-producing enzymes are actually the endotoxins (waste products) of these pathogenic bacteria.

Dr. Goldin and his research teams studied the difference between these enzyme levels in omnivores and vegetarians. In one study, the researchers removed meat from the diets of a group of omnivores for 30 days. An immediate reduction of steroid 7-alpha-dehydroxylase was found. When the probiotic *L. acidophilus* was supplemented to their diets, this group also showed a significant reduction in beta-glucuronidase and nitroreductase.

In other words, two dietary connections were found regarding these disease-causing enzymes: animal-based diets and a lack of intestinal probiotics. The two are actually related, because probiotics thrive in prebiotic-rich plant-based diets and suffer in animal-rich diets.

Two years later, Dr. Goldin and associates (Goldin *et al.* 1982) studied 10 vegetarian and 10 omnivore women. He found that the vegetarian women maintained significantly lower levels of beta-glucuronidase than did the omnivorous women.

The association between colon cancer and diets heavy in red meat has been shown conclusively in a multiple studies over the years. For example, an American Cancer Society cohort study (Chao *et al.* 2005) examined 148,610 adults between the ages of 50 and 74 living in 21 states of the U.S. They found that higher intakes of red and processed meats were associated with higher levels of rectal and colon cancer after other cancer variables were eliminated.

Other studies have confirmed that vegetarian diets result in a reduction of these carcinogenic enzymes produced by pathogenic bacteria. Researchers from Finland's University of Kuopio (Ling and Hanninen 1992) tested 18 volunteers who were randomly divided into either a conventional omnivore diet or a vegan diet for one month.

The vegan group followed the month with a return to their original omnivore diet. After only one week on the vegan diet, the researchers found that fecal urease levels decreased by 66%, cholylglycine hydrolase levels decreased by 55%, beta-glucuronidase levels decreased by 33% and beta-glucosidase levels decreased by 40% in the vegan group. These reduced levels continued through the month of consuming the vegan diet. Serum levels of phenol and p-cresol—also inflammation-producing endotoxins of pathogenic bacteria—also significantly decreased in the vegan group.

Within two weeks of returning to the omnivore diet, the formerly-vegan group's pathogenic enzyme levels returned to the higher levels they had before converting to the vegan diet. After one month of returning to the omnivore diet, serum levels of toxins phenol and p-cresol returned to their previously higher levels prior to the vegan diet. Meanwhile, the higher levels of inflammation-producing enzymes remained among the conventional omnivore diet (control) group.

A study published two years earlier by Huddinge University researchers (Johansson *et al.* 1992) confirmed the same results. In this study, the conversion of an omnivore diet to a lacto-vegetarian diet significantly reduced levels of beta-glucuronidase, beta-glucosidase, and sulphatase (more tumor-implicated, inflammation-producing enzymes) from fecal samples.

Another study illustrating this link between vegetarianism, pathogenic bacterial enzymes and cancer was conducted at Sweden's Huddinge University and the University Hospital (Johansson *et al.* 1998) almost a decade later. Dr. Johansson and associates measured the effect of switching from an omnivore diet to a lacto-vegetarian diet and back to an omnivore diet with respect to mutagenicity—by testing the body's fluid biochemistry to determine the tendency for tumor formation.

In this extensive study, 20 non-smoking and normal weight volunteers switched to a lacto-vegetarian diet for one year. Urine and feces were examined for mutagenicity (cancer-causing bacteria and their endotoxins) at the start of the study, at three months, at six months and at twelve months after beginning the vegetarian diet. Following the switch to the lacto-vegetarian diet, all mutagenic parameters significantly decreased among the urine and feces of the subjects. The subjects were then followed-up and tested three years after converting back to an omnivore diet (four years after the study began). Their higher mutagenic biochemistry levels had returned.

In another of Dr. Johansson's studies (Johansson and Ravald 1995)—this from Sweden's Karolinska Institute—29 vegetarians and 28 omnivores were tested. The tests revealed that the vegetarians secreted more salivary juices than did the omnivores. Adequate salivation is critical to the health of the mucosal membranes among the oral cavity and airways.

Arachidonic Acid

To add to these issues is the problem of consuming too much arachidonic acid in the diet. Arachidonic acid is an essential fatty acid naturally converted from other fatty acids by the body. However, diets rich in red meats can directly overload the body with arachidonic acid, producing a pro-inflammatory condition.

This subject has been studied extensively by researchers from Wake Forest University School of Medicine, led by Professor Floyd Chilton, Ph.D. Dr. Chilton has published a wealth of research data that have uncovered that foods high in arachidonic acid can produce a pro-inflammatory metabolism, especially among adults. Dr. Chilton's research also confirmed that a pro-inflammatory metabolism is trigger-happy and hypersensitive: creating the systemic inflammatory conditions prevalent in allergic hyperresponsiveness.

In research headed up by Dr. Darshan Kelley from the Western Human Research Center in California, diets high in arachidonic acid stimulated four times more inflammatory cells than diets low in arachidonic acid content. And this problem increases with age. In other words, the same amount of arachidonic acid-forming foods will cause higher levels of arachidonic acid as we get older (Chilton 2006).

According to the USDA's Standard 13 and 16 databases, red meats and fish produce the highest levels of arachidonic acid in the body. Diary, fruits and vegetables produce little or no arachidonic acid. Grains, beans and nuts produce none or very small amounts. Processed bakery goods produce a moderate amount of arachidonic acid.

Phytanic Acid

Another association we can make between inflammation and diets rich in animal-based foods relates to phytanic acid. Phytanic acid (tetramethylhexadecanoic acid) is a byproduct of plant food digestion inside the intestinal tracts of ruminating animals such as cows, goats, sheet and so on. While phytanic acid can be derived from plant-based foods, greater concentrations of nonesterified phytanic acid are formed in animals when chlorophyll is degraded within the stomachs of ruminants, along with mammalian peroxisomes. This is the result of these animals' unique multiple-stomach digestion process of grasses and other plant material. Humans, of course, do not digest food in the same manner, so we do not produce these concentrated levels of nonesterified phytanic acid from plant-based diets.

Otto-von-Guericke University (Germany) professor Dr. Peter Schönfeld has showed that the nonesterified phytanic acids from ruminants directly damage the membranes of our cell's mitochondria. The end result, his research found, is a corruption of the mitochondrial ATP energy production process (Schönfeld 2004).

This corruption in turn damages cell function, stimulating inflammation.

Asthma and the Vegan Diet

In 1985, researchers (Lindahl *et al.*) studied 35 asthma patients. Each of them had clinical asthma for an average of 12 years, and they were all consistently taking asthma medication—with many on oral cortisone. The patients switched to a vegan diet for one year. After four months on the vegan diet, 71% had a significant reduction of asthma symptoms.

After one year on the vegan diet, 92% had a significant reduction of asthma symptoms. Lung function also increased among all the patients. Vital capacity, forced expiratory volume (FEV1) levels all improved. Blood analyses were performed to measure levels of IgE, IgM, haptoglobin, cholesterol and triglycerides. These levels all significantly improved in all the patients.

The researchers also reported that the patients all began to take more responsibility for their health, and their overall health care costs decreased dramatically.

Problems with Processed Foods

Food processing consists of one or a combination of the following actions on food:

> ➤ chopping or pulverizing
> ➤ heating to high temperatures
> ➤ distilling or extracting its constituents
> ➤ otherwise isolating some parts by straining off or filtering
> ➤ clarifying or otherwise refining

Most consider food processing a good thing, because we humans like to focus on one or two characteristics or nutrients within a food. The idea is that we want the essence of the food, and don't want to fool around with the rest. In most cases—in terms of commercial food—it is a value proposition, because all the energy and work required to produce the final food product must equal or be greater than the increase in the processed food's financial value. Therefore, the more concentrated or isolated the attractive portion is, the more financial value is added.

Typically, this increase in financial value is due to the food being sweeter, smoother or simply easier to eat or mix with other foods. In the case of oils or flours, the food extract is used for baking purposes, for example. In the case of sugar—which is extracted and isolated from cane and beets—it is added to nearly every processed food recipe.

Ironically, what is left behind in this extraction is the food's real value. The healthy fiber and nutrients are stripped away in most cases. Plant fiber is a necessary element of our diet, because it renders sterols that aid digestion and reduce LDL cholesterol. Many nutrients are also attached to and protected by the plant's fibers. Once the fiber is stripped away, the remaining nutrients are easily damaged by sunlight, air, and the heat of processing.

What is being missed in the value proposition of food processing is that nature's whole foods have their greatest value—nutritionally—prior to processing. When a food is broken down, the molecular bonds that attach nutrients to the food's fibers and complex polysaccharides are lost. As these bonds are lost, the remaining components can become unstable in the body. When these components—such as refined sugar and simple polysaccharides (starches)—become unstable, they can form free radicals in the body. They thus add to our body's toxic burden because they can damage our cells.

In other words, whole foods provide the nutrients our bodies need in the combinations our bodies recognize. Nutrients are bonded within a matrix of structure and fiber. This allows our body to break the bonds and derive these nutrients as our bodies require them.

In some cases, we might need to physically peel a food to get to the edible part. In other cases, such as in the case of beans and grains, we may need to heat or cook them to soften the fibers to enable chewing and digestion. In the case of wheats, we can mill the whole grain (including the bran) to deliver the spectrum of fibrous nutrients. In other words, the closer we match the way our ancestors ate foods, the more our bodies will recognize them, and the better our bodies will utilize them.

Because many of our processed foods have been in our diet for many decades, it is difficult to prove that our modern diet of overly-processed foods produces greater levels of systemic inflammation and allergies. This doesn't mean that it is impossible, however.

To test this hypothesis, French researchers (Fremont *et al.* 2010) studied the effects of processed flax. Foods containing processed flax are a new addition to our diet—although our ancestors certainly ate raw or cooked whole flax. So they studied the introduction of modern processed flax into the French diet. In a study of 1,317 patients with allergies, they found that those who were allergic to flax could be identified by their sensitivity to extruded, heated flax, rather than raw flax seed. This of course indicates that the increase in flax allergies among the French is due to the increase in *processed flax* rather than the increased availability of flax. Certainly, over time, as flax allergies proceed, there will be more crossover allergies to raw flax. Because exposure to processed flax is fairly recent, allergies to processed flax but not raw flax indicates that the extrusion processing is what causes the identification of flax protein as an allergen.

What does processing do to create more sensitivity? Our digestive enzymes and probiotics have evolved to break down (or not) certain types of molecules. Imbalanced or denatured molecules can be considered foreign.

We can also see how processing increases diseases when we compare the disease statistics of developing countries with those of developed countries.

For example, like many developing countries, India has more heart disease in recent decades because of increased consumption of processed and fried foods. In the same way, the Chinese thrived for thousands of years on a rice-based diet. But when modern processing machines introduced white dehulled rice, malnutrition diseases began to occur. This is because the dehulling process results in the loss of important lignans, B vitamins E vitamins and others.

Processed and refined foods damage intestinal health and promote free radicals. They are nutrient-poor. They burden and starve our probiotics. Frying foods also produces a carcinogen called acrylamide (Ehling *et al.* 2005).

Processed Salt

Salt is included in this section because not only is it refined: Processed salt is stripped of important mineral nutrients. And processed foods typically contain incredible amounts of refined salt.

Salt is sometimes also referred to as sodium. However, it is not technically sodium. It is actually sodium chloride. Sodium is an essential trace element that helps balance blood pressure and the kidneys. Guidelines for maximum salt levels range from 2,200 milligrams a day to 2,300 milligrams. Adults who eat processed foods at every meal can consume from 3,000 milligrams to 5,000 mg per day.

Researchers from Indiana University (Mickleborough *et al.* 2005) studied dietary salt among 24 patients with exercise-induced asthma. The asthmatics were given either a low-salt diet or a high-salt diet for two weeks. The high-salt diet group experienced lower forced expiratory volumes (FEV1) and reduced lung function in general. Levels of pro-inflammatory neutrophils, eosinophils, eosinophil cationic protein (ECP), leukotrienes, prostaglandins, and inflammatory cytokines interleukin (IL)-1beta and IL-8 were all significantly higher in the high-salt diet group.

We will discuss salt alternatives in the next chapter.

Glycation

The rates of peanut allergies nearly doubled during the 1990s (Sicherer *et al.* 2003), and have continued to slowly rise among industrialized nations. As discussed earlier, peanut allergies have been known to crossover with hay fever and other allergies.

Not surprisingly, as peanut allergies have risen, so has allergic rhinitis incidence: And as we've discussed, peanut allergies are often expressed as allergic rhinitis, and other allergies often crossover from peanut allergies.

So what changed during this period? Did industrialized counties eat more peanuts during the 1990s? There is no evidence of that.

What changed during this period was the way peanuts are produced and packaged. Dry-roasted and sugar-coated ("honey roasted") peanuts became more popular among consumers in Western industrialized countries due to the fact that manufacturers developed new technologies for dry-roasting processing.

While trying to understand the associations, researchers from the Mount Sinai School of Medicine (Beyer *et al.* 2001) determined that even though the Chinese also eat a significant amount of peanuts, there are significantly fewer peanut allergies in China. Since the Chinese primarily eat boiled or minimally fried peanuts—while Western countries are now eating mostly dry-roasted peanuts—the researchers decided to compare the allergenicity of dry-roasted peanuts with boiled and fried versions.

First they found that the *Ara h1* protein content in peanuts—a primary allergen—was significantly reduced when peanuts are fried or boiled, as compared with the dry-roasted. Secondly, they found that the IgE binding ability of the *Ara h2* and *Ara h3* proteins was reduced when peanuts were boiled or fried—again compared with dry-roasting. This protein-IgE binding affinity is directly associated with the allergenicity of a food, as we discussed earlier.

A couple of years later, researchers from the USDA's Agricultural Research Service (Chung *et al.* 2003) confirmed these findings when their tests revealed that mature dry-roasted peanuts produced an increase in IgE binding—along with glycation end products.

This research was also duplicated later by other USDA researchers (Schmitt *et al.* 2004). However, in this study, the researchers also established that all three methods—frying, boiling and dry-roasting—increase the allergenicity of peanuts when compared to raw peanuts.

One of the leading researchers in the 2001 Mount Sinai study was Dr. Hugh Sampson. Dr. Sampson has since commented:

> *"The Chinese eat the same amount of peanut per capita as we do, they introduce it early in a sort of a boiled/mushed type form, as they do in many African countries, and they have very low rates of peanut allergies. All the countries that have westernized their diet are now seeing the same problem with food allergy as we see. Countries that have introduced peanut butter are now starting to see a rise in the prevalence of peanut allergies akin to the high rates al-*

ready found in the UK, Australia, Canada and some European countries."

We would add to his point regarding peanut butter that many peanut butter producers use dry-roasted peanuts. Additionally, there are generally two ways to manufacture peanut butter. Many commercial peanut butters are produced through a complex heating and blending process that includes blending the peanut butter with sugar and hydrogenated oils.

Alternatively, peanut butter can simply be made using a natural grinding process where the whole peanuts are ground and packed into jars without heating or blending. This process typically produces a separation of the oil on top, which is why so many manufacturers over-process and blend their peanut butters. However, the oil stirs back in quite easily.

Researchers from France's University of Burgundy (Rapin and Wiernsperger 2010) have confirmed that protein or lipid glycation produced by modern food manufacturers is linked to allergies.

In general, food manufacturing glycation is produced when sugars and protein-rich foods are combined and heated to extremely high temperatures. This is a typical process used for the manufacture of many commercial packaged foods on the grocery shelves today. During the process, sugars bind to protein molecules. This produces a glycated protein-sugar complex and glycation end products, both of which have been implicated in cardiovascular disease, diabetes, some cancers, peripheral neuropathy and Alzheimer's disease (Miranda and Outeiro 2010).

With regard to Alzheimer's disease, one of the end products of the glycation reaction is amyloid protein. Amyloid proteins have been found among the brain tissues and cerebrospinal fluids of Alzheimer's disease patients. Glycation is implicated in the amyloid plaque buildup found in Alzheimer's.

Glycation also takes place within the body. This occurs especially with diets with greater consumption of refined sugars and cooked or caramelized high-protein foods.

The western diet contains extraordinary levels of processed protein compared to traditional diets. Americans eat far beyond the amount of protein required for health. Studies indicate that Americans eat an average of 80-150 grams of protein a day. This is significantly higher than the 25-50 grams of protein recommended by nutritionists and health experts (Campbell 2006; McDougall 1983).

This amount of protein in the American diet is also significantly higher than even U.S. RDA levels. The U.S. recommended daily allowance for protein is 0.8 grams per 2.2 lbs of body weight. This converts to 54 grams for a person weighing 150 pounds. Americans eat on average nearly double that amount.

The western diet is also laden with refined sugars. Today, nearly every pre-cooked recipe found in mass market grocery stores contains refined sugar. Many brands now try to white-wash the massive sugar content of their products by calling their sugar content "all natural." This is a deception, because nature in the form of fiber has been unnaturally stripped away from their refined sugars. This is hardly a "natural" proposition. Nature attaches sugars to complex fibers, polysaccharides and nutrients in such a way that prevents them from easily attaching to proteins. Sugars that are cooked and stripped of these complexes become immediate glycation candidates within the body.

As our digestive system combines these sugars with proteins, many of the glycated proteins are identified as foreign by IgA or IgE antibodies in immune-burdened physiologies. Why are they considered foreign? Because glycated proteins and their AGE end products damage blood vessels, tissues and brain cells. In this case, the immune system is launching an inflammatory attack in an effort to protect us from our own diet!

There is no surprise that glycation among foods and in the body is connected with systemic inflammation. It is also no accident that the increased consumption of overly-processed foods and manufacturing processes that pulverize and strip foods of their fiber; and blend denatured proteins and sugars using high-heat processes has increased as our rates of inflammatory diseases have increased over the past century.

In fact, this connection between inflammatory diseases and processed foods has been observed clinically by natural physicians over the years. They may not have understood the precise mechanics, however. Many of these reputable health experts have categorized the effect of processed foods as one of acidifying the bloodstream. The concept was that denatured and over-processed foods produced more acids in the body.

This thesis did not go over too well among scientific circles, because the acidification mechanism was not scientifically confirmed, and there was no concrete mechanism.

Well this can now change, as we are providing the science showing both the mechanism and the evidence that glycation end products do produce acidification in terms of peroxidation radicals that damage cells and tissues.

We should note that a healthy form of natural glycation also takes place in the body to produce certain nutrient combinations. Unlike the radical-forming glycation produced by food manufacturing and refined sugar intake, this type of glycation is driven by the body's natural enzyme processes, resulting in molecules and end products the body uses and recognizes. When glycation is driven by the body's own enzyme processes, it is termed *glycosylation*, however.

Hydrolyzed Proteins

Proteins are composed of very long chains of amino acids. Sometimes hundreds and even thousands of amino acids can make up a protein. The body typically breaks apart these chains through an enzyme reaction called *proteolysis*.

Proteolysis breaks down proteins into amino acids and small groups of aminos called polypeptides. This is also called *cleaving*. As enzymes break off these polypeptides or individual amino acids from proteins, they replace the protein chain linkages with water molecules to stabilize the peptide or amino acid. This process is called *enzymatic hydrolysis*. Breaking away the peptides or amino acids allows the body to utilize the amino acid or polypeptide to make new proteins within the body.

The body then assembles its own proteins from these amino acids and small polypeptide combinations. The body's protein assembly is programmed by DNA and RNA. For this reason, the body must recognize the aminos and polypeptide combinations. The body produces a variety of enzymes to naturally break apart multiple proteins and polypeptides. Protein-cleaving enzymes are called *proteases*.

For this reason, strange or large polypeptide combinations can burden the body, especially if the body does not have the right enzymes to break those peptide chains apart.

Food manufacturers can synthetically break down proteins by extrusion, heating and blending with processing aids—including commercially produced enzymes. These enzymes force the break down of the proteins in the food. As water is integrated into the process, synthetic hydrolysis occurs. This produces foods that contain hydrolyzed proteins. These synthetically hydrolyzed protein foods may not be recognized by the body's immune system, and may stimulate an inflammatory response.

Illustrating this, French laboratory researchers (Bouchez-Mahiout *et al.* 2010) found by using immunoblot testing that hydrolyzed wheat proteins from skin conditioners produced hypersensitivity, which eventually crossed over to wheat protein food allergies. In other words, hydrolyzed wheat proteins in skin treatments are not necessarily recognized by the immune system. Once the body becomes sensitized to these hydrolyzed wheat proteins from skin absorption, this sensitivity can cross over to sensitivity to similar wheat proteins in foods.

Researchers from France's Center for Research in Grignon (Laurière *et al.* 2006) tested nine women who had skin contact sensitivity to cosmetics containing hydrolyzed wheat proteins (HWP). Six were found to react with either allergic skin hives or anaphylaxis to different products (including foods) containing HWP. The whole group also had IgE sensitivity to wheat flour or gluten-type proteins. The tests showed that they had become sensitive to HWP, and then later to unmodified grain proteins. As they tested further, they found that reactions often occurred among larger wheat protein peptide aggregates. The researchers concluded that the use of HWP in skin products can produce hypersensitivity to HWP, followed by a crossover to inflammatory responses to the wheat proteins in foods.

Spanish researchers (Cabanillas *et al.* 2010) found that enzymatic hydrolysis of lentils and chickpeas produced allergens for four out of five allergic patients in their research.

The commercial enzymes used by many food manufacturers can also stimulate allergic responses. Danish researchers (Bindslev-Jensen *et al.* 2006) tested 19 commercially available enzymes typically used in the food industry on 400 adults with allergies. It was found that many of the enzymes produced histamine responses among the patients.

Hydrolyzing proteins through manufacturing processes can create epitopes that the immune system does not recognize. Once the immune system launches an immune response to the epitope, it will remember those as allergens, even if they are part of foods once accepted by the body. Once sensitive to these allergens, the body can become cross-reactive to pollens and other food-related protein epitopes.

The Wholesome Diet

Dr. Raja Jabar, M.D. from the State University of New York Hospital and Medical Center reviewed this and other research regarding the role of diet in allergic rhinitis. He confirmed that diet has a significant effect. Dr. Jabar concluded:

"Patients with asthma and allergic rhinitis may benefit from hydration and a diet low in sodium, omega-6 fatty acids, and trans fatty acids, but high in omega-3 fatty acids, onions, and fruits and vegetables (at least five servings a day)."

Let's discuss the essentials of a wholesome diet in greater detail. Diets high in fruits and vegetables:

- ➤ increase antioxidant levels
- ➤ increase detoxification
- ➤ lower the burden on the body's immune system
- ➤ provide a host of bioavailable nutrients
- ➤ provide fiber, reducing LDL lipid peroxidation
- ➤ feed our probiotic colonies
- ➤ increase the strength of the liver
- ➤ alkalize and help purify the blood
- ➤ provide the body with trace and macro minerals
- ➤ lower inflammation

All of these effects work together to reduce and even reverse allergic hypersensitivity, as was evidenced in the study above and the studies we laid out in the previous chapter. Note that a serving is actually quite small. An apple is a typical serving. A cup of broccoli is a serving. Given this, it is pretty easy to eat five servings of fruits and vegetables per day.

Whole Food Antioxidants

A plethora of research has confirmed that damage from free radicals is implicated in many health conditions, including allergic hypersensitivity. Free radicals damage cells, cell membranes, organs, blood vessel walls and airways—producing hypersensitivity and causing systemic inflammation—as the immune system responds to an overload of tissue-damaging radicals.

Free radicals are produced by toxins, pathogens, trans fats, fried foods, red meats, radiation, pollution and various chemicals that destabilize within the body. Free radicals are molecules or ions that require stabilization. They reach stabilization by 'stealing' atoms from the cells or tissues of our body. This in turn destabilizes those cells and tissues—producing damage.

Antioxidants serve to stabilize free radicals before our cells and tissues are robbed—by donating their own atoms. A diet with plenty of fruits and vegetables supplies numerous antioxidants. Although antioxidants cannot be considered treatments for any disease, many studies have proved that increased antioxidant intake supports immune function and detoxification. These effects allow the immune system to respond with greater tolerance.

Antioxidant constituents in plant-based foods are known to significantly repeal free radicals, strengthen the immune system and help detoxify the system. These include *lecithin* and *octacosanol* from whole grains; *polyphenols* and *sterols* from vegetables; *lycopene* from tomatoes and watermelons; *quercetin* and *sulfur/allicin* from garlic, onions and peppers; *pectin* and *rutin* from apples and other fruits; *phytocyanidin flavonoids* such as *apigenin* and *luteolin* from various greenfoods; and *anthocyanins* from various fruits and oats.

Some sea-based botanicals like kelp also contain antioxidants as well. Consider a special polysaccharide compound from kelp called *fucoidan*. Fucoidan has been shown in animal studies to significantly reduce inflammation (Cardoso *et al.* 2009; Kuznetsova *et al.* 2004).

Procyanidins are found in apples, currants, cinnamon, bilberry and many other foods. The extract of *Vitis vinifera* seed (grapeseed) is one of the highest sources of bound antioxidant *proanthocyanidins* and *leucocyanidines* called *procyanidolic oligomers* or PCOs. Pycnogenol® also contains significant levels of these PCOs. Blueberries, parsley, green tea, black currant, some legumes and onions also contain PCOs and similar proantho-cyanidins.

Research has demonstrated that PCOs have protective and strengthening effects on tissues by increasing enzyme conjugation (Seo *et al.* 2001). PCOs have also been shown to increase vascular wall strength (Robert *et al.* 2000).

Oxygenated carotenoids such as *lutein* and *astaxanthin* also have been shown to exhibit strong antioxidant activity. Astaxanthin is derived from the microalga *Haematococcus pluvialis*, and lutein is available from a number of foods, including spirulina.

Most of these phytonutrients specifically modulate the immune system. For example, the flavonoids *kaempferol* and *flavone* have been shown to block mast cell proliferation by over 80% (Alexandrakis *et al.* 2003). Sources of kaempferol include Brussels sprouts, broccoli, grapefruit and apples.

Furthermore, *resveratrol* from grapes and berries modulate nuclear factor-kappaB and transcription/Janus kinase pathways—which strengthens immunity. Good sources of resveratrol include peanuts, red grapes, cranberries and cocoa (wine is not advisable for allergic conditions due to the damaging effects of ethanol upon the liver).

Nearly every plant-food has some measure of phytonutrients discussed above and more. These phytonutrients alkalize the blood and increase the detoxification capabilities of the liver. They help clear the blood of toxins.

Foods that are particularly detoxifying and immunity-building include fresh pineapples, beets, cucumbers, apricots, apples, almonds, zucchini, artichokes, avocados, bananas, beans, collard greens, berries, casaba, celery, coconuts, cranberries, watercress, dandelion greens, grapes, raw honey, corn, kale, citrus fruits, watermelon, lettuce, mangoes, mushrooms, oats, broccoli, okra, onions, papayas, parsley, peas, whole grains, radishes, raisins, spinach, tomatoes, walnuts, and many others.

These plant-based foods are also our primary source of soluble and insoluble fiber. Diets with significant fiber help clear the blood and tissues of toxins, and lipid peroxidation-friendly LDL cholesterol. Fiber is also critical to a healthy digestive tract and intestinal barrier. Fiber in the diet should range from about 35 to 45 grams per day according to the recommendations of many diet experts. Six to ten servings of raw fruits and vegetables per day should accomplish this—which is even part of the USDA's recommendations. This means raw, fibrous foods should be present at every meal.

Good fibrous plant sources also contain healthy *lignans* and *phytoestrogens* that help balance hormone levels, and help the body make its own natural corticoids. Foods that contain these include peas, garbanzo beans, soybeans, kidney beans and lentils.

Plant-based foods provide these immune-stimulating factors because these vary same factors make up the plants' own immune systems. For example, the red, blue and green flavonoid pigments in plants and fruits help protect the plant from oxidative damage from radiation. The proanthocyanidins in grains like oats, for example, help protect the oat plant from crown rust caused by the *Puccinia coronata* fungus. So the same biochemicals that stimulate immunity in humans are part of plants' immune systems.

These same whole food phytonutrients also neutralize oxidative radicals in our bodies—the reason they are called antioxidants. How do we know this? Scientists can measure the ability of a particular food to neutralize free radicals with specific laboratory testing. One such test is called the *Oxygen Radical Absorbance Capacity Test* (ORAC). This technical laboratory study is performed by a number of scientific organizations that include the USDA, as well as specialized labs such as Brunswick Laboratories in Massachusetts.

Research from the USDA's Jean Mayer Human Nutrition Research Center on Aging at Tufts University has suggested that a diet high in ORAC value may protect blood vessels and tissues from free radical damage that can result in inflammation (Sofic *et al.* 2001; Cao *et al.* 1998). These tissues, of course, include the airways. Research has confirmed that consuming 3,000 to 5,000 ORAC units per day can have protective benefits.

ORAC Values (100 grams) of Selected (raw) Fruits (USDA, 2007-2008)

Cranberry	9,382		Pomegranate	2,860
Plum	7,581		Orange	1,819
Blueberry	6,552		Tangerine	1,620
Blackberry	5,347		Grape (red)	1,260
Raspberry	4,882		Mango	1,002
Apple (Granny)	3,898		Kiwi	882
Strawberry	3,577		Banana	879
Cherry (sweet)	3,365		Tomato (plum)	389
Gooseberry	3,277		Pineapple	385
Pear	2,941		Watermelon	142

There is tremendous attention these days on two unique fruits from the Amazon rain forest and China called *açaí* and *goji berry* (or wolfberry) respectively. A recent ORAC test documented by Schauss *et al.* (2006) gives açaí a score of 102,700 and tests documented by Dr. Paul Gross gives goji berries a total ORAC of 30,300. However, subsequent tests done by Brunswick Laboratories, Inc. gave these two berries 53,600 (açaí) and 22,000 (goji) total-ORAC values.

In addition, we must remember that these are the dried berries being tested in the latter case, and a concentrate of açaí being tested in the former case. The numbers in the chart above are for fresh fruits. Dried fruits will naturally have higher ORAC values, because the water is evaporated—giving more density and more antioxidants per 100 grams.

For example, in the USDA database, dried apples have a 6,681 total-ORAC value, while fresh apples range from 2,210 to 3,898 in total-ORAC value. This equates to a two-to-three times increase from fresh to dried. In another example, fresh red grapes have a 1,260 total-ORAC value, while raisins have a 3,037 total-ORAC value. This comes close to an increase of three times the ORAC value following dehydration.

Part of the equation, naturally, is cost. Dried fruit and concentrates are often more expensive than fresh fruit. High-ORAC dried fruits or concentrates from açaí or gogi will also be substantially more expensive than most fruits grown domestically (especially for Americans and Europeans). Our conclusion is that local or in-country grown fresh fruits with high total-ORAC values produce the best value. Local fresh fruit offers great free radical scavenging ability, support for local farmers, and pollen proteins we are most likely more tolerant to.

By comparison, spinach—an incredibly wholesome vegetable with a tremendous amount of nutrition—has a fraction of the ORAC content of some of these fruits, at 1,515 total ORAC. Spinach, of course, contains many other nutrients, including proteins lacking in many high-ORAC fruits.

Dehydrated spices can have incredibly high ORAC values. For example, USDA's database lists ground Turmeric's total ORAC value at 159,277 and oregano's at 200,129. However, while we might only consume a few hundred milligrams of a spice per day, we can eat many grams—if not pounds—of sweet colorful fruit every day.

Quercetin Foods

A number of foods and herbs that benefit allergies contain quercetin. This is no coincidence. Multiple studies have shown that quercetin inhibits the release inflammatory mediators histamine and leukotrienes. Foods rich in quercetin include onions, garlic, apples, capers, grapes, leafy greens, tomatoes and broccoli. In addition, many of the herbs listed earlier contain quercetin as an active constituent. Many of the herbs listed in the herbal section also contain quercetin. Onions, garlic and apples contain some of the highest levels.

Quercetin stimulates and balances the immune system. In an *in vivo* study, four weeks of quercetin reduced histamine levels and allergen-specific IgE levels. More importantly, quercetin inhibited anaphylaxis responses (Shishehbor *et al.* 2010).

Cairo researchers (Haggag *et al.* 2003) found that among mast cells exposed to allergens and chemicals in the laboratory, quercetin inhibited histamine release by 95% and 97%.

Over the past few years, an increasing amount of evidence is pointing to the conclusion that foods with quercetin slow inflammatory response and autoimmune derangement. Researchers from Italy's Catholic University (Crescente *et al.* 2009) found that quercetin inhibited arachidonic acid-induced platelet aggregation. Arachidonic acid-induced platelet aggregation is seen in allergic inflammatory mechanisms.

Researchers from the University of Crete (Alexandrakis *et al.* 2003) found that quercetin can inhibit mast cell proliferation by up to 80%. Onions have also been shown *in vivo* tests to reduce bronchoconstriction.

Organic foods contain higher levels of quercetin. A study from the University of California-Davis' Department of Food Science and Technology (Mitchell *et al.* 2007) tested flavonoid levels between organic and conventional tomatoes over a ten-year period. Their research concluded that quercetin levels were 79% higher for tomatoes grown organically under the same conditions as conventionally-grown tomatoes.

Root Foods

It is no coincidence that many of the herbs used for the airways—which we'll discuss more in the next chapter—have been roots, such as khella, ginger, turmeric, onions garlic and many others. In fact, herbalists have long recognized that roots tend to have many benefits for respiratory conditions.

The observation that particular plant portions tend to stimulate healing in certain parts of the body has been detailed in the *Doctrine of Signatures*. The concept of particular signatory plants and their benefits has been part of traditional medicine for centuries and recorded among various *Materia Medica*. The Swiss physician Paracelsus documented the concept for western medicine during the Sixteenth century.

Other root foods considered helpful for hypersensitivity include beets, carrots, turnips, parsnips and others. These root foods are known for their ability to alkalize the bloodstream and stimulate detoxification. They are also known to help rejuvenate the liver and adrenal glands.

Practical Antioxidant Strategies

We've seen the research that diets with a greater amount of fruits and vegetables—and antioxidants in general—can reduce allergic hypersensitivity and systemic inflammation. Does this mean that if we change our diet we will immediately get relief?

218

It is not that simple. Multiple issues should be considered along with nutrition, as we'll discuss further in this and coming chapters.

For one thing, nutrients lighten the body's inflammatory load, but do not eliminate it. For example, researchers from the Human Nutrition Research Center on Aging at Tufts University (Tucker *et al.* 2004) studied the relationships between homocysteine and B vitamins. They studied 189 healthy volunteers between 50 and 85 years old. They gave the subjects either one cup daily of fortified cereal (with 440 micrograms of folic acid, 1.8 milligrams of vitamin B-6, and 4.8 micrograms of vitamin B-12) or an unfortified cereal (placebo). After twelve weeks, the fortified cereal eaters had significantly less homocysteine levels than did the placebo cereal.

So while the cereal decreased the inflammatory load—illustrated by the reduction in homocysteine—it did not eliminate it. In fact, it is likely that while the inflammatory load was being decreased with the extra nutrients, the load was being added on by virtue of the sugar and milk in the cereal.

Do milk and eggs have any effect upon allergic hypersensitivity? Just consider research from Malaysia's University of Kebangsaan (Yusoff *et al.* 2004). The medical researchers studied the effects of avoiding eggs, milk and other dairy products in 22 children with asthma and allergies. After eight weeks of this single-blind study, 13 children eliminated the foods and 9 children did not.

After eight weeks, average anti-ovalbumin IgGs and anti-beta lactoglobulin IgG levels were significantly lower in the elimination group. Throughout the eight-week period, peak expiratory flows among the elimination group were significantly better. The researchers concluded: *"These results suggest that even over the short time period of eight weeks, an egg- and milk-free diet can reduce atopic symptoms and improve lung function in asthmatic children."*

In addition, research has found that diets high in processed salts stimulate more allergic hyperactivity, and as we've discussed at length, diets heavy in animal-based foods produce a number of acidic elements and free radicals that can increase systemic inflammation.

These foods, of course, form the backbone of the western diet. In other words, the western diet is a pro-inflammatory diet, and the plant-food oriented Mediterranean diet is an anti-inflammatory diet.

The question then simply becomes: How badly do we want to reverse our systemic inflammation and allergic symptoms? Enough to make some significant changes in our diet?

This dialog certainly contrasts to the allergy strategies promoted by western medicine: *Avoid all allergens, take all the medications, but don't worry about your diet.*

The Alkaline Diet

This discussion of nutrients should also include the reflective effects of a healthy diet: The proper acid-alkaline balance among the blood, urine and intercellular tissue regions. The reference to acidic or alkaline body fluids and tissues has been made by numerous natural health experts over the years. Is there any scientific validity to this?

Many nutritionists condemn an acidic metabolism and loosely call appropriate metabolism as a *state of alkalinity*. Strictly speaking, however, an alkaline environment is not healthy. The blood, interstitial fluids, lymph and urine should be *slightly acidic* to maintain the appropriate mineral ion balance. Let's dig into the science.

Acidity or alkalinity is measured using a logarithmic scale called pH. The term pH is derived from the French word *pouvoir hydrogene*, which means 'hydrogen power' or 'hydrogen potential.' pH is quantified by an inverse log base-10 scale. It measures the proton-donor level of a solution by comparing it to a theoretical quantity of hydrogen ions (H+) or H_3O+.

The scale is pH 1 to pH 14, which converts to a range of 10^{-1} (1) to 10^{-14} (.00000000000001) moles of hydrogen ions. This means that a pH of 14 maintains fewer hydrogen ions. It is thus *less acidic* and *more alkaline* (or basic).

The pH scale has been set up around the fact that water's pH is log-7 or simply pH 7—due to water's natural mineral content. Because pure water forms the basis for so many of life's activities, and because water neutralizes and dilutes so many reactions, water was established as the standard reference point or neutral point between what is considered an acid or a base solution. In other words, a substance having greater hydrogen ion potential (but lower pH) than water will be considered acidic, while a substance with less H+ potential (higher pH) than water is considered a base (alkaline).

Now the solution with a certain pH may not specifically maintain that many hydrogen ions. But it has the same *potential* as if it contained those hydrogen ions. That is why pH is hydrogen power or hydrogen potential.

In human blood, a pH level in the range of about 6.4 is considered healthy because this state is slightly more acidic than water, enabling the bodily fluids to maintain and transport minerals. It enables the *potential* for minerals to be carried by the blood, in other words. Minerals are critical to every cell, every organ, every tissue and every enzyme process occurring within the body. Better put, a 6.4 pH offers the appropriate *currency* of the body's fluids: This discourages acidosis and toxemia, maintaining a slight mineralized status.

Acidosis is produced with greater levels of carbonic acids, lactic acids, and/or uric acids among the joints and tissues. These acids are readily oxidizing, which produces free radicals. However, an overly alkaline state can precipitate waste products from cells, which also floods the system with radicals. For this reason, *toxemia* results from overly acidic blood and tissues or overly alkaline blood and tissues. In other words, pH *balance* is the key.

Ions from minerals like potassium, calcium, magnesium and others are usually positively oriented—with alkaline potential. But to be carried through a solution, the solution must have the pH potential to carry them.

Besides being critical to enzymatic reactions, these minerals bond with lipids and proteins to form the structures of our cells, organs and tissues—including our airways, nerves and mucosal membranes.

Natural health experts over the past century have observed among their patients and in clinical research that an overly acidic environment within the body is created by a diet abundant in refined sugars, processed foods, chemical toxins and amino acid-heavy animal foods. More recently, research has connected this acidic state to toxemia. The toxemia state is a state of free radical proliferation, which damages cells and tissues. It is also a state that produces systemic inflammation, because the immune system is over-worked as it tries to remove the cell and tissue damage.

As mentioned earlier, animals accumulate toxins within their fat tissues. They are bioaccumulators. Thus, animals exposed to the typical environmental toxins of smog and chemical pollutants in their waters and air—along with pesticides and herbicides from their foods—will accumulate those toxins within their fat cells and livers. And those who eat those animals will inherit (and further accumulate) these accumulated toxins. In addition, animals secrete significant waste matter as they are being slaughtered.

Plants are not bioaccumulators. While they can accumulate some pesticides and herbicide chemicals within their leaves and roots, they do not readily absorb or hold these for long periods within their cells. This is because many environmental toxins are, as mentioned, fat soluble. Because plants have little or no fat, they can more easily systemically rid their tissues of many of these toxins over time.

Further, as the research has shown, a diet heavy in complex proteins—which contain far more amino acids than our bodies require—increases the risk and severity of allergic hypersensitivity. Amino acids are the building blocks of protein. A complex protein can have tens of thousands of amino acids. While proteins and aminos are healthy, a diet too rich in them will produce deposits in our joints and tissues, burdening our immune system.

As we discussed in the last chapter, research also reveals that diets rich in red meats discourage the colonization of our probiotics, and encourage the growth of pathogenic microorganisms that release endotoxins that clog our metabolism and overload our immune system. Diets rich in red meats also produce byproducts such as phytanic acid and beta-glucuronidase that can damage our intestinal cells and mucosal membranes within the intestines. Greater levels of cooked saturated fats also raise cholesterol levels, especially lipid peroxidation-prone low-density lipoproteins (LDL).

The complexities of digesting complex proteins produce increased levels of beta-glucuronidase, nitroreductase, azoreductase, steroid 7-alpha-dehydroxylase, ammonia, urease, cholylglycine hydrolase, phytanic acid and others. These toxic enzymes deter our probiotics and produce systemic inflammation. Not surprisingly, they've been linked to colon cancer.

By contrast, plant-based foods contain many antioxidants, anti-carcinogens and other nutrients that strengthen the immune system and balance the body's pH. Plant-based foods also discourage inflammatory responses. Plant-based foods feed our probiotics with complex polysaccharides called prebiotics. They are also a source of fiber (there is little fiber in red meat)—critical for intestinal health.

Nutrition researchers from Portugal's University of Porto (Barros *et al.* 2008) studied the diets and asthma severity among 174 asthmatic adults. They used symptoms, lung function and exhaled nitric oxide to gauge asthma severity and control among the patients. After eliminating factors related to medications, age, sex, education and other factors; they found that those whose asthma was controlled had a 23% higher aMED Score (a diet score denoting higher intake of fruits, vegetables, fiber and healthy oils) and drank less alcohol—compared to more severe asthmatics.

They also found that significant adherence to the Mediterranean diet reduced the risk of uncontrolled asthmatic episodes by 78%. They concluded: *"High adherence to traditional Mediterranean diet increased the likelihood of asthma to be under control in adults."*

The Mediterranean diet does not completely eliminate meat, but it is focused on more plant-based foods, healthier oils and less red meat. However we configure our diet, there are choices we can make at every meal. The research shows that the greater our diet trends toward the Mediterranean diet, the lower our toxic load will be and the stronger our immunity will be. This will allow us to better combat and eventually lower systemic inflammation.

This also not a condemnation of dairy. Milk is a great food, assuming it contains what nature intended: probiotics. Real milk is inseparable from probiotics, and when probiotics are killed off by pasteurization, milk becomes a dubious food. We'll talk about this more later.

Anti-Allergic Fat Strategies

The types of fats we eat relate directly to allergic hypersensitivity because some fats are pro-inflammatory while others are anti-inflammatory—and allergies are an inflammatory condition. This doesn't mean that the pro-inflammatory fats are necessarily bad. Rather, we must have a *balance* of fats between the pro- and anti-inflammatory ones, with the balance trending towards the anti-inflammatory side.

The fat balance of our diet is also important because our cell membranes are made of different lipids and lipid-derivatives like phospholipids and glycolipids. An imbalanced fat diet therefore can lead to weak cell membranes, which leads to cells less protected and more prone to damage by oxidative radicals—and increased intestinal permeability.

Illustrating this, Danish researchers (Willemsen *et al.* 2008) tested the intestinal permeability/barrier integrity of incubated human intestinal epithelial cells with different dietary fats. (Remember the relationship between intestinal permeability and allergies verified by research given in the last chapter). The different fats included individual omega-6 oils linolenic acid (LA), gamma linolenic acid (GLA), DGLA, arachidonic acid (ARA); a blend of omega-3 oils alpha-linolenic acid (ALA), eicosapentaenoic acid (EPA), docohexaenoic acid (DHA); and a blend of fats similar to the composition of human breast milk fat.

The researchers found that the DGLA, ARA, EPA, DHA and GLA oils reduced interleukin-4 mediated intestinal permeability. LA and ALA did not. The blend with omega-3 oils, *"effectively supported barrier function,"* according to the researchers. They also concluded that DGLA, ARA, EPA and DHA—all long chain polyunsaturated fats—were *"particularly effective in supporting barrier integrity by improving resistance and reducing IL-4 mediated permeability."*

Certain fats also directly reduce allergic rhinitis. Researchers from the Technical University of Munich (Hoff *et al.* 2005) studied the diets of 568 adults and their serum levels of IgE. They also studied the cell membranes of the subjects—populated by the fatty acids provided by the diet.

They found that those with increased alpha-linolenic acid (ALA) in their diets were half as likely to have allergies, while those whose cell membranes had more eicosapentaenoic acid (EPA) were also about half as likely to have allergies and allergic rhinitis.

The processed oils in margarine are also problematic for asthmatic and allergic conditions. Researchers from the German Cancer Research Center in Heidelberg (Nagel and Linseisen 2005) studied 105 patients with asthma and allergies, matched with 420 healthy control subjects. The research found that heavy consumption of margarine increased the risk of adult-onset asthma and allergies by 73%.

So it is critical that we eat a balance of natural, unprocessed fatty acids. Here is a quick review of the major fatty acids and the foods they come from:

Major Omega-3 Fatty Acids (EFAs)

Acronym	Fatty Acid Name	Major Dietary Sources
ALA	Alpha-linolenic acid	Walnuts, soybeans, flax, canola, pumpkin seeds, chia seeds
SDA	Stearidonic acid	hemp, spirulina, blackcurrant
DHA	Docosahexaenoic acid	Body converts from ALA; also obtained from certain algae, krill and fish oils
EPA	Eicosapentaenoic acid	Converts in the body from DHA

Major Omega-6 Fatty Acids (EFAs)

Acronym	Fatty Acid Name	Major Dietary Sources
LA	Linoleic acid	Many plants, safflower, sunflower, sesame, soy, almond especially
ARA	Arachidonic acid	Meats, salmon
PA	Palmitoleic acid	Macadamia, palm kernel, coconut
GLA	Gamma-linolenic acid	Borage, primrose oil, spirulina

Major Omega-9 Fatty Acids

Acronym	Fatty Acid Name	Major Dietary Sources
EA	Eucic acid	Canola, mustard seed, wallflower
OA	Oleic acid	Sunflower, olive, safflower
PA	Palmitoleic acid	Macadamia, palm kernel, coconut

Major Saturated Fatty Acids

Acronym	Fatty Acid Name	Major Dietary Sources
Lauric	Lauric acid	Coconut, dairy, nuts
Myristic	Myristic acid	Coconut, butter
Palmitic	Palmitic acid	Macadamia, palm kernel, coconut, butter, beef, eggs
Stearic	Stearic acid	Macadamia, palm kernel, coconut, eggs

Essential fatty acids (EFAs) are fats the body does not form. Eaten in the right proportion, they can also lower inflammation and speed healing. EFAs include the long-chain polyunsaturated fatty acids—and the shorter chain linolenic, linoleic and oleic polyunsaturates. EFAs include omega-3s and omega-6s. The omega-3s include alpha linolenic acid (ALA), docosahexaenoic acid (DHA) and eicosapentaenoic acid (EPA). EPA and DHA are found in algae, mackerel, salmon, herring, sardines, sablefish (black cod). The omega-6s include linoleic acid, (LA), palmitoleic acid (PA), gamma-linoleic acid (GLA) and arachidonic acid (ARA). The term *essential* was originally given with the assumption that these types of fats could not be assembled or produced by the body—they must be taken directly from our food supply.

This assumption, however, is not fully correct. While it is true that we need *some* of these from our diet, our bodies can readily convert LA to ARA, and ALA to DHA and EPA as needed. Therefore, these fats can be considered essential in the sense that they are not generated by the body, but we do not necessarily have to consume each one of them.

Monounsaturated fats are high in omega-9 fatty acids like oleic acid. A monounsaturated fatty acid has one double carbon-hydrogen bonding chain. Oils from seeds, nuts and other plant-based sources have the largest quantities of monounsaturates. Oils that have large proportions of monounsaturates such as olive oil are known to lower inflammation when replacing high saturated fat in diets. Monounsaturates also aid in skin cell health and reduce atopic skin responses.

Monounsaturated fatty acids like oleic acid have been shown in studies to lower heart attack risk, aid blood vessel health, and offer anti-carcinogenic potential. They are typical among Mediterranean diets. The best sources of omega-9s are olives, sesame seeds, avocados, almonds, peanuts, pecans, pistachio nuts, cashews, hazelnuts, macadamia nuts, several other nuts and their respective oils.

Polyunsaturated fats have at least two double carbon-hydrogen bonds. They come from a variety of plant and marine sources. Omega-3s ALA, DHA and EPA simply have longer chains with more double carbon-hydrogen bonds. ALA, DHA and EPA are known to lower inflammation and increase artery-wall health. These *long-chain* omega-3 polyunsaturates are also considered critical for intestinal health.

The omega-6 fatty acids are the most available form of fat in the plant kingdom. Linoleic acid is the primary omega-6 fatty acid and it is found in most grains and seeds.

Saturated fats have multiple fatty acids without double bonds (the hydrogens "saturate" the carbons). They are found among animal fats, and tropical oils such as coconut and palm. Milk products such as butter and whole milk contain saturated fats, along with a special type of healthy linoleic fatty acid called CLA or *conjugated linoleic acid*.

The saturated fats from coconuts and palm differ from animal saturates in that they have shorter chains. This actually gives them—unlike animal saturates—an antimicrobial quality.

Trans fats are oils that either have been overheated or have undergone hydrogenation. Hydrogenation is produced by heating while bubbling hydrogen ions through the oil. This adds hydrogen and repositions some of the bonds. The "trans" refers to the positioning of part of the molecule in reverse—as opposed to "cis" positioning. The cis positioning is the bonding orientation the body's cell membranes work best with. Trans fats have been known to be a cause for increased radical species in the system; damaging artery walls; contributing to inflammation, heart disease, high LDL levels, liver damage, diabetes, and other metabolic dysfunction (Mozaffarian *et al.* 2009). Trans fat overconsumption slows the conversion of LA to GLA.

Conjugated linolenic acid (CLA) is a healthy fat that comes from primarily from dairy products. CLA is also a trans fat, but this is a trans fat the body works well with—it is considered a healthy trans fat.

Researchers from St Paul's Hospital and the University of British Columbia (MacRedmond *et al.* 2010) gave 28 overweight adults with milk-related asthma 4.5 g/day of CLA or a placebo for 12 weeks in addition to their conventional asthma treatment. After the twelve weeks, those in the CLA group experienced significantly reduced airway hyperreactivity compared to the beginning of treatment and compared to the placebo group. The CLA group also experienced a significant reduction of weight and BMI compared with the control group. The CLA group also had lower leptin/adiponectin ratios—associated with balanced metabolism.

Arachidonic acid (ARA): The science and research on arachidonic acid was discussed in the previous chapter. ARA is considered an essential fatty acid, and research has shown that it is vital for infants while they are building their intestinal barriers. However, as we discussed, ARA is pro-inflammatory and stimulates inflammatory mediators like leukotrienes and histamines. While ARA is healthy for children, and we do need ARA, too much of it as we age burdens our immune systems, pushing our bodies towards hypersensitivity.

As we discussed, ARA content is highest in red meats, oily fish, fried foods and processed foods. Plant-based foods contain little or no ARA.

Interestingly, carnivorous animals cannot or do not readily convert linoleic acid (found in many common plants) to arachidonic acid, but herbivore animals do convert linoleic acid to arachidonic acid, as do humans. This conversion—on top of a red meat-heavy diet—results in high arachidonic acid levels for red-meat heavy diets. In contrast, a diet that is balanced between plant-based monounsaturates, polyunsaturates and some saturates (such as the Mediterranean diet) will balance arachidonic acids with the other fatty acids.

Gamma linoleic acid (GLA): As mentioned earlier, a wealth of studies have confirmed that GLA reduces or inhibits the inflammatory response. Leukotrienes produced by arachidonic acid stimulate inflammation, while leukotrienes produced by GLA block the conversion of polyunsaturated fatty acids to arachidonic acid. This means that GLA lowers inflammation.

A healthy body will convert linoleic acid into GLA readily, utilizing the same delta-6 desaturase enzyme used for ALA to DHA conversion.

From GLA, the body produces *dihomo-gamma linoleic acid,* which cycles through the body as an eicosinoid. This aids in skin health, healthy mucosal membranes, and down-regulates inflammatory hypersensitivity.

In addition to conversion from LA, GLA can also be obtained from the oils of borage seeds, evening primrose seed, hemp seed, and from spirulina. Excellent food sources of LA include chia seeds, seed, hempseed, grapeseed, pumpkin seeds, sunflower seeds, safflower seeds, soybeans, olives, pine nuts, pistachio nuts, peanuts, almonds, cashews, chestnuts, and their respective oils.

The conversion of LA to GLA (and ALA to DHA) is reduced by trans fat consumption, smoking, pollution, stress, infections, and various chemicals that affect the liver.

Docosahexaenoic acid (DHA), obtained from algae, fish and krill, has significant therapeutic and anti-inflammatory effects according to the research.

Researchers from the University of Southampton School of Medicine (Kremmyda *et al.* 2009) studied the connection between DHA and allergies. They investigated five epidemiological studies that associated fish consumption during pregnancy and allergic outcomes of their children. They found that studies have indicated that some protection is afforded by the pregnant mother's fish or fish oil consumption, to reduce levels of hay fever and asthma. However, there were mixed results regarding lasting protection. DHA supplementation during infancy may decrease the risk of developing some allergies, but any lasting therapeutic benefits are still unclear according to the research.

Researchers from Germany's Research Center for Environmental Health (Schnappinger *et al.* 2009) studied fatty acids and allergies among 388 adults. RAST results found that those with higher DHA supplementation or fish consumption had nearly 75% less incidence of allergies. This, however, occurred among the women and not the men. The researchers attributed this to better fatty acid metabolism among women.

It appears that the anti-inflammatory effects of DHA in particular relate to a modulation of a gene factor called NF-kappaB. The NF-kappaB is involved in signaling among cytokine receptors. With more DHA consumption, the transcription of the NF-kappaB gene sequence is reduced. This appears to reduce inflammatory signaling (Singer *et al.* 2008).

DHA readily converts to EPA by the body. EPA degrades quickly if unused in the body. It is easily converted from DHA as needed. Our bodies store DHA and not EPA.

Because much of the early research on the link between fatty acids and inflammatory disease was performed using fish oil, it was assumed that both EPA and DHA fatty acids reduced inflammation. Recent research from the University of Texas' Department of Medicine/Division of Clinical Immunology and Rheumatology (Rahman *et al.* 2008) has clarified that DHA is primarily implicated in reducing inflammation. DHA was shown to inhibit RANKL-induced pro-inflammatory cytokines, and a number of inflammation steps, while EPA did not.

The process of converting ALA to DHA and other omega-3s requires an enzyme produced in the liver called delta-6 desaturase. Some people—especially those who have a poor diet, are immune-suppressed, or burdened with toxicity such as cigarette smoke—may not produce this enzyme very well. As a result, they may not convert as much ALA to DHA and EPA.

For those with low levels of DHA—or for those with problems converting ALA and DHA—low-environmental impact and low toxin content DHA from microalgae can be supplemented. Certain algae produce significant amounts of DHA. They are the foundation for the DHA molecule all the way up the food chain, including fish. This is how fish get their DHA, in other words. Three algae species—*Crypthecodinium cohnii, Nitzschia laevis* and *Schizochytrium spp.*—are in commercial production and available in oil and capsule form.

Microalgae-derived DHA is preferable to fish or fish oils because fish oils typically contain saturated fats and may also—depending upon their origin—contain toxins such as mercury and PCBs (though to their credit, many producers also carefully distill their fish oil). However, we should note that salmon contain a considerable amount of arachidonic acid as well (Chilton 2006). And finally, algae-derived DHA does not strain fishery populations.

One study (Arterburn *et al.* 2007) measured pro-inflammatory arachidonic acid levels within the body before and after supplementation with algal DHA. It was found that arachidonic acid levels decreased by 20% following just one dose of 100 milligrams of algal DHA.

In a study by researchers from The Netherlands' Wageningen University Toxicology Research Center (van Beelen *et al.* 2007), all three species of commercially produced algal oil showed equivalency with fish oil in their inhibition of cancer cell growth. Another study (Lloyd-Still *et al.* 2007) of twenty cystic fibrosis patients concluded that 50 milligrams of algal DHA was readily absorbed, maintained DHA bioavailability immediately, and increased circulating DHA levels by four to five times.

In terms DHA availability, algal-DHA is just as good as fish. In a randomized open-label study (Arterburn *et al.* 2008), researchers gave 32 healthy men and women either algal DHA oil or cooked salmon for two weeks. After the two weeks, plasma levels of circulating DHA were bio-equivalent.

Alpha-linolenic acid (ALA) is the primary omega-3 fatty acid the body can most easily assimilate. Once assimilated, the healthy body will convert ALA to omega-3s, primarily DHA, at a range of about 7-40%, depending upon the health of the liver. One study of six women performed at England's University of Southampton (Burdge *et al.* 2002) showed a conversion rate of 36% from ALA to DHA and other omega-3s. A follow-up study of men showed ALA conversion to the omega-3s occurred at an average of 16%.

We should include that ALA, which comes from plants, has been shown to halt or slow inflammation processes, similar to DHA. In fact, we discussed a study earlier from the Technical University of Munich (Hoff *et al.* 2005) that showed that a diet with higher levels of ALA decreased allergy incidence by about half among their large study population.

In addition, studies at Wake Forest University (Chilton *et al.* 2008) showed that ALA-rich flaxseed oil produced anti-inflammatory effects, along with borage oil and echium oil (the latter two also containing GLA).

Furthermore, we probably should mention that flaxseed has been recommended specifically for respiratory ailments by traditional herbalists for centuries. This is not only because of its omega-3 levels: it is also because flaxseed contains mucilage, which helps strengthen our mucosal membranes.

The healthy fat balance: In a meta-study by researchers from the University of Crete's School of Medicine (Margioris 2009), numerous studies showed that long-chain polyunsaturated omega-3s tend to be anti-inflammatory while omega-6 oils tend to be pro-inflammatory.

This, however, simplifies the equation too much. Most of the research on fats has also shown that most omega-6s are healthy oils. Balance is the key. Let's look at the research:

Researchers from the University of Colorado School of Medicine (Covar *et al.* 2010) gave a nutritional formula enriched with eicosapentaenoic acid (EPA) and gamma-linolenic fatty acid (GLA) together with antioxidants or a placebo to 43 children with asthma between the ages of six and fourteen. After twelve weeks, the fatty acid formula group had more asthma-free days. Those on the fatty acid formula also exhaled lower nitric oxide levels, and had better forced expiratory volume (FEV1) levels than the placebo group as well. PBMC cells showed increase anti-inflammatory activity among the treated group, as well as lower disease biomarkers in general.

Research has also illustrated that reducing animal-derived saturated fats reduces inflammation, cardiovascular disease, high cholesterol and diabetes (Ros and Mataix 2008). What should replace the saturated fat consumption, however?

The relationships became clearer from a study performed at Sydney's Heart Research Institute (Nicholls *et al.* 2008). Here fourteen adults consumed meals either rich in saturated fats or omega-6 polyunsaturated fats. They were tested following each meal for various inflammation and cholesterol markers. The results showed that the high saturated fat meals increased inflammatory activities and decreased the liver's production of HDL cholesterol; whereas (good) HDL levels and the liver's anti-inflammatory capacity were increased after the omega-6 meals.

What this tells us is that the omega-3/omega-6 story is complicated by the saturated fat content of the diet and subsequent liver function. High saturated fat diets increase (bad) LDL (lipid peroxidation) content and reduce the anti-inflammatory and antioxidant capacities of the liver. Diets lower in saturated fat and higher in omega-6 and omega-3 fats encourage antioxidant and anti-inflammatory activity.

We also know that diets high in monounsaturated fats—such as the Mediterranean diet—are also associated with significant anti-inflammatory effects. Mediterranean diets contain higher levels of monounsaturated fats like oleic acids (omega-9) from foods like olives and avocados (and their oils); as well as higher proportions of fruits and vegetables, and lower proportions of saturated fats.

High saturated fat diets are also associated with increased obesity, and a number of studies have shown that obesity is directly related to inflammatory diseases—including allergies as we've discussed. High saturated fat diets and diets high in trans fatty acids have also been clearly shown to accompany higher levels of inflammation—illustrated by increases in inflammatory factors such as IL-6 and CRP (Basu *et al.* 2006).

To maximize anti-inflammatory factors, the ideal proportion of omega-6s to omega-3s is recommended at about two to one (2:1). The western diet has been estimated by researchers to up to thirty to one (30:1) of omega-6s to omega-3s. This large imbalance (of too much omega-6s and too little omega-3s) has also been associated with inflammatory diseases, including allergies, asthma, arthritis, heart disease, ulcerative colitis, Crohn's disease, and others. When fat consumption is out of balance, the body's metabolism will trend towards inflammation. This is because in the absence of omega-3s and GLA, omega-6 oils convert more easily to arachidonic acid. Remember also that ARA is pro-inflammatory (Simopoulos 1999).

Noting the research showing the relationships between the different fatty acids and inflammation, and the condition of the liver (which can be burdened by too much saturated fat), scientists have logically arrived at a model for dietary fat consumption for a person who is either dealing with or wants to prevent inflammation-oriented conditions such as allergies:

Omega-3	20%-25% of dietary fats
Omega-6+Omega-9	40%-50% of dietary fats
Saturated	5%-10% of dietary fats
GLA	10%-20% of dietary fats
Trans fats	0% of dietary fats

Nuts, seeds, grains, beans, olives and avocados can provide the bulk of these healthy fats in balanced combinations. Walnuts, pumpkin seeds, flax, chia, soy, canola and algal-DHA can fill in the omega 3s. Healthy saturated fats can be found in coconuts, palm and dairy products. These foods are typical of the Mediterranean diet.

The Importance of Raw Foods

Most nutrients are heat-sensitive. Vitamin C, fat-soluble vitamins A, E and B vitamins are reduced during pasteurization. Many fatty acids are transformed by high heat to unhealthy fats. Important plant nutrients, such as anthocyanins and polyphenols, are also reduced during pasteurization, along with various enzymes. Proteins are denatured or broken down when heated for long. While this can aid in amino acid absorption, it can also form unrecognized peptide combinations. In milk, for example, some of the nutritious whey protein, or lactabumin, will denature into a number of peptide combinations that are not readily absorbed.

A 2008 study on strawberry puree from the University of Applied Sciences in Switzerland showed a 37% reduction in vitamin C and a significant loss in antioxidant potency after pasteurization. A 1998 study from Brazil's Universidade Estadual de Maringa determined that Barbados cherries lost about 14% of their vitamin C content after pasteurization. During heat treatment, vitamin C will also convert to dehydroascorbic acid together with a loss of bioflavonoids.

A 2008 study at Spain's Cardenal Herrera University determined that glutathione peroxidase—an important antioxidant contained in milk—was significantly reduced by pasteurization. In 2006, the University also released a study showing that lysine content was significantly decreased by milk pasteurization. A 2005 study at the Universidade Federal do Rio Grande determined that pasteurizing milk reduced vitamin A (retinol) content from an average of 55 micrograms to an average of 37 micrograms. A study at North Carolina State University in 2003 determined that HTST pasteurization significantly reduced conjugated linoleic acid (CLA) content—an important fatty acid in milk shown to reduce cancer and encourage good fat metabolism.

A 2006 study on bayberries at the Southern Yangtze University determined that plant antioxidants such as anthocyanins and polyphenolics were reduced from 12-32% following UHT pasteurization. Polyphenols, remember, are the primary nutrients in fruits and vegetables that render anti-carcinogenic and antioxidant effects.

One of the most important losses from pasteurization is its enzyme content. Diary and plant foods contain a variety of enzymes that aid in the assimilation or catalyzing of nutrients and antioxidants. These include xanthenes, lysozymes, lipases, oxidases, amylases, lactoferrins and many others contained in raw foods. The body uses food enzymes in various ways. Some enzymes, such as papain from papaya and bromelain from pineapples, dissolve artery plaque and reduce inflammation. While the body makes many of its own enzymes, it also absorbs many food enzymes or uses their components to make new ones.

Pasteurization also typically leaves the food or beverage with a residual caramelized flavor due to the conversation of the enzymes, flavonoids and sugars to other compounds. In milk, for example, there is a substantial conversion from lactose to lactulose (and caramelization) after UHT pasteurization. Lactulose has been shown to cause intestinal cramping, nausea and vomiting.

In the case of pasteurized juices, pasteurization can turn the alkaline nature of what comes from fruits and vegetables acidic. This pH change can alter the state of our mucous membranes.

As for irradiation, there is little research on the resulting nutrient content outside of a few microwave studies (which showed decreased nutrient content and the formation of undesirable metabolites). There is good reason to believe that irradiation may thus denature some nutrients.

Whole foods in nature's packages are significantly different from pasteurized processed foods. Fresh whole foods produced by plants contain various antioxidants and enzymes that reduce the ability of microorganisms to grow. The Creator also provided whole foods with peels and shells that protect nutrients and keep most microorganisms out. Microorganisms may invade the outer shell or peel somewhat, but the peel's pH, dryness and density—together with the pH of the inner fruit—provide extremely effective barriers to microorganisms and oxidation.

For this reason, most fruits and nuts can be easily stored for days and even weeks without having significant nutrient reduction. Once the peel or shell is removed, the inner fruit, juice or nut must be consumed to prevent oxidation and contamination—depending upon its pH and sugar content.

Whole natural foods also contain polysaccharides and oligosaccharides that combine nutrients and sugar within complex fibers. These combinations also help prevent oxidation and pathogenic bacteria colonization. With heat processing, however, the sugars are broken down into more simplified, refined form, which allows microbial growth and oxidation. Why? Because simple sugars provide convenient energy sources for aggressive bacteria and fungi colonies. By contrast, our probiotics are used to eating the complexed oligosaccharides in fibrous foods. In other words, heat-processing produces the perfect foods for pathogenic microorganism colonization.

As we discussed in the last chapter, pathogenic microorganisms provide the fuel for systemic inflammation. They can infect the body's (and airways') tissues directly, and/or their endotoxins—waste products—stream into our bloodstream to max out our immune system and detoxification processes. This causes systemic inflammation, and of course, allergic hypersensitivity.

Raw vs. Pasteurized Milk

Remember the asthma/allergy study by researchers at Switzerland's University of Basel (Waser *et al.* 2007). The researchers studied 14,893 children between the ages of five and 13 from five different European countries, including 2,823 children from farms, and 4,606 children attending a Steiner School (known for its farm-based living and instruction). The researchers found that drinking farm milk was associated with decreased incidence of allergies and asthma. In other words, the raw milk was found to be the largest single determinant of this reduced asthma and allergy incidence among farm children. Why?

Raw milk from the cow can contain a host of bacteria, including *Lactobacillus acidophilus*, *L. casei*, *L. bulgaricus* and many other healthy probiotics. Cows that feed from primarily grasses will have increased levels of these healthy probiotics. This is because a grass diet provides prebiotics that promote the cow's own probiotic colonies. A diet of primarily dried grass and dried grains will reduce probiotic counts and increase pathogenic bacteria counts. As a result, most non-grass fed herds must be given lots of antibiotics to help keep their bacteria counts low. Probiotics, on the other hand, naturally keep bacteria counts down.

As a result, the non-grass fed cow's milk will have higher pathogenic bacteria counts than grass-fed cows. This means that the milk itself will also have high counts. When the non-grass-fed cow's milk is pasteurized, the heat kills most of these bacteria. The result is milk containing dead pathogenic bacteria parts. These are primarily proteins and peptides, which get mixed with the milk and are eventually consumed with the milk.

In other words, pasteurization may kill the living pathogenic bacteria, but it does not get rid of the bacteria proteins. This might be compared to cooking an insect: If an insect landed in our soup, we could surely cook it until it died. But the soup would still contain the insect parts—and proteins.

Now the immune system of most people, and especially infants with their hypersensitive immune system, is trained to attack and discard pathogenic bacteria. And how does the body identify pathogenic bacteria? From their proteins.

In the case of pasteurized commercial milk, our immune systems will readily identify heat-killed microorganism cell parts and proteins and launch an immune response against these proteins as if it were being attacked by the microorganisms directly. This was shown in research from the University of Minnesota two decades ago (Takahashi *et al.* 1992).

It is thus not surprising that weak immune systems readily reject pasteurized cow's milk. In comparison, healthy cow raw milk has fewer pathogenic microorganisms and more probiotic organisms. This has been confirmed by tests done by a California organic milk farm, which compared test results of their raw organic milk against standardized state test results from conventional milk farms.

In addition, pasteurization breaks apart or denatures many of the proteins and sugar molecules. This was illustrated by researchers from Japan's Nagasaki International University (Nodake *et al.* 2010), who found that when beta-lactoglobulin is naturally conjugated with dextran-glycylglycine, its allergenicity is decreased. A dextran is a very long chain of glucose molecules—a polysaccharide. The dextran polysaccharide is naturally joined with the amino acid glycine in raw state. When pasteurized, beta-lactoglobulin is separated.

This is not surprising. Natural whole cow's milk also contains special polysaccharides called oligosaccharides. They are largely indigestible polysaccharides that feed our intestinal bacteria. Because of this trait, these indigestible sugars are called prebiotics.

Whole milk contains a number of these oligosaccharides, including oligogalactose, oligolactose, galactooligosaccharides (GOS) and transgalactooligosaccharides (TOS). Galactooligosaccharides are produced by conversion from enzymes in healthy cows and healthy mothers.

These polysaccharides provide a number of benefits. Not only are they some of the more preferred foods for probiotics: Research has also shown that they reduce the ability of pathogenic bacteria like *E. coli* to adhere to our intestinal cells.

These oligosaccharides also provide environments that reduce the availability of separated beta-lactoglobulin. This is accomplished through a combination of probiotic colonization and the availability of the long-chain polysaccharides that keep these complexes stabilized.

This reduced availability of beta-lactoglobulin has been directly observed in humans and animals following consistent supplementation with probiotics (Taylor *et al.* 2006; Adel-Patient *et al.* 2005; Prioult *et al.* 2003).

It is not surprising, given the information that people with allergies often benefit simply from withdrawing from pasteurized milk and cheese. Raw milk, yogurt, kefir, goat's milk and cheese, along with soy and almond milk are great alternatives.

Healthy Cooking

While raw whole foods are often more wholesome to the body, some foods must be cooked to make them more digestible. These include most grains, beans, and some vegetables. Our section on Chinese medicine in the next chapter will illustrate that some herbs require cooking to eliminate certain alkaloids.

The question is: how much cooking and processing do we need to do to our foods? How much cooking is necessary? Yes, cooking some foods often increases their digestibility. This is particularly important with grain-based foods and beans. Cooking these foods will help break down their fibers and complex carbohydrates into more digestible forms.

Also, many vegetables are more assimilable when they are cooked— or even better, steamed. Steaming vegetables in a pot with a covered lid will preserve most nutrients, while softening some of fibers that hold the nutrients. Foods such as beets, asparagus, broccoli, rhubarb, squash and many others are delicious and nutritious after being steamed or lightly boiled in clean water.

Other plant foods are best eaten raw. These include lettuce, cucumbers, avocado, onions and many others. Because the nutrients in these foods are not so tightly bound within the cell walls of the plants, they can be destroyed by the heat and/or easily separated during cooking.

While the cell walls of plants do contain nutrients, they must be broken down during mastication and digestion. Some cell walls are tougher than others are, and require cooking or processing to break their cell walls. Chlorella—a blue-green algae—is a good example. Many nutrients in chlorella are bound within tightly-packed cell walls, so chlorella is more nutritious when the cell walls have been broken prior to ingestion.

A healthy diet strikes a balance between raw and cooked foods. A perfect way to accomplish this is a dinner that includes a salad topped with seeds, yogurt, olive oil and apple cider vinegar; and an entrée of cooked grains and/or beans with a nice sauce spiced with antioxidant herbs. Breakfast and lunch can include fresh fruit, nuts, raw cheese and fermented dairy; with lightly cooked grains such as oats and barley. Snacks can go raw with apples, nuts, raisins and seeds for sustained, slow-digesting energy and essential fats.

A plant-based food diet can be extremely creative and varied. It can also be extremely colorful and exotic. This is because there are so many different foods and spices to choose from. A flip through a Mediterranean diet cookbook will confirm this immediately.

Note also that eating or drinking extremely cold foods is not advisable for hypersensitivity. This means that water and drinks are better at room temperature or slightly cool—but never with ice. This also means that ice cream, snow cones, frozen yogurts and other such "foods" should be avoided (not to mention their grotesque refined sugar levels).

Adding Anti-inflammatory Spices to Our Meals

We can also spice our cooked foods with excellent and flavorful anti-inflammatory herbs. We discussed a number of herbs earlier that research has shown will reduce inflammation and strengthen the immune system. As a reminder, these include:

➢ Ginger (*Zingiber officinalis*)
➢ Cayenne (*Capiscium frutescens* or *Capiscium annum*)
➢ Turmeric (*Curcuma longa*)
➢ Basil (*Osimum basilicum*)
➢ Rosemary (*Rosmarinus officinalis*)
➢ Oregano (*Origanum vulgare*)
➢ Reishi mushroom (*Ganoderma spp.*)
➢ Garlic (*Allium sativum*)
➢ Onions (*Allium cepa L.*)

It should be noted that there is a great difference between a spice dose and a therapeutic dose. A therapeutic dose of one or more of these spices will typically be larger than a spice dose. The sign of a therapeutic dose of these spices within a dish is when the spice can be readily tasted. That is, the pungent flavor of the spice stands out in the food. If the amount of spice simply flavors the food a little, then it will probably not be enough to stimulate any immune response. If the spice can be specifically tasted (for example, *"that dish tastes garlicy"* or *"tastes peppery"*) then the spice will likely be enough to stimulate a therapeutic response.

That said, if multiple spices are used, the dose of each spice can be smaller. After all, the meal should also taste good. This, however, is why traditional Chinese and Indian food is so spicy. The recipes come from therapeutic traditions.

Another element of the therapeutic dose is consistency. It is not enough to have one or more of these spices once a week with a particular dish. The spice(s) should be added to at least one meal every day.

In addition, care must be taken to protect therapeutic spices from degradation. This can occur when spices are left in the light or sun for an extended period, or when spices are left open to oxygen. Often spices are left in kitchen racks exposed to the lights of the kitchen and window, or left in unsealed containers or shakers. Oxygen and light degrade the biochemical constituents that give these spices their therapeutic properties.

This latter point is likely one of the main reasons our culinary spices cannot be considered therapeutic. Leaving the spice exposed can take place during processing, packaging and shipping; as well as in the kitchen. Therefore, we should consider purchasing our therapeutic spices from a bulk herb store, or from suppliers or brands that respect their therapeutic nature.

By far the best way to consume or add these foods to our diet is in their fresh form. Many of these herbs can be grown in our garden or purchased from a local farmers' market or grocery store as fresh. As discussed earlier, fresh foods maintain more bioactive nutrients. This is because their beneficial constituents are naturally sealed within the food's peel, shell or cell walls.

Note also that these anti-inflammatory herbal spices (and most of the other natural products contained in this chapter) will typically not stimulate a therapeutic response immediately. Depending upon the status of our immune system, it may take weeks or months before the daily dosing of these natural elements is seen in the form of modulating the immune response.

Anti-Allergy Nutritional Supplement Strategies

A strategy to boost the immune system with a variety of plant-based fresh foods of sufficient quantity may require supplementation. Even if we eat only organically-grown foods and/or foods grown in healthy soils, we could still be deficient in some nutrients. This is because over the last century, our soils have slowly been eroded by a combination of chemical fertilizers, commercial farming, run-off, and acidification from pollution.

What this all means is that even the best diet may be lacking in some nutrients.

We may be eating a narrow range of foods and/or exposed to a significant amount of toxins or infections. In other words, because toxins and infections 'burn up' nutrients and antioxidants—as the body requires these to neutralize radicals and produce enzymes—a person with systemic inflammation living in a toxic modern environment will likely require more nutrients than a healthy person living in a natural environment.

There are a number of isolated nutrients that have been shown to help allergies and asthma. A few, like vitamins C, A, D, and E and others have been shown to reduce inflammation by modulating inflammatory mediators and balancing Th1 and Th2—to help reduce hypersensitivity

(Mainardi *et al.* 2009). Others, such as selenium—as we discussed in the last chapter—directly relate to the liver's glutathione processes for reducing toxins and radicals.

At the same time, nutritional supplement research has been plagued with inconsistent data. Why is this? Some studies show results while others have contradicted those results. Why is this?

The problem is that only some—but not all—hypersensitivities are caused by, complicated by, and/or worsened by deficiencies in certain nutrients. When a person's diet is lacking in an important nutrient, the body sometimes responds with critical weaknesses in immunity and inflammation. This can, for those prone to hypersensitivity, produce the potential for allergic response.

Many people are deficient in some or many nutrients, depending upon their diet. Even people who regularly take multi-vitamins become deficient in some nutrients. Why is this? This is an extremely complicated subject—one that could take an entire book to fully explore. To summarize, there are a number of reasons why people don't get the nutrients their body needs. These range from the more obvious—of poor diet choices—to the less obvious—of not being able to absorb certain nutrients due to enzyme issues, probiotic deficiencies and/or intestinal defects.

As has been shown in a number of studies, especially regarding B vitamins, a person may take a good multivitamin yet still be deficient because they lack the intrinsic factors that help assimilate those nutrients. In other cases, there is a chelation problem, where the nutrient is not absorbed because it doesn't have the right intestinal biofactors available within either the diet or the intestines. In still other cases, a nutrient may not be in a form that the body recognizes. This is often the case with synthetic multivitamins. In some cases, the body might treat the particular nutrient as a foreign molecule, and possibly even decide to break it down and expel it.

For those who are deficient in one or more nutrients, a good supplement source or change in the diet can immediately help their inflammatory hypersensitivity. Yet for those not deficient in that nutrient or nutrients, supplementing the same nutrient will offer little benefit for their condition.

In other words, if a person is not deficient in the nutrient, taking more of the nutrient will likely not help them at all. Furthermore, overloading on isolated nutrients that have been shown to help those who are deficient can lead to a worsening of inflammation. This is due to the fact that synthesized, isolated nutrients can overload our livers and detoxification systems, as they are metabolized. Some vitamins, such as vitamin A, can be directly toxic if over-supplemented. The bottom line is that for the most part, more is not necessarily better when it comes to nutrients.

So it is essential that we engage in a supplement strategy very logically. First, we need to have a healthy amount of plant-based foods in our diet, with raw, fresh foods with plenty of fiber and phytonutrients. This will create a solid foundation.

Secondly, we can add a food-based multivitamin as a sort of insurance policy to make sure we get enough of the most important nutrients. A food-based multivitamin is one where the nutrients are sourced directly from foods, or grown on food substrates such as spirulina. These sorts of multivitamins are more recognized by the body's processes and immune system.

Thirdly, we can pay closer attention to certain nutrients that have been shown in some research to decrease the severity or incidence of allergy episodes. For these nutrients, we may decide to take a focused combination or isolated nutrient. But here we need to understand that many isolated nutrients can imbalance our body and create other deficiencies. Therefore, we need to approach isolated nutrient supplementation with caution. Best to err on the side of nature's balance of whole food sources, in other words.

For example, if we are taking more vitamin C, we can use a food-based or mineral ascorbate vitamin C supplement that offers chelated versions, and bioflavonoids that help the body assimilate and utilize the vitamin C.

If we are taking a mineral supplement like magnesium, we can take one that offers a chelated version together with calcium and trace minerals—offered by coral or mined sources, for example. The point here is that taking excess magnesium without the supporting and balancing minerals can exhaust the body of calcium, zinc and other essential, supporting elements.

We can also consult with a nutritionally-oriented health professional who can test our body's nutrient levels. Tests range from urine tests to blood tests and hair analyses—the latter of which may be appropriate to establish cellular mineral levels (Wilson 1998). This can be very helpful when trying to determine if we have a particular nutrient deficiency.

With that said, let's discuss a few nutrients and their relationship with allergies and asthma. Most of these first nutrients have been well-researched for their effects over the past few decades and need little support or reference:

Choline: Choline is a B vitamin that has in some research, been shown to help reduce allergy and asthma severity and frequency. High doses tested have been in the range of three grams per day.

Magnesium: We discuss magnesium in a separate section later that includes other minerals. Magnesium supplements have been shown in some research to specifically benefit allergies and asthma. Other research has shown intravenous magnesium to be effective for asthma episode emergency treatment.

Omega-3 fatty acids: We illustrated the full breadth of fatty acid foods previously. It is important to have a balance of fatty acids, rather than to just eat a poor fatty food diet and then simply add a DHA or ALA supplement on top. Note that one study found fish oil may not be good for aspirin-allergic asthma. Algae-sourced DHA supplements provide an effective way to supply mercury-free and pollution-free DHA.

Quercetin: We also discussed quercetin foods previously. Quercetin supplements may be appropriate if the diet is lacking in plant-based foods. As mentioned earlier, this flavonoid inhibits histamine and leukotrienes—inflammatory mediators—in the body.

Selenium: Research has suggested that many asthmatics tend to be deficient in selenium, as discussed earlier. Selenium supplements have been shown to help reduce allergy symptoms as well. While selenium supplements might offer generous amounts, one brazil nut will supply about 120 micrograms of selenium. This is 170% of the recommended daily value.

Vitamin C is considered by researchers as one of the "first line of defense" antioxidants, because it is readily available to neutralize free radicals at mucosal membranes and tissue fluids. A number of studies have shown that vitamin C can lower histamine and leukotriene levels.

Vitamin C supplement doses typically range from one to three grams per day. As mentioned, chelated versions and versions with bioflavonoids help the potency of vitamin C. Some health researchers have also noted that vitamin C and quercetin tend to work well together. This is why apples and onions are so healthy. While fruits and many vegetables offer readily-assimilable doses of vitamin C with bioflavonoids, vitamin C drink powders with chelated ascorbates also provide a good way to supplement extra vitamin C.

Coenzyme Q10 (CoQ10): Many health proponents swear by CoQ10, but there is little research to confirm that CoQ10 can reduce allergy or asthma symptoms. Furthermore, many plant foods and other foods contain CoQ10. CoQ10 stimulates mitochondria activities, which can help support immunity.

Lycopene: This phytonutrient, usually isolated from tomatoes, has been shown in some research to reduce allergies and asthma hypersensitivity.

Beta-carotene and other Carotenoids: These vitamin A precursors are essential antioxidants often lacking in many diets. Some research has shown that carotenoids can prevent exercise-induced asthma and allergies.

Vitamin E: Vitamin E supplementation has been shown to help prevent cardiovascular and respiratory diseases. A few studies have shown inconclusive findings, however. One note to make about this is that there are several types of tocopherols and tocotrienols, and many vitamin E supplements are limited to one or two types. Subsequent study has shown that combinations of multiple tocopherols and tocotrienols have significant benefit. This means combinations of tocopherols and tocotrienols obtained from whole foods (grains and palms have high levels) or their derived supplements. The bottom line is that the E vitamins are essential antioxidants that help prevent lipid peroxidation.

B Vitamins: B vitamins, especially B6 and B12, are key factors as the body deals with toxins and medications—such as theophylline, which has produced B6 deficiencies. This is because most B vitamins donate *methyl* groups, used to neutralize radicals in the bloodstream.

For people with intrinsic factor problems, the assimilation of B vitamins may be difficult. For this reason, the injection of B vitamins has been shown to help improve allergies and asthmatic hypersensitivity. However, we should note that sublingual B vitamins have also been shown to be readily assimilated into the bloodstream—in a manner similar to injections. Sublingual dosing is also less expensive and painful to administer. There are several good sublingual B vitamin supplements available.

Magnesium, Sulfur, Zinc and Other Minerals

Magnesium deficiency has been found to be at the root of a number of conditions, especially those related to anxiety, spasms and muscle cramping. Not surprisingly, allergies and asthmatic hypersensitivity can be significantly reduced with magnesium supplementation.

Magnesium, along with calcium, is critical for mucosal membrane integrity, smooth muscle tone and nerve conduction. Magnesium is part of the calcium ion channel system. Magnesium regulates calcium infusion into the nerves, which helps keep them stabilized and balanced. This is why magnesium deficiencies within the calcium ion channel system causes overstrain among muscles. This translates to spasms, cramping and muscle fatigue.

Magnesium is also a critical element used by the immune system. A body deficient in magnesium will likely be immunosuppressed. Animal studies have illustrated that magnesium deficiency leads to increased IgE counts, and increased levels of inflammation-specific cytokines. Magnesium deficiency is thus also associated with increased degranulation among mast/basophil/neutrophil cells, which of course release the his-tamines, leukotrienes and prostaglandins responsible for allergic rhinitis.

It is no surprise that magnesium has also been shown to benefit anxi-ety, as it helps balance nerve firing. Magnesium has also been shown to have anti-asthmatic effects when combined with dosing with larger (one gram or more) doses of vitamin C.

Foods high in magnesium include soybeans, kidney beans, lima beans, bananas, broccoli, Brussels sprouts, carrots, cauliflower, celery, cherries, corn, dates, bran, blackberries, green beans, pumpkin seeds, spinach, chard, tofu, sunflower seeds, sesame seeds, black beans and navy beans, mineral water and beets.

Calcium, is also critical for the functioning of nerves and muscles. Every cell utilizes calcium, evidenced by calcium ion channels present in every cell membrane. Therefore, calcium is necessary for healthy lungs and airways. Thus, calcium deficiency results in more than bone problems. Muscle cramping and airway constriction are also side effects of calcium deficiency. Low calcium levels also result in deranged nerve firing, which can produce anxiety and depression. Supplementing calcium should also be accompanied by magnesium supplementing. For example, a supple-ment with 1,000 mg of calcium can be balanced by 600 mg of magnesium along with trace minerals.

Good calcium foods include dairy, bok choy, collards, okra, soy, beans, broccoli, kale, mustard greens and others.

Zinc is another important mineral for the hypersensitivity condition. Researchers from Italy's INRAN National Research Institute on Food and Nutrition (Devirgiliis *et al.* 2007) have investigated the relationship be-tween zinc and chronic diseases including allergies and asthma. Their research determined that an "imbalance in zinc homeostasis" can impair protein synthesis, cell membrane transport and gene expression. These factors, they explained, stimulate imbalances among hormones and tissue systems, producing inappropriate hyperresponsiveness.

Researchers from Australia's University of Adelaide (Lang *et al.* 2011) found that poor zinc nutrition is associated with lung disorders. They also found that low zinc is linked to a loss of appetite. This of course relates to mucosal membrane health. They found that smoke exposure increased bronchial inflammation, and dietary zinc reduced lung inflammatory macrophages by 50-60%. They concluded that: *"Zinc is an important anti-inflammatory mediator of airway inflammation."*

As zinc ions pass through the cell membrane, they assist the cell in the uptake of nutrients. Zinc transporters interact with genes to regulate the transmission of nutrients within the cell, and the pathways in and out of the cell. Zinc concentration within the cell is balanced by proteins called metallothioneins. These proteins require copper and selenium in addition to zinc. Metallothioneins are critical to the cell's ability to scavenge various radicals and heavy metals that can damage the cells. Deficiencies in metallothioneins have been seen among chronic inflammatory conditions such as allergies, as well as fatal diseases such as cancer.

Research has also shown that zinc modulates T-cell activities (Hönscheid *et al.* 2009).

Dr. Jabar (2002) commented that, *"patients with upper respiratory tract infections can expect a shorter duration of symptoms by taking high doses of vitamin C (2g) with zinc supplements, preferably the nasal zinc gel, at the onset of their symptoms."*

Good zinc foods include cowpeas, beans, lima beans, milk, brown rice, yogurt, oats, cottage cheese, bran, lentils, wheat and others.

Sulfur: Research has also confirmed that dietary sulfur can significantly relieve allergy symptoms. In a multi-center open label study by researchers from Washington state (Barrager *et al.* 2002), 55 patients with allergic rhinitis were given 2,600 mg of methylsulfonylmethane (MSM)—a significant source of sulfur derived from plants—for 30 days. Weekly reviews of the patients reported significant improvements in allergic respiratory symptoms, along with increased energy. Other research has suggested that sulfur blocks the binding of histamine among receptors.

Good sources of sulfur include avocado, asparagus, barley, beans, broccoli, cabbage, carob, carrots, Brussels sprouts, chives, coconuts, corn, garlic, leafy green vegetables, leeks, lentils, onions, parsley, peas, radishes, red peppers, soybeans, shallots, Swiss chard and watercress.

Potassium is lowered by theophylline medications and some other asthma medications. Low potassium levels will contribute to imbalances in blood pressure and the kidneys. These issues also relate directly airway constriction.

Good potassium foods include bananas, spinach, sunflower seeds, tomatoes, pomegranates, turnips, lima beans, navy beans, squash, broccoli and others.

Trace minerals: These should not be ignored in this discussion. Trace elements are important to nearly every enzymatic reaction in the body.

While minerals have been shown to provide therapeutic results, we must be careful about mineral supplements, especially those that provide single or a few minerals. Minerals co-exist in the body, and a dramatic increase in one can exhaust others as the body depletes the oversupply. Thus, an isolated macro-mineral supplement can easily produce a mineral imbalance in the body, which can produce a variety of hypersensitivity issues.

Better to utilize natural sources of minerals. These include, first and foremost, mineral-intensive vegetables. Nearly all vegetables contain generous mineral content in the combinations designed by nature. Best to eat a mixed combination of vegetables to achieve a healthy array of trace minerals.

Whole food mineral sources also contain many trace minerals in their more-digestible *chelated* forms. Chelation is when a mineral ion bonds with another nutrient, providing a ready ion as the body needs it.

Most organically-grown plant-based foods provide a rich supply of trace minerals, assuming we are eating enough of them. Other good sources of full spectrum trace minerals include natural mineral water, whole (unprocessed) rock salt, coral calcium, spirulina, AFA, kelp and chlorella. These sources will typically have from 60 to 80 trace elements, all of which are necessary for the body's various enzymatic functions. See the author's book, *Pure Water*.

We should also note that research by David Brownstein, M.D. (2006) has illustrated that whole unprocessed salt does not affect the body—high blood pressure, asthma and allergy severity and so on—like refined salts (often called sodium).

These naturally-chelated mineral sources also prevent the side effects known for mineral supplements. For example, magnesium can easily produce diarrhea in the 2,000-5,000 milligram level. While this might be considered a minor side effect, diarrhea can also produce dehydration.

Numerous holistic doctors now prescribe full-spectrum mineral combinations for allergic conditions. Many have attested to their clinical successes in recommending minerals to balance the inflammatory response and stimulate healthy mucosal membranes. Full range supplements that have RDA levels of the macrominerals combined with trace levels of the other minerals can provide a good foundation. Eating more than 5-6 servings a day of fruits and vegetables can provide the rest.

Greenfood/Superfood Supplements

While taking isolated supplements might offer some relief in some cases, we should also realize that some isolated nutrients may not be readily assimilable. Isolated nutrients in large doses can also throw off the body's balance of other nutrients, as we've discussed. Many nutrients are called cofactors because their effectiveness requires the presence of other nutrients. This sort of cooperative character of nutrients is simply because the body's processes are heavily related to each other. As opposed to a lot of research, very little occurs in the body within a vacuum.

Superfood supplements offer nature's balance of nutrients. Superfoods are quite simply, extremely nutritious foods. Many are available as supplements, as they may be dehydrated and encapsulated or pressed into tablets—or simply taken as a powder. Many superfoods—primarily nutritious fruits and vegetables such as noni, mangosteen and wheat grass—may also be eaten raw. Here we will quickly summarize some of the most credible superfoods and their effect upon inflammation:

Chlorella: A virtually complete food. This microalga is cultivated in pools or tanks under controlled conditions. Chlorella contains numerous antioxidant nutrients, B vitamins, lots of chlorophyll, beta-carotene and trace minerals. It is an excellent source of protein. It also contains Chlorella Growth Factor, (CGF) which helps stimulate growth and immunity.

Spirulina: This microalga grows in hot climates; typically in pools or tanks. It contains most of the antioxidant vitamins, prebiotics, beta-carotene, every essential amino acid, GLA, phycocyanin, B12 and many other nutrients.

Wheatgrass: This is the young plant of the wheat, picked when it is several inches high. Wheatgrass is a concentrated source of greenfood nutrients, and contains many of the phytonutrients and trace minerals found in vegetables. Wheatgrass is also known to help detoxify the blood and liver due to its high levels of chlorophyll and alkalizing mineral content.

Sprouts: Sprouts from beans and wheats contain numerous enzymes, along with high levels of phytonutrients. Sprouts can be homegrown easily, but can now also be found in powder form.

Aloe: Aloe vera has been used traditionally for inflammation, constipation, wound healing, skin issues, ulcers and intestinal issues for at least five thousand years. Aloe's constituents include anthraquinones and mucopolysaccharides, which help replenish the mucosal membranes.

Mushrooms: We discussed Reishi mushroom and Hoelen mushroom (*Wolfiporia extensa*) in the Chinese herbal medicine section earlier. Other mushrooms, such as Maitake (*Grifola frondosa*), Shiitake (*Lentinula elodes*), Turkey Tails (*Coriolus versicolor or Trametes versicolor*), Agaricus (*Agaricus blazeil*), Cordyceps (*Cordyceps sinensis*) and Lion's Mane (*Hericium erinaceus*) all have the distinction of stimulating the immune system and increasing tolerance. Blends of mushrooms are readily available in encapsulated supplement form.

Lecithin: This is derived primarily from brewer's yeast and soy, and is known to contain choline and inositol—two nutrients beneficial for cell membranes and nerve cells. Lecithin has been shown to relax nerves and help smooth muscle function.

Kelp is a microalga that contains a host of nutrients and phytonutrients, including fucoidan—shown to be a significant antioxidant. Kelp is also a good source of iodine—a critical trace element for thyroid health. Kelp powder is salty, and can replace refined salt as a condiment.

Green Papaya: This superfood has been used to help rebuild weakened mucosal membranes. It contains a special enzyme called papain, as well as vitamins A, C, E and Bs. In fact, it contains more vitamin A than carrots and more vitamin C than oranges on a per-content basis.

Bee Pollen has been recommended by traditional practitioners for allergic hypersensitivity because it contains a variety of antioxidant nutrients, enzymes, and proteins—many of which are derived from pollen. Many traditional physicians and clinicians have documented observing that bee pollen can increase allergic tolerance and immunity in many of their patients. Bee pollen is best used from hives and honeybees harvesting pollens from the same plants the person is sensitive to. For example, if a person is sensitive to ragweed, bee pollen from honeybees that harvest orange blossoms will likely not help create tolerance as much as bee pollen coming from *Ambrosia* sp., or other 'ragweed' species.

It should also be noted that local bees are more likely to be harvesting the pollens that we are sensitive to.

This strategy uses concepts similar to immunotherapy, discussed earlier. Thus, someone with a pollen allergy should approach bee pollen with care, starting with only very minute amounts, and increasing over time. A dose that produces an allergic response should be cut back to the dose that does not produce an allergic response. Those with severe allergies or a history of anaphylaxis should take bee pollen in the presence of a health professional or someone trained in anaphylaxis treatment.

Royal Jelly: This superfood, made by the Queen, supplies similar nutrients as bee pollen, along with others. Royal jelly supplies vitamins A, C, D, E, Bs, enzymes, steroid hormones, trace minerals and all the essential amino acids. Royal jelly is also a rare source for natural acetylcholine. Royal jelly has been recommended for asthma and bronchitis for many centuries. It is also reputed to stimulate the adrenal and thyroid glands— which increase tolerance.

Royal jelly can also contain very minute levels of pollen proteins as well. Thus it can provide a good entry point to bee pollen.

Manuka Honey: Raw honey in general has been shown to be antimicrobial and soothing to the mucosal membranes. Thus, it is often used in cough syrups and sore throat remedies as we've described. Manuka honey is a special honey that comes from honeybees that harvest from the flowers of the Manuka bush (*Leptospermum scoparium*). This particular honey is thought to exert stronger immunity-building effects than normal raw honey. It is also reputed to be a remedy for ulcers, sinus infections and irritable bowels. Most of the world's supply comes from New Zealand, where the Manuka tree flourishes. This honey is also typically treated very gently to preserve its antioxidant and antimicrobial properties.

Note also that honey also contains minute portions of pollen proteins. Therefore, we can also choose a local raw honey from bees that harvest flowers from plants we are allergic to in order to increase our tolerance.

Super Vegetables: Extraordinary vegetables include parsley, broccoli, spinach, kale and cabbage. Cabbage is also excellent for rebuilding mucosal membranes, supplying what is now termed vitamin U, as we will discuss later in more detail.

Super Brans, Fibers and Seeds: These include psyllium seed, oat bran, rice bran, fennel seed, flax seed, sesame seed, sunflower seeds and others. These supply mucilage, lignans and important plant fibers that stimulate mucosal membrane health. They also decrease lipid peroxidation and lower LDL cholesterol.

Plant Gums: These include guar gum and glucomannan. Most gums derived from plants provide mucilage and glucuronolactone, and other healthy polysaccharides. These constituents help maintain the health of our mucosal membranes. They also bind to toxins. Glucuronolactone is also a key component in many of the body's flexible connective tissues, which include the nasal tissues.

Special Yeast Supplements

Mold is a type of fungi. So are yeasts. Some yeast can be infective, but many are probiotic. The nutritional yeast species we discuss here, which include Brewer's yeast, Nutritional Yeast and EpiCor®, are all derived from an organism called *Saccharomyces cerevisiae*. This organism is used in brewing and baking. It is thus considered a healthy and probiotic organism, unless of course it overpopulates the body and begins to dominate probiotic bacteria colonies.

For this reason, EpiCor®, Brewer's Yeast or Nutritional Yeast come in dehydrated forms. In other words, the yeast colonies are killed by heat before packaging. This heat kills and preserves their nutrients, and prevents their overgrowth in the body. (However, a person who has mold allergies might still have a reaction to even heat-killed yeast, because those proteins are still present. At the same time, minute portions gradually increased may increase tolerance.)

So what is the difference between EpiCor®, Brewer's Yeast and Nutritional Yeast? The answer lies in their unique processes of fermentation.

Brewer's Yeast is a byproduct of the brewing industry, thus it typically does not have the higher levels of nutrients that the other two have. Brewer's yeast still has a variety of nutrients, including many trace elements (such as chromium and selenium), B vitamins (but not B12 as many assume), many antioxidants and proteins.

Nutritional Yeast, on the other hand, does contain vitamin B12, as well as higher levels of the same nutrients and even more, according to leading manufacturer, Red Star®. Nutritional Yeast has been grown in substrate specifically to enhance its nutrient levels—in a proprietary process. This type of yeast is often found in health food stores.

EpiCor® is another yeast derivative that is produced using a proprietary method. EpiCor® may have even more enhanced levels of certain nutrients, which include those mentioned above, along with nucleotides and possibly additional antioxidants and immune factors. The reason that EpiCor® may have additional immune factors is because during fermentation, the yeast is *stressed.* Like any organism, when the yeasts are stressed, they produce immune factors to protect themselves.

After EpiCor® has been stressed, it is then heat-killed, dehydrated and powdered, rendering those immune factors and nutrients.

EpiCor® has been the subject of focused research, which has found that it significantly lowers systemic inflammation and increases tolerance.

In one study (Robinson *et al.* 2009), 500 milligrams of EpiCor® or a placebo was given to 80 healthy volunteers with seasonal grass allergies during pollen season. After six and twelve weeks, the EpiCor® group experienced a significant reduction of allergy symptoms compared to the placebo group.

Other EpiCor® studies have shown that it increases salivary IgA (mucosal immunity), and reduces serum IgE (pro-allergy sensitivity).

While there are others, these nutritional supplements have been chosen to maximize the body's antioxidant capacities, increase tolerance, and stimulate detoxification processes. They also have considerable research backing up these claims. A consistent program of these whole nutritional supplements in addition to a predominantly plant-based diet is a solid strategy for stemming systemic inflammation.

Coffee and Tea

As for coffee and tea, there is a good amount of evidence that coffee can ease asthmatic and allergic symptoms. This has been shown to be primarily due to their theobromine and theophylline content, in addition to some stimulant effects from the caffeine. These natural bronchodilators have been known to open airways and stop bronchial spasms. Thus, many have used coffee or black tea for immediate asthmatic episode relief.

The problem, however, is that processed coffees and black teas also contribute significant acidity to the system when considerable amounts are consumed. This is evidenced by research showing that people who drink too much coffee experience more ulcers and acid reflux issues.

The solution comes down to the processing. When coffee beans are roasted, a number of radicals are produced as they oxidize, exposing their unbuffered tannic acid content. With storage and shipping, they further oxidize. This is why coffee is typically black, and bitter.

This said, black coffee and black tea can still provide antioxidants—more than many western diets do. These include chlorogenic acid and caffeic acid.

The consistent use of black coffee and black tea also comes with a price in terms of caffeine, which can disrupt sleep and increase anxiety.

A better strategy to utilize coffee's beneficial properties is to lightly home-roast green beans, rendering less oxidation. Soaking the green beans in hot water prior to roasting will also decrease their caffeine content.

As for tea, green tea and black tea come from the leaves of the same plant (*Camellia sinensis*). However, green teas are prepared quite differently. Black tea leaves are typically cooked in ovens, whereas green teas are typically air dried with minimal heat. Some exotic black teas will also be sun-dried, but the sun is typically very hot and the drying times are longer. These techniques concentrate the tannins and deplete many of the antioxidants in the plant.

We should mention that the anti-asthmatic rescue medication and bronchodilator theophylline was originally derived from *Camellia sinensis*. One might wonder, then, why theophylline has adverse side effects. This is because the theophylline was isolated without the other buffering constituents provided by the whole leaf of the plant.

At any rate, green tea, green coffee and cola berry extracts all contain natural theophylline and theobromine. So assuming we were able to get these with less processing and adulteration, we could have a healthy source of natural airway dilators.

Early Anti-Allergy Diet Strategies

In the last chapter we discussed the significant effect that breastfeeding has on reducing the risk of allergies among infants and children. The bottom line is that breast milk gives the child a host of immune cells and immunoglobulins that fine tune the baby's immune system. Additionally, breast milk gives the child a host of probiotics that help colonize the intestinal tract and mucosal membranes of the airways. Breast milk also delivers special nutrients and fatty acids that stimulate tolerance and balance. While there are some fine replacements for breast milk available today, nothing is quite as good as the real thing—from a healthy mother.

We might suggest that if the mother is unable to supply milk, there are breast milk banks that supply donated breast milk to mothers who cannot breast feed. Currently there are eleven banks in the U.S. and Canada. They require a prescription from a pediatrician, but this should not be difficult because most pediatricians advocate breast milk. These breast milk banks accept and store donated breast milk from lactating mothers under the rules and guidelines of the *Human Milk Banking Association of North America*. Banks within the association medically screen donations and providers for diseases, alcohol and nutritional quality.

In addition, there are several natural lactation inducement strategies to consider. Unfortunately, these are outside the scope of this text.

A healthy mother's diet is also critical. Research from Japan's Fukuoka University (Miyake *et al.* 2010) on 763 Japanese mother-child teams found that the mother's higher dietary intake of dairy products, milk, cheese and calcium during pregnancy significantly reduced the risk of wheeze among the infants—due likely because of the prebiotic content that dairy provides. They also found that vitamin D supplementation during pregnancy also significantly reduced the rates of wheeze among the children.

When Can Cow's Milk be Introduced?

The research we laid out in Chapter Four illustrates that cow's milk or solid foods should not be introduced too early. This is because an infant's intestinal wall barrier has not matured enough, leaving the intestinal cells exposed to larger peptides and proteins that can stimulate hypersensitivity.

At the same time, some early exposure has benefits, especially when it comes to cow's milk. Early exposure can mean the immune system becomes more tolerant, but that is only if the intestinal barrier has matured to a point where the mucosal membrane, IgAs and desmosomes are all in place to prevent allergen exposure to the tissues and bloodstream.

For these reasons, many physicians suggest that mothers should wait four months before introducing cow's milk to their babies. Is this advice backed up by clinical evidence? Let's look at some of the research, remembering that early allergies often turn into allergic rhinitis and even asthma later in childhood:

Researchers from Israel's Allergy and Immunology Institute and the Assaf-Harofeh Medical Center (Katz *et al.* 2010) surveyed the feeding history of 13,019 infants. Those children with apparent milk allergies were challenged and tested with skin prick testing. They found that .5% or 66 of the 13,019 children had active milk allergies. They also found that those children with milk allergies were introduced to milk at an average age of 116 days, while the infants without milk allergies were introduced to milk at an average age of 62 days.

Furthermore, the risk of becoming allergic to milk among infants who were introduced to milk in the first 14 days was .005%, while the risk of developing milk allergies when given milk between 105 days and 194 days was 1.75%. The researchers concluded that the early introduction of milk along with breastfeeding can help prevent milk allergies.

This research may lie in contradiction to the exclusive breastfeeding research we quoted in the last chapter. We should add that these results may likely depend upon the nature of the milk given. They also did not study the effects of natural raw milk from grass-fed cows or even goats. These sources of milk provide natural probiotics and a host of immune factors that more closely match mother's breast milk. Extrapolating from this and the research we'll lay out shortly, raw cow's or goat's milk will likely provide more protection to the intestinal barrier than pasteurized cow's milk.

Infant Formula Considerations

This brings us to an often temporary, yet common problem for parents: Their infant or young child becomes sensitive to milk or other formula ingredient. Or perhaps their child has increased risk because the mother has allergies or asthma.

Scientists around the world have focused a great amount of research upon this problem. This has resulted in several options, depending upon the sensitivity. Here we will lay out the research, and let the parent and their health professional apply the specific situation. Remember that parents should also consult their health professional prior to implementing any of these feeding strategies.

For children with milk sensitivities, there are several choices. Here are some of the choices we'll discuss in this section:

> Soy formulas
> Rice milk formulas
> Almond milk formulas
> Goat milk
> Donkey milk
> Sheep milk
> Hydrolyzed formulas (milk, soy, rice, casein)
> Partially-hydrolyzed formulas
> Amino acid formulas
> Omega-3 additives (with any formula)

Not all, but the majority of children with milk sensitivities will tolerate soy formula. Finish researchers (Klemola *et al.* 2002) found from testing 170 milk-allergic children that all but about 10% tolerated the soy formula. The other 10% tested sensitive to the soy formula.

Soy formulas are typically rich in protein. Still, some believe that they simply do not provide the nutrition for subtle brain development. The newest solution has been hydrolyzed formulations. Here the proteins are broken down in a way that approximates what is done in a healthy intestinal tract. Because larger macromolecules can seep through immature intestinal barriers and stimulate sensitivity, hydrolyzed proteins can provide a possible temporary feeding solution for an allergic child.

Hydrolyzed milk formulas are now recommended for babies with high allergy risk, especially if breastfeeding is impossible. Partially hydrolyzed formulas will also break down larger allergen-proteins like beta-LG into smaller peptides. When they are broken down enough, they become indistinguishable to the immune system because they are in amino acid or smaller peptide form. These partially hydrolyzed formulas appear to significantly reduce allergenicity to casein protein as well (Nentwich *et al.* 2001).

Hydrolyzed milk formulations may also reduce allergy risk in general, especially among those who are genetically susceptible. Researchers from the Marien-Hospital in Wesel, Germany (von Berg *et al.* 2003) studied 2,252 infants between 1995 and 1998 who had higher risk of allergies. For one year, the infants were fed cow's milk, a partially hydrolyzed whey formula, an extensively hydrolyzed whey formula, or an extensively hydrolyzed casein formula. Both the hydrolyzed casein formula and the partially hydrolyzed whey formula caused less allergies among the children compared to the cow's milk formula.

Finnish researchers (Seppo *et al.* 2005) gave 168 milk-allergic infants with an average age of eight months either hydrolyzed whey formula or soy formula. Both groups tolerated the two formulas quite well. They also found that both supported normal growth and nutritional status through two years of age.

Spanish hospital researchers (Ibero *et al.* 2010) fed hydrolyzed casein milk formula to 67 milk-allergy children aged between one month and one year old. The formula was tolerated by 98.5% of the children.

Italian researchers (Fiocchi *et al.* 2003) found that children who were both allergic to cow's milk and soy tolerated and thrived from a hydrolyzed rice formula.

Another group of Italian researchers (D'Auria *et al.* 2003) studied 16 milk-allergic infants. They also found that rice hydrolysate formula renders normal growth and nutrition, along with *"adequate metabolic balance"* using standardized growth indices (Z scores) and biochemical nutrient testing.

Pediatric researchers from The Netherlands' Wilhelmina Children's Hospital (Terheggen-Lagro *et al.* 2002) gave thirty milk-allergic children extensively hydrolyzed casein-based formula. They found that this was well tolerated by the children.

Italian researchers (Giampietro *et al.* 2001) found, in a two-center study of 32 milk-allergic children, that the majority successfully tolerated two extensively hydrolyzed whey-based formulas.

Researchers from Brazil's San Paolo Hospital (Agostoni *et al.* 2007) tested four different types of feeding with 125 infants with allergies. After being fed breast milk for four months or more, the infants were weaned to either soy formula, a casein hydrolysate formula, a rice hydrolysate formula, or were exclusively breastfed for the remainder of the year. Both the hydrolysates (casein- and rice-based) were accompanied by better weight compared to the soy formula—which fared the worst out of the feeding strategies.

In a recent review (Alexander and Cabana 2010) of multiple studies, infants fed with partially hydrolyzed whey protein formula had a 44% reduced likelihood of developing allergic symptoms, as compared with children who fed with milk formula.

Hydrolyzed formulas have proved to reduce allergy risk better than partially-hydrolyzed formulas, however. In a study from Denmark (Halken *et al.* 2000), 595 children were either breastfed or given formula from June 1994 to July 1995. Of the 595, 478 children finished the study. Of these, 232 ended up being breastfed; 79 were fed a hydrolyzed casein formula; 82 were fed an extensively hydrolyzed whey formula; and 85 were fed a partially hydrolyzed whey formula. Cow's milk allergy rates were highest among those fed partially hydrolyzed formula. Extensively hydrolyzed formula was more effective in preventing milk allergies.

Researchers from the University of Milan Medical School (Terracciano *et al.* 2010) tested 72 children with an average age of 14 months, and followed up over a 26 month period. They gave the children either hydrolyzed rice formula, extensively hydrolyzed milk formula or a soy formula. Surprisingly, they found that children not exposed to milk protein residue become tolerant to milk earlier than children fed hydrolyzed milk. The researchers felt that this was due to the substantial change in the protein among hydrolyzed milks.

Researchers from Italy's University of Palermo (Carroccio *et al.* 2000) divided up a group of infants who were sensitive to cow's milk and/or hydrolyzed proteins into two groups. The 21 hydrolyzed protein-intolerant infants were fed donkey milk. The 70 cow's milk-intolerant infants were given casein-hydrolyzed milk.

The children were followed up after four years to see if either method produced more or less allergic sensitivities. All of the donkey milk infants suffered from multiple sensitivities, whereas 28% (20) of the hydrolyzed-casein milk drinkers had sensitivities. Four out of seven of the patients receiving donkey milk were also intolerant to sheep milk. Three of the 21 donkey milk drinkers became intolerant to the donkey milk. The good news is that 52% of the donkey milk drinkers became tolerant to milk over the four year period. Even better, 78% of the hydrolyzed-casein group became milk-tolerant over the four years.

Almond milk may also be a good alternative. Researchers from Italy's University of Messina (Salpietro *et al.* 2005) tested almond milk feeding on a group of 52 infants aged five to nine months who had milk allergies. They compared this to soy milk formula. They found that while supplementation with soy-based formula and hydrolyzed milk protein formulas both caused sensitivities in 23% and 15% respectively, none of the children developed sensitivities to almond milk. The researchers also found the almond milk to be safe and nutritious.

A newer option is the amino acid formula. An amino formula contains an array of individual amino acids rather than hydrolyzed proteins. Amino acids are the fundamental building blocks for protein production. Mount Sinai School of Medicine researchers (Sicherer *et al.* 2001) tested 31 children with milk allergies with a pediatric amino acid-based formula and compared this with tolerance to hydrolyzed milk formula. Of the 31 children, 13 did not tolerate the hydrolyzed formula, while almost all of the children tolerated the amino acid formula. The amino formula also maintained normal growth rates among the children.

A newer development is an amino acid-based formula combined with docosahexaenoic acid (DHA) and arachidonic acid—at levels that closely resemble those of breast milk. In a study of 165 allergic infants, Duke University Medical Center researchers (Burks *et al.* 2008) found that this amino acid/EFA formula was hypoallergenic, and provided a safe alternative to breast milk.

Swedish researchers (Furuhjelm *et al.* 2009) also found that consuming DHA during pregnancy decreased the risk of childhood allergy.

Milk formulations with algae-derived omega-3s have shown to reduce allergy risk compared to other non-omega-3 formulations. Dallas researchers (Birch *et al.* 2010) gave a formula supplemented with docosahexaenoic acid (DHA) and arachidonic acid (ARA) or placebo to 179 children through the first year of infancy. The formula significantly reduced the risk of wheezing, asthma and hay fever/allergies through three years of age.

Note: The American Academy of Pediatrics, the European Society of Pediatric Gastroenterology and Nutrition, and the European Society of Pediatric Allergy and Clinical Immunology all concur that prior to using any of these alternative formulas, they should be tested using the double-blind placebo-controlled challenges for allergic children or children with a high risk of milk or other allergies.

Solid Food Introduction Strategies

Introducing solid foods to the baby is an important milestone. This text will not profess the best method. Rather, we'll lay out some of the research. While some suggest that the order of foods introduced is important, others have shown that the order is not that important.

What is known is that most children are exposed to sensitivities at home or through breastfeeding, and early solid food exposure can often lead to sensitivity. This means that early solid foods are probably better being low-sensitivity, easily-digested plant-based foods such as squashes, fruits and other simple foods—rather than the more common allergen foods. This is supported by research. Also, introducing common allergenic solid foods into children's diets is best done a bit later, gradually and in small increments (Vlieg-Boerstra *et al.* 2008).

Illustrating this, Dutch researchers (Kiefte-de Jong *et al.* 2010) found that by two years of age, about 12% of children are constipated. Furthermore, those children with constipation were more likely to have been introduced to gluten prior to six months of age.

Feeding solid foods prior to three months old appears to increase allergies, but so does feeding any solid foods after seven months old. Researchers have confirmed, for example, that feeding grains before three months or after seven months increases the child's risk of celiac disease and/or wheat allergies (Guandalini 2007). From this we can assess from the research that a safe strategy is to gradually increase solid foods during the fifth or sixth month, accompanied by breast milk feeding through the first year.

Researchers from Finland's University of Tampere (Nwaru *et al.* 2010) related the introduction of solid foods with the incidence of allergies and asthma at five years old. They studied 994 children and found that the average length of exclusive breastfeeding was 1.8 months among the children. They calculated late introductions of potatoes, rye, meat, and fish was significantly linked to bronchial hyperreactivity and allergies. The research discovered that diets higher in potatoes and fish were most related to allergic hyperreactivity among the children. They concluded that late solid food introduction increased the risk of allergies and asthmatic hypersensitivity.

Chapter Six
Herbal Medicine for Allergies

There are numerous herbs that have been utilized in traditional medicine for modifying allergic hypersensitivity. While each herb works in a unique manner, various herbs stimulate similar mechanisms in the body. Herbal medications have been shown to:

- ➤ Strengthen the immune system
- ➤ Increase tolerance
- ➤ Stimulate detoxification processes
- ➤ Donate key nutrients
- ➤ Balance and strengthen the adrenal glands
- ➤ Subdue anxious nervous response
- ➤ Strengthen mucous membranes
- ➤ Feed probiotics
- ➤ Reverse systemic inflammation
- ➤ Alkalize the bloodstream
- ➤ Rebuild the airways
- ➤ Relax smooth muscles
- ➤ Neutralize free radicals
- ➤ Rejuvenate the liver

A significant amount of research and clinical experience has verified that herbal medicines accomplish these effects and more. This is generally because nature's herbs will typically contain tens if not hundreds of bioactive constituents—each stimulating our metabolism and immune system in synergistic ways.

Herbal medicine works differently than most pharmaceuticals, which are typically designed to shut off or inhibit a particular symptom or physiological mechanism in an isolated manner. Herbal medicine, in contrast, produces body-wide systemic changes, which generally boost immunity and stimulate multiple mechanisms.

Here we will summarize some of the herbs that traditional healers from different disciplines have utilized to curb allergic hypersensitivity by reversing the underlying physiological conditions.

This presentation of the science and traditional use of medical herbs is not simply the personal opinion of the author. Rather, this discussion utilizes the medical science and research of numerous researchers, scientists and physicians trained in herbal medicines. Here traditional uses of herbal medicine have been derived from various formularies and *Materia Medica* texts from different traditions, as well as from documented clinical application of these herbs upon significant populations over centuries—

some even over thousands of years. This discussion also includes formulations and herbs that have been used for asthma, some for respiratory infections (such as sinusitis) and some for food allergies. We include these, because not only do these conditions often accompany allergic rhinitis: They also share the same underlying conditions, as we've discussed.

We should note that because allergic rhinitis is a relatively new condition that developed first among the aristocratic classes over the past century—which have typically avoided traditional herbal medicine—the usage of herbs for allergic rhinitis is not as well documented as that of asthma. But since the two share similar underlying conditions—with the addition that allergic rhinitis is also responding to the extreme overloading of modern toxins and a poor diet—and the resulting destruction of the body's immune system, probiotics and mucosal membranes. Fortunately, the rebuilding of the immune system, increased tolerance to allergens, and the rebuilding of the airway mucosal membranes is precisely what traditional asthmatic herbal formulations have been shown to accomplish. So they are perfectly applicable to allergic rhinitis. In addition, asthmatic herbs also offer a strengthening of the body's various detoxification functions.

Unless otherwise noted, the information in this chapter utilizes the following reference materials (see reference section for complete citation): Bensky *et al.* 1986; Bisset 1994; Blumenthal 1998; Blumenthal and Brinckmann 2000; Bruneton 1995; Chevallier 1996; Chopra *et al.* 1956; Christopher 1976; Clement *et al.* 2005; Duke 1989; Ellingwood 1983; Fecka 2009; Foster and Hobbs 2002; Frawley and Lad 1988; Gray-Davidson 2002; Griffith 2000; Gundermann and Müller 2007; Halpern and Miller 2002; Hobbs 2003; 1997; Hoffmann 2002; Hope *et al.* 1993; Jensen 2001; Kokwaro 1976; Lad 1984; LaValle 2001; Lininger *et al.* 1999; Mabey 1988; Mehra 1969; Mindell and Hopkins 1998; Murray and Pizzorno 1998; Nadkarni and Nadkarni 1908/1975; Newall *et al.* 1996; Newmark and Schulick 1997; O'Connor and Bensky 1981; Potterton 1983; Schulick 1996; Schauenberg and Paris 1977; Schulz *et al.* 1998; Shi *et al.* 2008; Shishodia *et al.* 2008; Tierra 1992; Tierra 1990; Tiwari 1995; Tisserand 1979; Tonkal and Morsy 2008; Weiner 1969; Weiss 1988; Williard 1992; Williard and Jones 1990; White and Foster 2000; Wood 1997.

Chinese Herbal Formulations

Chinese medicine differentiates the power of the body into three driving elements: *Jing, Shen* and *Qi.*

Jing energy is considered the basic genetic or primordial programming of the body.

Shen energy is considered the psyche of the body.

Qi energy is the active and vital element of the body.

Chinese medicinal formulary utilizes a four-step combination process. The four steps are: *Jun, Chen, Zuo* and *Shi*. Jun is the key herb(s) intended to correct the specific condition. Chen is supportive to *Jun,* either by increasing Jun's effects or by reducing *Jun's* side effects. *Zuo* supports both *Jun* and *Chen*—increasing their efficacy and reducing any relative side effects. Meanwhile, *Shi* is intended to synergize the formulation, increasing its assimilation and ability to work in a balanced manner.

As we'll find in this section, Chinese herbal medicine has been validated traditionally by its clinical use on billions of patients over thousands of years; as well as scientifically through modern controlled research.

For example, illustrating Chinese herbs' ability to halt the inflammatory process, researchers from the Taiwan's China Medical University (Chang *et al.* 2010) investigated the effects of 83 Chinese herbs on eosinophil cationic protein. Remember that ECP build-up in the lungs is a sign of systemic inflammation, and it often accompanies severe allergic rhinitis. ECP also accompanies airway hypersensitivity and remodeling damage to the airways.

Of the 83 Chinese herbs, numerous herbs were found to decrease ECP. Among these, eight herbs, (Tao Ren, Sie Cao, Wei Ling Sian, Gan Cao, Jhih Mu, Dang Guei, Sheng Di Huang, and Mu Tong) also specifically reduced the ability of ECP to bind to cells. In other words, many of the 83 herbs protected the airway cells from ECP damage in one respect or another.

The researchers also extracted key constituents of the eight herbs and tested their ability to decrease ECP binding. The researchers also found that several regularly-prescribed herbal formulations also significantly inhibited ECP. The researchers found that extracts of Heng Di Huang, Dang Guei and Mu Tong significantly inhibited ECP binding and damage to airway cells. Some of the most significant reduction in ECP damage to the cells took place with Gang Cao and Sheng Di Huang; and their constituents glycyrrhizic acid and verbascose.

This of course, is one study of many that have illustrated the effects of Chinese herbs. Remember that numerous herbs of the 83 reduced ECP to different degrees. The research zoomed in on those that were most effective.

Here we will describe many of the most effective and successful Chinese anti-allergy and anti-asthma herbal formulas, followed by a listing and description of the individual herbs common among these formulas. Note that some of the Chinese names refer to a specific part of the plant and a specific process to prepare it for the formulation. We'll try to break these down for easier understanding for the reader.

The Saiboku-To Formula

Saiboku-To, or TJ-96 as it is termed by researchers, is a well-known anti-asthma herbal medication used for hundreds if not thousands of years in China and Japan. It is a blend of 10 herbal extracts from the following plants:

> Gan Cao (*Glycyrrhiza uralensis*) (Chinese Licorice)
> Sti Zi (*Perilla frutescens*) (Perilla)
> Da Zao (*Ziziphus zizyphus*) (Jujube)
> Hou Po (*Magnolia officinalis*) (Magnolia)
> Huang Qin (*Scutellaria baicalensis*) (Baikal Skullcap)
> Fu Ling (*Wolfiporia extensas*) (Hoelen mushroom)
> Chai Hu (*Bupleurum chinense*) (Bupleurum)
> Ban Xia (*Pinellia ternata*) (Pinellia)
> Sheng Jiang (*Zingiber officinalis*) (Ginger)
> Ben Shen (*Panex ginseng*) (Ginseng)

Medical researchers from the Japan's Public Tamana Central Hospital (Egashira and Nagano 1993) tested the Saiboku-To formulation on 112 adults with oral steroid-dependent asthma. The Saiboku-To group had significantly fewer asthmatic symptoms and better quality of life results than did the placebo group.

Researchers from the Tokyo Metropolitan Fuchu Hospital (Urata *et al.* 2002) gave 2.5 grams of Saiboku-to (or TJ-96) to asthmatics or a placebo three times a day for four weeks. After the four weeks, the TJ-96 group had significantly lower counts of pro-inflammatory eosinophils and eosinophilic cationic protein. Symptoms also significantly improved among the TJ-96 group. The researchers concluded: *"Our results suggest that TJ-96 has an anti-inflammatory effect on bronchial eosinophilic infiltration. This study raises further interesting therapeutic possibilities and argues for further trials of new approaches to the treatment of asthma."*

Researchers from the Tokyo University of Pharmacy and Life Science (Taniguchi *et al.* 2000) tested urine metabolites after administering Saiboku-To to humans. They found that Saiboku-To produced flavonoids and lignans, along with their hydrogenated metabolites.

The individual extracts and some of their constituents were also tested. Medicarpin derived from *Glycyrrhiza glabra*, magnolol and 8,9-dihydroxydihydromagnolol from *Magnolia officinalis*, baicalein, wogonin and oroxylin A from *Suctellaria baicalensis* all inhibited lymphocyte proliferation. In other words, they reduced and/or blocked inflammation. The researchers calculated that the levels of inflammation inhibition provided by these extracts ranged from 20-100 times provided by a dose of prednisolone (oral steroid).

The researchers also found that the oral administration of Saiboku-To and constituent extracts significantly reduced allergic inflammation of the ear. These effects were quantified to be 53% of the effects of predniso-lone. The researchers concluded that these anti-inflammatory effects suggested that Saiboku-To significantly suppressed allergic reactivity.

The Sho-Seiryu-To/Xiao-Qing-Long-Tang Formula

Another popular asthma formula in traditional Chinese medicine and Japanese medicine (Kampo) is called Sho-Seiryu-To (or SST) in Japanese medicine and the Xiao-Qing-Long-Tang formula in Chinese medicine. This formula has proved successful in clinical settings for many centuries in both regions. This formula consists of:

- Ban Xia (*Pinellia ternata*) (Pinellia)
- Gan Cao (*Glycyrrhiza uralensis*) (Chinese Licorice)
- Xi Xin (*Herba asari*) (Chinese Wild Ginger)
- Gan Jiang (*Zingiberis officinalis*) (Ginger)
- Gui Zhi (*Cinnamomum cassia*) (Cinnamon)
- Ma Huang (*Ephedra sinica*) (Ephedra)
- Wu Wei Zi (*Schisandra chinensis*) (Shizandra)
- Bai Shao (*Paeonia lactiflora* Pall.) (Red Peony)

Researchers from Japan's Kitasato University (Nagai *et al.* 2004) researched the effects of SST among asthma patients. SST was found to reduce IgE antibodies among bronchial fluids after seven days of treatment. SST also reduced IL-4 and IL-5 production. In addition, IFN-gamma returned to normal levels. Nerve growth factor increases after SST suggested that airway remodeling and Th1/Th2 balances were modulated by the SST formulation.

One of the constituents, pinellic acid, proved to be one of the central ingredients, as it directly decreased IgE levels.

The STA-1 Formula

STA-1 has several herbs in common with other formulas. This is not a coincidence, as doctors of traditional Chinese medicine will often formulate slightly different blends to deal with specific symptoms and physiologies. Some of these, such STA-1 and the others we are describing here, have been standardized and used extensively over the centuries.

Researchers from Taiwan's China Medical University (Chang *et al.* 2006) gave the STA-1 formula, the STA-2 formula (same herbs with slightly different extraction methods) or a placebo to 120 patients with asthma for six months. After the six month period, the STA-1 and the STA-2 groups exhibited significantly better symptoms and lung function compared with the placebo group. The STA-1 group also showed significantly reduced allergen-specific IgE levels.

This formula contains ten herbs:

> Gan Cao (*Glycyrrhiza uralensis*) (Chinese Licorice)
> Mai Men Dong (*Ophiopogon japonicus*) (Japonica)
> Xi Yang Shen (*Panax quinquefolium L*) (American Ginseng)
> Ban Xia (*Pinellia ternata*) (Pinellia)
> Shu Di Huang (*Rehmannia glutinosa*) (Cooked Rehmannia root)
> Mu Dan Pi (*Paeonia moutan*) (Peony tree root)
> Shan Zhu Yu (*Cornus officinalis*) (Dogwood)
> Fu Ling (*Wolfiporia extensas*) (Hoelen fungus)
> Ze Xie (*Alisma orientale*) (Alisma)
> Shan Yao (*Dioscorea opposita*) (Chinese Yam)

The Anti-Asthma Herbal Medicine Intervention Formula

The ASHMI herbal formulation is a blend of herbs studied by Dr. Xiu-Min Li and Dr. Hugh Sampson from New York's Mount Sinai School of Medicine. It is a derivative of a traditional Chinese formulation of fourteen Chinese herbs, named MSSM-002 by the Shandong Weifang Pharmaceutical Factory Co., Ltd of China. Like the FAHF formula, the ASHMI formula has undergone rigorous animal and laboratory testing, including phase I testing with humans. ASHMI has also undergone rigorous human testing in China. The ASHMI studies have all shown great success in all of this research.

ASHMI contains three herbal extracts:

> Ling Zhi (*Ganoderma lucidum*) (Reishi)
> Ku Shen (*Sophora flavescens*) (Sophora)
> Gan Cao (*Glycyrrhiza uralensis*) (Chinese Licorice)

This formula has been shown to modulate the TH1/TH2 balance and reduce hypersensitivity (Li *et al.* 2000). Mount Sinai researchers also found that ASHMI significantly reduced inflammatory cytokines IL-4 (Bolleddula *et al.* 2007).

Chinese researchers (Wen *et al.* 2005) gave the ASHMI formula or prednisone treatment to 91 allergic asthmatic patients, and compared their effects. They found that after four weeks, the ASHMI group had significantly improved lung function. Furthermore, the ASHMI group's IgE levels, eosinophil levels and inflammatory cytokine levels dropped. Unlike the adverse side-effects known in steroid treatment, ASHMI dosing produced no significant side effects.

One notable result as the two treatment groups were compared was that serum IFN-gamma and cortisol levels were significantly increased in the ASHMI group, while those two levels were lower in the prednisone group. They also found that ASHMI lowered allergic IgE levels, eosinophil counts, and Th2 cytokines IL-5 and IL-13.

This illustrates that ASHMI strengthened the immune system while it lowered symptoms of allergic asthma among the patients. Pharmaceuticals, on the other hand, often weaken the immune system because they can break down into toxic byproducts.

Other laboratory and animal studies out of the Mount Sinai School of Medicine have also confirmed the ability of the ASHMI formula to reduce asthma symptoms, lung hyperreactivity and inflammation (Srivastava *et al.* 2010; Zhang *et al.* 2010).

The evidence is quite conclusive that this herbal formula specifically reduces not only asthma symptoms, but the body's inclination for inflammation. The inflammatory process is halted by virtue of a rich combination of natural constituents that modify cytokines while stimulating the repair of a deranged immune system.

This result is actually quite typical among herbal medicines. The problem is that herbal combination research has simply not been given adequate research funding. Because herbs contain a wide variety of constituents that work in balance, they affect a number of physiological results in the body. They also typically have few adverse side effects, assuming they are properly prepared and dosed.

These results were enough for the FDA to approve phase I and phase II drug trials for the ASHMI herbal combination. In 2009, Mount Sinai researchers (Kelly-Peiper *et al.* 2009) reported that they had given ASHMI to 20 patients with allergic asthma in the phase I drug trial. This study proved ASHMI's safety. Its phase II trial is underway.

The Modified Mai Men Dong Tang Formula

This formula, also termed nMMDT, was modified from the traditional Chinese Mai Men Dong Tang formula used for centuries for allergic asthma in Chinese medicine. Researchers from Taiwan's China Medical University Hospital (Hsu *et al.* 2005) gave the mMMDT formula to 100 asthmatic patients for four months. After the treatment period, asthma symptoms significantly improved, lung capacity significantly increased, and IgE levels significantly decreased among the mMMDT group.

This formula contains five herbs:

> Gan Cao (*Glycyrrhiza uralensis*) (Chinese Licorice)
> Mai Men Dong (*Ophiopogon japonicus*) (Japonica)
> Xi Yang Shen (*Panax quinquefolium* L) (American Ginseng)
> Ban Xia (*Pinellia ternata*) (Pinellia)
> Herba Tridacis procumbentis (*Cercospora tridacis-procumbentis*) (Procuben)

Mount Sinai Medical School researchers (Li and Srivastava 2006) found in their research that the mMMDT formulation showed positive effectiveness as an asthma treatment.

The Ravan Napas Formula

This formulation, utilized by the ancient Uighur peoples of what is now considered Northern China, has been studied sparsely of late, but it had a glorious reputation for healing asthma among the Uighur peoples for many centuries.

In a recent study from researchers from China's First Affiliated Hospital and Xinjiang Medical University (Abdureyim *et al.* 2011), Raven napas was studied extensively in the laboratory and it was found that Ravan napas significantly reduced asthma symptoms *in vivo*.

In this study, it was found that Raven napas blocked allergic asthma from several perspectives. These included rebalancing the Th1/Th2 mechanisms and cytokines, blocking eosinophil and neutrophil proliferation, inhibiting the release of histamine and leukotrienes by mast cells, and modulating the genetic expression of allergic asthma.

This all resulted in significant reductions of all these inflammatory components, and a reduction of symptoms of inflammation, allergies and asthma.

The Ravan napas formulation contains the following herbs:

➢ *Hyssopus cuspidatus* (Hyssop)
➢ *Foeniculum vulgare* Mill. (Fennel)
➢ *Carthamus tinctorius* L (Safflower seed)
➢ *Brassica rapa* L (Mustard/Rapeseed/Turnip seed)
➢ *Malva verticillata* L. (Mallow)
➢ *Astragalus mongholicus* (Astragalus)
➢ *Ziziphus jujuba* (Red Date)
➢ *Viola tianshanica* (Violet)

The Xia-Bai-San Formula

This formula contains extracts from four herbs:

➢ *Morus alba* L. (Mulberry Bark)
➢ *Lycium chinense* Mill. (Gogi berry)
➢ *Glycyrrhiza uralensis* (Chinese Licorice)
➢ *Oryzae sativa* (Oryza seed)

Researchers from Taiwan's Council of Agriculture (Lee *et al.* 2009) studied Xia-Bai-San's anti-inflammatory properties.

The researchers found that the XBS formula significantly reduced lipopolysaccharides that induced lung inflammation *in vivo*. The mechanism related to the suppression of NF-kappaB activation. They concluded that Xia-bai-san, *Morus alba*, and *Glycyrrhiza uralensis* specifically inhibit airway inflammation, explaining some of the formula's anti-asthma and anti-allergic effects.

An earlier study from the College of Chinese medicine (Yeh *et al.* 2006) found that XBS reduced levels of pro-inflammatory TNF-alpha, IL-1beta, IL-6, KC, MIP-2, and MCP-1, while it increased anti-inflammatory IL-10. XBS also decreased leukocytes, nitric oxide and NF-kappaB, thus reducing inflammation. The researchers concluded: *"These results suggest that XBS could be a useful adjunct in the treatment of acute respiratory distress syndrome."*

The Shinpi-To Formula

Another Chinese herbal formula is Shinpi-To, which has also been called *Formula divinita* and TJ-8532. This blend of seven Chinese herbs has also been used traditionally for centuries to treat childhood allergies and asthma. The formula contains:

> ➤ Ma Huang (*Ephedra sinica*) (Ephedra)
> ➤ Xing Ren (*Prunus armeniaca* L) (Bitter Apricot Seed)
> ➤ Hou Po (*Magnolia officinalis*) (Magnolia)
> ➤ Chen Pi (*Citrus reticulata* Blanco) (Tangerine Peel)
> ➤ Gan Cao (*Glycyrrhiza uralensis*) (Chinese Licorice)
> ➤ Chai Hu (*Bupleurum chinense*) (Bupleurum)
> ➤ Sti Zi (*Perilla frutescens*) (Perilla)

Researchers from Japan's Saga Medical School (Hamasaki *et al.* 1993) tested Shinpi-To and found that it significantly inhibited the process of IgE-mediated leukotriene production—involved in the hypersensitive asthmatic and allergic response. This effect was found to occur together with a reduction of pro-inflammatory arachidonic acid. The pro-inflammatory enzyme phospholipase A2 was also inhibited by the Shinpi-To formula.

The Ding-Chuan-Tang Formula

This traditional Chinese medicine formula also has herbs common to other formulas, and is also focused upon airway hypersensitivity. Pediatric medical researchers from Taiwan's Chang Gung University (Chan *et al.* 2006) gave this Ding Chuan Tang formula or a placebo to 52 asthmatic children for 12 weeks. At the end of the treatment period, symptoms improved among the asthmatic group; and serum inflammatory mediators also improved. Hypersensitivity also improved (decreased) among the herbal treatment group.

The formula contains nine herbs:

> ➤ Gang Cao ((*Glycyrrhiza uralensis*) (Chinese Licorice)
> ➤ Ban Xia (*Pinellia ternata*) (Pinellia)
> ➤ Ying Xing (*Gingko biloba*) (Gingko)
> ➤ Ma Huang (*Ephedra sinica*) (Ephedra)
> ➤ Kuan Dong Hua (*Tussilago farfara*) (Coltsfoot flower)

> Sang Bai Pi (*Morus alba, L.*) (Mulberry root bark)
> Sti Zi (*Perilla frutescens*) (Perilla)
> Xing Ren (*Prunus armeniaca L*) (Bitter Apricot Seed)
> Huang Qin (*Scutellaria baicalensis*) (Baikal Skullcap)

A similar formula—with the addition of *Lonicera japonica*—was studied by researchers from China's Qingdao Institute of Clinical Medicine (Li *et al.* 1992). The researchers gave this formula or a placebo to 60 children with severe asthma. The formula-treated group experienced a *"cure rate"* of 27%, and the treatment eliminated asthma symptoms (*"effective rate"*) in 93% of the group. The researchers concluded that the herbal formulation *"had potent pharmacological action."*

In vitro tests by the researchers confirmed that the herbal formula relaxed the smooth muscles around the airways by inhibiting the effects of histamine and acetylcholine. Furthermore, they found that the herbal formula was able to significantly extend symptom-free periods among asthmatics.

Microorganism testing *in vitro* also illustrated that the DCT herbal formulation inhibited a number of bacteria and viruses, including *Streptococcus hemolyticus* (causes strep throat), *Staphylococcus aureus* (causes "staph" and MRSA), *Flexners Dysentery bacillus* (causes dysentery), *Diplococcus pneumoniae* (causes pneumonia) and *Pseudomonas aeruginosa*. They found that the herbs could also inhibit the respiratory syncytial virus—known for its etiology in sinus and respiratory infections.

The Xin-Cang Formula

This formulation contains:

> Xin Yi (*Magnolia officinalis*) (Magnolia flower)
> Can Go Erzi (*Xanthium sp.*) (Cocklebur fruit)

Researchers from China's Yueyang Hospital of Integrated Traditional Chinese and Western Medicine and the Shanghai University of Traditional Chinese Medicine (Zhu *et al.* 2005) studied the Xin-Cang formula on chronic asthmatic children.

The researchers divided sixty asthmatic children into two groups. One group was treated with Xin-cang and the other group was treated with the pharmaceutical asthma medication ketotifen fumarate.

After three months of treatment, "total response"—which included measures of airway inflammatory eosinophil levels, IgEs, interleukin-4 (IL-4)s, IL-5s and lung function, including and forced expiratory volumes (FEV1)—significantly improved among the Xin-cang group.

The Food Allergy Herbal Formula (FAHF)

Mount Sinai School of Medicine researchers have been testing this traditional anti-allergy formula made of Chinese medicine herbs for over a decade. The blend, dubbed FAHF, has undergone a parade of cruel studies on mice, even though the formula and its derivatives have been used in human treatment for centuries and probably even thousands of years in Chinese medicine.

The FAHF formula contains the following herbs:

➤ Ling Zhi (*Ganoderma lucidum*) (Reishi)
➤ Fu Zi (*Aconitum carmichaelii*,) (Aconitum)
➤ Wu Mei (*Prunus mume*) (Black plum)
➤ Chuan Jiao (*Zanthoxylum simulans*) (Szechwan Pepper)
➤ Xi Xin (*Herba asari*) (Chinese Wild Ginger)
➤ Huang Lian (*Coptis chinnensis*) (Gold Thread)
➤ Huang Bai (*Phellodendron amurense*) (Phellodendron)
➤ Gan Jiang (*Zingiberis officinalis*) (Ginger)
➤ Gui Zhi (*Cinnamomum cassia*) (Cinnamon)
➤ Ren Shen (*Panex ginseng*) (Ginseng)
➤ Dang Gui (*Angelica sinensis*) (Dong Quai)

FAHF-2 is the above formula, *minus* Fu-Zi and Xi-Xin.

As we discuss this formulation's research, remember that traditional Chinese physicians have safely prescribed the complete FAHF formula or similar formulations using many of the same herbs for many centuries—*and still do.*

The first Mount Sinai study (Li *et al.* 2001) cruelly sensitized mice to fresh whole peanuts by introducing the cholera toxin, followed by a boosting. They then fed the mice the FAHF-1 herbal formula for seven weeks. After the seven weeks, the FAHF-1 completely halted peanut-induced anaphylactic reactions in the mice. It also significantly reduced histamine release and lymphocyte proliferation, and reduced peanut-specific IgEs within two weeks of treatment. These tolerance levels remained for four weeks after the treatment was stopped. Cytokines IL-4, IL-5, and IL-13 synthesis were also decreased in the FAFH-1 mice.

The second published Mount Sinai study on FAFH (Srivastava *et al.* 2005) came four years later. It also tested mice with peanut allergies. This study used the revised FAHF-2 herbal formula, which removed two herbs, Fuzi and Xixin, as noted earlier. They found that the FAHF-2 also successfully blocked peanut allergy anaphylaxis, as well as rendered long term peanut tolerance. Among the FAHF-2 mice, there were no anaphylactic reactions, and histamine/body core temperatures decreased. They also observed a down-regulation of the pro-inflammatory Th-2 response.

Another Mount Sinai study, this one two years later (Qu *et al.* 2007), found that, once again, peanut-specific IgE levels fell while IgG2a levels increased after dosing with FAHF-2. Reduced IL-4 and IL-5, and a modulation of the balance between Th1 and Th2 within the intestines illustrated how this herbal combination modulated the immune system and increased tolerance.

Yet another FAHF-2 study by Mount Sinai Medical School researchers followed three years later (Kattan *et al.* 2008). Once again, the FAHF-2 formula proved successful in mice by reducing peanut anaphylaxis. This time, they also tested the individual herbs to see if they could isolate a single herb or constituent responsible for the activity.

This proved unsuccessful. Although most of the herbs had some positive effects upon histamine, cytokines and allergic symptoms, the formula worked best in combination. In the end, the researchers admitted that the formula, *"may work synergistically to produce the curative therapeutic effects produced by the whole formula."* In other words, the herbs alone did not have the same effect the combination formula had.

Now let's think about this for a second. Here is a team of medical researchers from one of the world's most respected medical schools, failing to understand precisely what part of a formula—that has undergone ten years of laboratory and animal research—is the active element. What does this tell us about nature, and the wisdom of those traditional Chinese medicine physicians who devised these formulas?

Furthermore, remember that these research teams did not fall off the turnip truck. They were experienced researchers with M.D. degrees and Ph.D.s. Some were professors of medicine at one of the world's most prestigious medical schools. Why did these physicians have to resort to an ancient Chinese herbal remedy? Perhaps these traditional Chinese medicine physicians and healers had an understanding about the body and the application of herbal medicine that modern medicine has yet to comprehend.

Perhaps, in other words, conventional western medicine should not be so high-minded about their pharmaceutical approach to health. Perhaps the institution needs a little humility and respect for the knowledge and wisdom of our ancestors.

The next Mount Sinai study focused on the mechanisms of the formulation (Srivastava *et al.* 2009). This time, mice with peanut allergies received FAHF-2 each day for seven weeks, while receiving periodic oral challenges with peanuts over a period of 36 weeks. They also gave some mice T-cell- or IFN-gamma-reducing antibodies during that period. Once again, they found that the FAHF-2 treatment protected mice from anaphylaxis, this time for more than 36 weeks after the treatment was stopped.

Furthermore, their testing revealed up to a 50% reduction of peanut-specific IgE levels, and up to a 60% increase in IgG levels, which continued long after the treatment period. In other words, the FAHF-2 formula modified their immune systems. The conclusion of the researchers: *"Food Allergy Herbal Formula-2 provides long-term protection from anaphylaxis by inducing a beneficial shift in allergen-specific immune responses mediated largely by elevated CD8(+) T-cell IFN-gamma production."*

Finally, nearly ten years after beginning research on the formula, human clinical studies have begun. Researchers from New York's Mount Sinai School of Medicine (Wang *et al.* 2010) tested 19 food allergy patients with FAHF-2. The herbal formula significantly decreased interleukin (IL-5) levels among the active treatment group after seven days of treatment. In culture, FAHF-2 also increased interferon gamma and IL-10 levels.

We should note—given the research from Chapter Three on allergy crossover between foods and pollens—that FAHF-2 should also have similar effects upon tolerance to pollens.

Individual Chinese Anti-Allergy Herbs

We can see that many of the above formulas have herbs in common. Here are some of the active herbs contained in the formulas above. Several of these herbs are also popular in Ayurvedic and/or Western herbalism, as we'll discuss.

Ban Xia (Pinella)

This is the root of the plant called *Pinellia ternata*, and also commonly called Pinellia. There are also a number of related species called Pinellia, with similar properties. It is a grassy bush that grows primarily in Asia. The raw herb is poisonous and should never be consumed. Herbalists have also applied the raw herb and root to the skin for rheumatic pain.

The Ban Xia used in Chinese medicine is Pinellia root that has been carefully fried in fresh Ginger. This removes its toxic effect, and only this version is added to the formulas discussed earlier.

Ban Xia has been used for centuries in formulation and also alone for respiratory conditions. Triterpenoid saponins and benzoic acid are two primary constituents. *In vivo* studies have confirmed its ability to increase mucosal membrane secretions and thus reduce airway sensitivity.

In one, researchers from South Korea's Sangji University (Ok *et al.* 2009) found that *Pinellia ternata* in formulation reduced eosinophils, histamine and allergen-specific IgEs, along with notable Th2 pro-inflammatory cytokine (IL-5 and IL-13) expression within the lungs.

Chai Hu (Bupleurum)

Bupleurum (*Bupleurum chinense* or *Bupleurum falcatum*) has also been called Hare's Ear, Saiko and Thorowax. Bupleurum belongs in the Umbelliferae family, and thus is related to fennel, dill, cumin, coriander and others—and exerts similar medicinal effects.

The root is typically used, and its constituents include triterpenoid saponins called saikosides, flavonoids such as rutin, and sterols such as bupleurumol, furfurol and stigmasterol. The saikosides in Bupleurum have been known to boost liver function and reduce liver toxicity. In general, Bupleurum appears to also stimulate detoxification.

Bupleurum is used to stimulate the spleen, purify the blood and rejuvenate the liver—and has been used to treat hepatitis. As it relates to the allergy and asthmatic conditions, Bupleurum was studied by researchers at the Beijing University of Traditional Chinese Medicine (Chen *et al.* 2005) on 58 patients with spleen deficiency. After one month of treatment, tests showed that levels of epinephrine and dopamine were decreased and beta-endorphin levels had increased substantially among the Bupleurum-treated group. They concluded that Bupleurum significantly *"regulates nervous and endocrine systems."*

Chuan Jiao (Szechwan Pepper)

This is the fruit from *Zanthoxylum simulans* which is also sometimes referred to as *Fructus Zanthoxyli Bungeani* or *Pericarpium zanthoxyli bungeani* in traditional Chinese medicine. More precisely, this herb is also referred to as Sichuan pepper. The tree is also called Prickly ash, and is grown around the world. The small peppers that come from the Prickly ash tree can be dried and ground or used fresh.

Chuan Jiao is also referred to as Fagara, Sansho, Nepal pepper or Szechwan pepper.

Because it is very spicy and hot, it is often used in Sichuan dishes—known for their spiciness. Chuan Jiao contains limonene, geraniol and cumic alcohol, among with a number of other medicinal constituents.

In traditional Chinese medicine, Chuan Jiao is known to remove abdominal pain, vomiting, nausea and parasites—especially roundworm. It is also used as a skin wash for eczema, and has a mild diuretic effect.

Dang Gui (Dong Quai)

This is *Angelica sinensis,* also referred to as *Corpus radix angelicae sinensis* in traditional Chinese medicine. The roots and rhizomes are used. In Western herbology, it is sometimes referred to simply as Angelica. It is also called Dong quai.

This herb contains courmarins and a number of volatile oils. Thus it is known to lower blood pressure, relax tense muscles and improve circulation, as it inhibits platelet aggregation. It is also known as a potent anti-inflammatory, and is known to rejuvenate the adrenal glands.

Dong quai is also considered antispasmodic, which means it reduces hypersensitivity. It stimulates tolerance. It is a very popular herb for balancing the female reproductive system and irregular menstruation. It is considered a tonic in general, and has been used in traditional medicine for colds, fevers, inflammation, arthritis, rheumatic issues and anemia.

Fu Zi (Aconitum)

Fuzi's botanical name is *Aconitum carmichaelii*, and it is also referred to as *Radix Aconiti Carmichaeli Praeparata* among Chinese medicine. It is also commonly called Aconitum or Monkshood by herbalists. It is a well-known herb in both Chinese medicine and Ayurveda. There are many related species. The rationale for excluding this herb from the FAHF formula is likely because unprocessed Aconitum can be poisonous.

However, Ayurvedic and Chinese herbal formulations utilize Aconitum only after it has been thoroughly steamed with Ginger. This precise process of extraction makes Aconitum a safe herbal medicine as prescribed by traditional doctors.

This toxin-extracted Aconitum has been used for thousands of years for clearing obstructions and blockages among the organs and channels. It is used for chills, colds and congestion.

A number of traditional texts have documented its anti-inflammatory and anti-arthritic effects.

In its raw form, Aconitum is used among herbalists strictly for external purposes. As a liniment, Aconitum is considered useful for rheumatism and neuralgia.

It is also used in homeopathy in infinitesimal (significantly diluted) doses.

The type of Aconitum utilized in the original FAHF formula is the processed version. It was also extremely diluted to reduce any potential of toxicity. Nonetheless, we should issue the appropriate warning about Aconitum: *This can be a lethal poison and should only be prescribed by a health professional expert in its safe usage.*

Gan Cao (Chinese Licorice) and Licorice

Glycyrrhiza uralensis is also called Chinese Licorice. It is not the common Licorice (*Glycyrrhiza glabra*) known in Western and Ayurvedic herbalism. However, the two plants have nearly identical uses and constituents. So this discussion also serves *Glycyrrhiza glabra*.

Chinese Licorice is known in Chinese medicine as giving moisture and balancing heat to the lungs. It has thus been extensively used to stop coughs and wheezing. It is also known to clear fevers. Taken either internally or topically, it is known to ease carbuncles and skin lesions. It is also soothing to the throat and eases muscle spasms. The root is thus described as antispasmodic.

Researchers from New York's Mount Sinai School of Medicine (Jayaprakasam *et al.* 2009) extensively investigated the properties of *Glycyr-*

rhiza uralensis. They found that *G. uralensis* had five major flavonoids: liquiritin, liquiritigenin, isoliquiritigenin, dihydroxyflavone, and isoononin. Liquiritigenin, isoliquiritigenin, and dihydroxyflavone were found to suppress airway inflammation via inhibiting eotaxin. Eotaxin stimulates the release of eosinophils to hypersensitive airways during inflammation.

Licorice also contains glactomannan, triterpene saponins, glycerol, glycyrrhisoflavone, glycybenzofuran, cyclolicocoumarone, glycybenzofuran, cyclolicocoumarone, licocoumarone, glisoflavone, cycloglycyrrhisoflavone, licoflavone, apigenin, isokaempferide, glycycoumarin, isoglycycoumarin, glycyrrhizin and glycyrrhetinic acid (Li *et al.* 2010; Huang *et al.* 2010).

One of its main active constituents, isoliquiritigenin, has been shown to be a H2 histamine antagonist (Stahl 2008). Chinese Licorice has been shown to prevent the IgE binding that signals the release of histamine. This essentially disrupts the histamine inflammatory process while modulating immune system responses (Kim *et al.* 2006).

Another important constituent, glycyrrhizin, is a potent anti-inflammatory biochemical. It has also been shown to halt the breakdown of cortisol produced by the body. Let's consider this carefully. Like cortisone, cortisol inhibits the inflammatory process by interrupting interleukin cytokine transmission. If cortisol is prevented from breaking down, more remains available in the bloodstream to keep a lid on inflammation.

This combination of constituents gives Licorice aldosterone-like effects. This means that the root stimulates the production and maintenance of steroidal corticoids. Animal research has confirmed that Licorice is anti-allergic, and decreases anaphylactic response. It also balances electrolytes and inflammatory edema (Lee *et al.* 2010; Gao *et al.* 2009).

Gan Jiang (Ginger)

This is *Zingiberis officinalis*, also called *Rhizoma zingiberis officinalis* in traditional Chinese medicine. It is quite simply common Ginger root.

Ginger is extensively used in both Chinese and Ayurvedic medicine. It is also commonly used in Western herbalism and a number of other traditional medicines around the world.

Ginger is one of the most versatile food-spice-herbs known to humanity. In Ayurveda—the oldest medical practice still in use—Ginger is the most recommended botanical medicine. Ginger is referred to as *vishwabhesaj*—meaning "universal medicine"—by Ayurvedic physicians.

An accumulation of studies and chemical analyses has determined that Ginger has at least 477 active constituents. As in all botanicals, each constituent will stimulate a slightly different mechanism—often moderating the mechanisms of other constituents. Many of Ginger's active constituents have anti-inflammatory and/or pain-reducing effects. These include a number of gingerols and shogaols.

Clinical evaluation has documented that Ginger blocks inflammation by inhibiting lipoxygenase and prostaglandins in a balanced manner. This allows for a gradual reduction of inflammation and pain without the negative GI side effects that accompany NSAIDs. Ginger also stimulates circulation, inhibits various infections, and strengthens the liver.

Properties of Ginger supported by traditional clinical use include being analgesic, anthelmintic, anticathartic, antiemetic, antifungal, antihepatotoxic, antipyretic, antitussive, antiulcer, cardiotonic, gastrointestinal motility, hypotensive, thermoregulatory, analgesic, tonic, expectorant, carminative, antiemetic, stimulant, anti-inflammatory, antimicrobial and more.

Ginger has therefore been used as a traditional treatment for inflammatory conditions, sinusitis, bronchitis, rheumatism, asthma, colic, nervous disorders, colds, coughs, migraines, pneumonia, indigestion, respiratory ailments, fevers, nausea, colds, flu, ulcers, hepatitis, liver disease, colitis, tuberculosis and many digestive ailments to name a few.

Gui Zhi (Cinnamon)

This is *Cinnamomum cassia*, also referred to as *Ramulus cinnamomi cassiae* in traditional Chinese medicine. It is commonly called cinnamon—a delicious culinary spice present in most kitchens.

Cinnamon is used in just about every traditional medicine. The bark is often used, although the twigs are also utilized. Its constituents include limonene, camphor, cineole, cinnamic aldehyde, gums, mannitol, safrole, tannins and oils.

According to Western herbalism, Ayurvedic medicine and traditional Chinese medicine, it is useful for colds, sinusitis, bronchitis, dyspepsia, asthma, muscle tension, toothaches, the heart, the kidneys, and digestion. It is also thought to strengthen circulation in general. Its properties are described as expectorant, diuretic, stimulating, analgesic and alterative. In other words, it is an immune-system modulator. It is also thought to dilate the blood vessels and warm the body according to these traditional disciplines.

Huang Qi (Astragalus)

Astragalus (*Astragalus mongholicus* or *Astragalus membranaceus*) root is a well-known immune system adaptogen. In other words, it strengthens the immune system, allowing it to become more tolerant. Astragalus has also been proven to be calming, anti-inflammatory and anti-microbial.

In Chinese medicine, Astragalus is known to treat *qi* deficiency. Remember, *qi* (or *chi*) is the vigor of the body, expressed in circulation, heat, detoxification and immunity. Thus, Astragalus invigorates the body. Astragalus is often used to treat exhaustion, adrenal deficiency, spleen deficiency and circulation issues. Laboratory and *in vivo* research has shown it can reduce blood pressure and increase circulatory health.

Astragalus contains a number of constituents, such as astragalosides, isoastragalosides, astramembrannin, afrormosin, catycosin, daucosterol, formononetin, ononin, pinitol, sitosterol, and various flavonoids, including methoxyisoflavone. It also contains two polysaccharide glucans, heteroglycans, and calycosin.

Researchers from China's Sichuan University (Wang *et al.* 2010) gave *Astragalus membranaceus* to 15 asthma patients and 15 healthy volunteers. They found that Astragalus reduced IL-4 cytokines and modulated the Th1/Th2 ratio, reducing pro-inflammatory processes—evidenced by changes in genetic signalling.

Researchers from Shanghai's Huashan Hospital of Fudan University (Xie *et al.* 2006) found that Astragalus reduced the production of TNF-alpha and inhibited NF-kappa B activity. This illustrated its adaptogenic properties and ability to inhibit inflammation.

Astragalus root may not be a major airway modifying herb as some others are, but its use as an adaptogen can support the powerful effects of airway-oriented herbs.

For example, researchers from China's Huai Ning County Hospital (Wang *et al.* 1998) studied the effects of a combination of *Astragalus membranceus, Codonpsis pilosula* and *glycyrrhiza uralensis* on 28 asthmatic patients for six weeks. After the treatment period, their lung functions, measured by FVC, FEV1 and PEF, were significantly improved. They also found that the herbs significantly decreased airway responsiveness following the treatment period.

Huang Lian (Gold Thread)

This is from the species *Coptis chinnensis*. It is often referred to as *Rhizoma coptidis* in Chinese medicine. Its common names include Gold thread or Golden thread. In Ayurveda, other species of *Coptis* spp. are also considered Gold thread.

Materia Medica of traditional Chinese medicine have documented that Gold thread removes heat associated with histamine responses affecting the eyes, throat and skin. It has also proved helpful for digestion. Applied topically, it has been used to calm skin rash, and has been used to treat boils and abscesses.

In Ayurveda, Gold thread is considered a bitter and tonic herb that reduces fever (antipyretic). It is also reputed to belong in the same category as Goldenseal.

Huang Bai (Phellodendron)

This is from the plant with the botanical name *Phellodendron amurense* or *Phellodendron chinense*. It is also called *Cortex phellodendri* in traditional Chinese medicine. One of Huang bai's most common Western names is the Amur cork tree. Others have simply called this tree the Cork tree.

In a study by researchers from Taiwan's National Changhua University (Tsai *et al.* 2004), Huang bai in combination with another herb, Qian niuzi (Pharbitis), was found to significantly affect the ion transport mechanisms within the cells of the intestinal wall. Other clinical documentation has confirmed that it can reduce blood pressure, slow contraction reflexes within the intestines, and modulate the central nervous system. Ointments of Huang bai have been used traditionally for treating eczema as well.

Jujube

The *Ziziphus zizyphus* plant produces a delicious sweet date that tastes very much like a sweet apple. The fruit has many different properties in traditional medicine. It has been used to stimulate the immune system. It has been used to reduce stress, reduce inflammation, sooth indigestion, and repeal GERD.

Jujube contains a variety of constituents, including mucilage, ceanothic acid, alphitolic acid, zizyberanal acid, zizyberanalic acid, zizyberanone, epiceanothic acid, ceanothenic acid, betulinic acid, oleanolic acid, ursolic acid, zizyberenalic acid, maslinic acid, tetracosanoic acid, kaempferol, rutin, quercetin and others.

These constituents suggest the extensive support that this fruit can render for asthma sufferers with regard to rebuilding the mucosal membranes, reducing inflammation, relaxing the mind and nerves, and soothing the airways.

Ku-Shen (Sophora)

The small shrub *Sophora flavescens* is known to substantially modulate the immune system. It has also been shown to slow tumor progression (Li *et al.* 2010).

Among other constituents, it contains prenylated flavonoids, quinolizidine alkaloids (such as matrine), dehydromatrine, flavascensine and a number of other alkaloids (Liu *et al.* 2010; Jung *et al.* 2010). Research has shown it to inhibit several cytokines involved in the inflammatory sequence, notably IL-6 and TNF-alpha. It also blocks the release of the pain precursor, substance P (Liu *et al.* 2007; Xiao *et al.* 1999).

This herb has also been extensively used in traditional Hawaiian herbal medicine for asthma and other airway issues. In further research as a Polynesian medicine, it has been shown to significantly reduce allergy responses among the airways (Massey *et al.* 1994).

Ling Zhi (Reishi)

This is none other than *Ganoderma lucidum*, also known as Reishi—a popular medicinal mushroom. Reishi has been shown in numerous studies to significantly stimulate the immune system, increase tolerance and moderate inflammation.

Reishi contains many constituents, including steroids, triterpenes, lipids, alkaloids, glucosides, coumarin glycoside, choline, betaine, tetracosanoic acid, stearic acid, palmitic acid, nonadecanoic acid, behenic acid, tetracosane, hentriacontane, ergosterol, sitosterol, ganoderenic acids, ganolucidic acids, lucidenic acids, lucidone and many more.

Ling Zhi strengthens immunity and modulates the body's tolerance and responses to allergens. Reishi has been shown to increase production of IL-1, IL-2 and natural killer cell activity. A number of studies have shown that Reishi can significantly lower IgE levels specific to allergens, and reduce inflammatory histamine levels. It has also been shown to improve lung function and has been used traditionally for bronchitis and asthma.

Recently, researchers from Japan's University of Toyama (Andoh *et al.* 2010) found that Reishi also relieves skin itching and rash *in vivo*.

Ma Huang (Ephedra)

Ephedra (*Ephedra sinica, E. vulgaris* and related species) has received some unfair restrictions and negative press over the past few years as a result of unscrupulous product formulators combining refined Ephedra with caffeine, refined sugar, taurine and other inappropriate ingredients.

Ephedra in fact is a very popular herbal remedy in traditional Chinese medicine and Japanese medicine—where it is called Mao. However, it also grows all over the world, and thus has also been a part of North American Indian folk medicine and Western herbalism, as well as other indigenous medicines around the world. Among North American traditional herbalists, Ephedra has been called Mormon tea, Desert tea, Brigham tea, Mexican tea and Nevada fir. It should be noted that some of these species of Ephedra differ slightly in constituents with the Asian variety, but still share some of the same effects.

Two primary constituents, ephedrine and norephedrine/pseudo-ephedrine, have been isolated and synthesized into decongestants and weight loss pharmaceutical drugs. These have been proven in multiple drug trials to curb allergic response, open the airways, and curb the appetite. However, as isolated constituents, they have also been known to cause side effects, which include nausea, flushing, insomnia, blood vessel constriction and restlessness. In contrast, whole herb Ephedra contains many other constituents that help balance and buffer these side effects. And for this reason, it has been used safely for thousands of years in traditional medicines around the world.

These other constituents include tannins, flavones, phosphorus, calcium and volatile oils. These work synergistically with ephedrine and pseudoephedrine to reduce inflammation, dilate airways, clear the nasal passages, purify the bloodstream and increase urination. Ephedrine and pseudoephedrine make up anywhere from 30% to 90% of the alkaloid content of Ephedra.

Japanese researchers (Shibata *et al.* 2000) have found that these two constituents in Ephedra inhibit mast/basophil/neutrophil cell degranulation. As we discussed in the immune chapter, mast/basophil/neutrophil cell degranulation releases leukotrienes, histamine and other mediators that stimulate the allergic and asthmatic response.

In the 1990s, Ephedra began being used by adolescents to achieve intoxication. There were complaints of side effects and a few fatalities as a result of overdosing. Due to the confusion regarding how to utilize Ma huang, Ephedra should be prescribed by a knowledgeable herbalist or medical professional.

Ren Shen (Panex Ginseng)

Panex ginseng is a traditional remedy for allergies and hypersensitivity with thousands of years of use. Panax ginseng will come in white forms and red forms. The color depends upon the aging or drying technique used.

The Ginseng in the FAHF formula is termed *Radix* Ginseng or Ren shen but it is *Panex ginseng*. Depending upon how the Ginseng is cured, there are several types of Ren shen.

When Ginseng is cultivated and steamed, it is called 'red root' or Hong Shen. Ginseng root will turn red when it is oxidized or processed with steaming. Some feel that red root is better than white, but this really depends upon its intended use, the age of the root, and how it was processed. Soaking Ginseng in rock candy produces a white Ginseng that is called Bai shen. This soaking seems odd, but this has been known to increase some of its constituent levels such as superoxide and nitric oxide. When the root is simply dried, it is called 'dry root' or Sheng shaii shen. Korean Red Ginseng is soaked in a special herbal broth and then dried.

There are a number of species within the *Panax* genus, most of which also contain most of the same adaptogens, referred to as gensenosides. Most notable in the *Panex* genus is American Ginseng, *Panax quinquefolius*.

Ginseng contains camphor, mucilage, panaxosides, resins, saponins, gensenosides, arabinose and polysaccharides, among others.

Eleutherococcus senticosus, often called Siberian Ginseng, is actually not Ginseng. While it also contains adaptogens (eleutherosides), these are not the gensenoside adaptogens within Ginseng that have been observed for their ability to relieve hypersensitivity.

Researchers from Italy's Ambientale Medical Institute (Caruso *et al.* 2008) tested an herbal extract formula consisting of *Capparis spinosa, Olea europaea, Panax ginseng* and *Ribes nigrum* (Pantescal) on allergic patients. They found that allergic biomarkers, including basophil degranulation CD63 and sulphidoleukotriene (SLT) levels were significantly lower after 10 days. They theorized that these biomarkers explain the herbal formulation's *"protective effects."*

Researchers from Japan's Ehime University Graduate School of Medicine (Sumiyoshi *et al.* 2010) tested *Panax ginseng* on mice sensitized to hen's eggs. After the oral feedings, they found that the Ginseng significantly reduced allergen-specific IgG Th2 levels. It also increased IL-12 production, and increased the ratio of Th1 to Th2 among spleen cells. In addition, it enhanced intestinal CD8, IFN-gamma, and IgA-positive counts. The researchers concluded that, *"Red Ginseng roots may be a natural preventative of food allergies."*

Ginseng has been found to stimulate circulation and improve cognition. It is also known to reduce fatigue, and stress. Herbalists also use it to improve appetite, and as a mild stimulant and potent antioxidant.

Wu Mei (Black Plum)

Prunus mume (Seib et Zucc) is also referred to as *Fructus pruni mume* in Chinese medicine. It is also called *Omae* in Korea, *Ume* or *Umeboshi plum* in Japan, which translates, quite simply, to 'Dark plum' or 'Black plum.' It is also referred to as Mume. It is, quite simply, the fruit of a special variety of plums.

This plum is treasured for its immune-stimulating properties. The Chinese *Materia Medica* describes it as able to alleviate coughing and lung deficiencies. It has a strongly astringent property, and thus helps to cleanse the digestive tract and halt diarrhea. Research documented in the *Medica* has indicated that it stimulates bile production, is anti-microbial, and has been able to relieve fever, nausea, abdominal pain and vomiting.

Xi Xin (Chinese Wild Ginger)

Xi xin's botanical name is *Herba asari.* It is also called Chinese Wild Ginger (not to be confused with common Ginger). The entire plant is used, but its roots have significant usefulness. It is pungent and warming, and widely used in Chinese and Ayurveda medicine to provide heat and help clear the body of phlegm and congestion. It is said to slow the histamine response while stimulating the immune system's detoxification routines. TCM doctors often prescribe it alone with Aconitum to help relieve congestion. It is also sometimes combined with peppermint herb to help clear headaches and nasal congestion.

Yin Xing (Gingko)

The extracts or powders from the leaves of the *Gingko biloba* plant are now popular all over the world. Ginkgo's standardized extracts are part of many formulas, from brain tonics to blood purification formulations. It also has a long history of use in Chinese medicine for expanding the airways.

Gingko contains numerous flavonoids and terpenoids, including ginkgolide, amentoflavone, biolobetin, bilobalide, ginkgetin, glycosides, ginkgolic acids, quercetin, isorhamnetins, kaempferol and others. Ginkgolide, for example has been shown to inhibit platelet aggregating factor (PAF), which means that it helps prevent clotting events within the arteries. This has been suspected as being one of its mechanisms that enable it to open the airways.

In a study by British researchers (Guinot *et al.* 1987), Gingko was shown to be protective against exercise-induced bronchospasm; and decreased the subjects' sensitivity to dust mites.

Researchers from China's Qingdao Hospital of Integrated Traditional and Western Medicine (Li *et al.* 1997) tested a liquid Gingko leaf concentrate or a placebo on 61 asthmatic patients. They found the Gingko concentrate reduced asthmatic hyperactivity symptoms and increased lung function significantly better than the placebo.

A study from researchers at Germany's Hannover School of Pharmacy and Medicine (Wilkens *et al.* 1990) studied six asthmatic patients using the Ginkgo extract BN 52063. Intake of the extract resulted in an almost immediate reduction in platelet factor 4 (PF4) and beta-thromboglobulin (beta-TBG). PF4 and beta-TBG are instigated in asthmatic hypersensitivity and bronchial spasm as we've mentioned earlier.

Ayurvedic Anti-Allergy Herbs and Formulations

Ayurvedic doctors have been prescribing herbal medicine to their patients with airway conditions for thousands of years. There is a wealth of information provided in the Vedic and *Materia Medica* texts that have been passed down through the centuries. Ancient texts that include tenets on Ayurveda include the *Arshnashaka, Kricch-Hridroganashak, Mehnashaka, Kasaswasahara, Pandunashaka, Kamla-Kushta-Vataraktanashaka, Rasayana, Sangrahi, Balya, Agnideepana, Tridoshshamaka, Dahnashaka, Jwarhara, Krimihara* and *Prameha.*

This information has had a tradition of acceptance and clinical application among literally hundreds of millions of patients over the centuries.

Ayurvedic doctors were highly esteemed and respected around the world for thousands of years. In fact, the medicines of Arabia, China, Europe, Greece and Rome borrowed many of their basic principles and herbal medicine applications from Ayurveda. And of course, these medical traditions also practiced those principles on millions of patients over the centuries. We can thus conclude that Ayurveda has had a rich history of clinical use, success and safety.

Because of this history of safety, little thought was given to double-blind studies until recent years. This history of thousands of years of success and safety of Ayurvedic herbs did not indicate the need for clinical research until Ayurveda was challenged by modern medicine. The age of pharmaceuticals has challenged Ayurvedic formulations, just as they have challenged Chinese formulations. And just as Chinese formulations are proving successful in double-blind, placebo-controlled research, Ayurvedic medicine has also proved successful and safe in clinical research.

For example, clinical researchers from Richmond, VA (Singh *et al.* 2007) extensively reviewed a variety of databases including numerous studies of Ayurvedic herbs for airway conditions. They eliminated studies on Chinese medicinal herbs. Forty-two articles were found and 37 studies were evaluated utilizing three independent evaluators and one arbitrator. They concluded that many Ayurvedic herbs appear to be useful in the treatment of airway hypersensitivity.

At the same time, Ayurvedic medicine research has been trailing research on Chinese medicine. Traditional Chinese medicine has enjoyed research funding over the past decade or so from the Chinese government, and more recently from a few Western medical schools. As a result, while Ayurvedic formulations have such a rich tradition of success, for many herbs we must rely primarily upon the traditional texts for clinical documentation, with only a smattering of clinical research for additional verification.

An ancient allergy formula developed by Ayurvedic physicians has been called Aller-7. This formula includes:

➢ *Phyllanthus emblica*
➢ *Terminalia chebula*
➢ *Terminalia bellerica*
➢ *Albizia lebbeck*
➢ *Piper nigrum*
➢ *Zingiber officinale*
➢ *Piper longum*

Ayurvedic researchers from the Natural Remedies Research Center in Bangalore, India (Amit *et al.* 2003) studied the Aller-7 formula *in vivo* and found that the formula blocked the lipoxygenase and hyaluronidase enzymes, which stimulate and maintain the rhinitis inflammatory condition.

Another traditional Ayurvedic formula has been used for asthmatic hypersensitivity (we'll call it the AAA Formula) contains the following herbs:

> *Boswellia serrata* (Boswellia)
> *Glycyrrhiza glabra* (Licorice root)
> *Curcuma longa* (Tumeric root)

School of Pharmacy researchers from Egypt's University of Beni Sueif (Houssen *et al.* 2010) gave 63 asthma patients either the AAA Formula or a placebo for four weeks. They found that inflammatory leukotrienes, nitric oxide and malondialdehyde were significantly reduced among the group treated with the AAA herbal combination. They also saw a significant improvement in symptoms among the AAA-treated group.

Here are these and other individual Ayurvedic herbs used for airway hypersensitivities:

Antamool (Tylophora)

Tylophora indica—also called *Tylophora asthmatica*—has been researched over the past four decades, yet surprisingly has received little attention from many herbalists and media texts.

Tylophora is a perennial shrub native to Southern and Eastern India. The plant has traditionally been used to treat asthma, rheumatism and dermatitis. It is known as being emetic, expectorant, bronchodilating and diaphoretic.

Tylophora contains several medicinal alkaloids, including tylophorine. These and other alkaloids have been described as phenanthroindalizidines.

A crossover study by Indian researchers (Shivpuri *et al.* 1969) gave 110 asthmatic patients either raw Tylophora (leaf) or a placebo (spinach). After one week, 62% of the Tylophora group had moderate to complete symptom relief, while the placebo group experienced 28% relief in comparison. The researchers then treated the placebo group with Tylophora and gave the group treated first with Tylophora the placebo. This time, 50% of the new Tylophora group experienced moderate to complete relief of asthma symptoms, while 11% of the new placebo group reported relief.

Three years later the same researchers (Shivpuri *et al.* 1972) followed up this study by testing 103 asthmatic patients with an alcoholic extract of Tylophora leaves. This time, 56% of the Tylophora group reported moderate to complete relief of asthma symptoms, compared to 32% in the placebo group.

A few years later, another Indian research team (Thiruvengadam *et al.* 1978) gave 350 milligrams of Tylophora leaf powder or a placebo plus anti-asthmatic medications each day to 30 asthmatic patients for two weeks. The Tylophora group had a significant improvement in lung function and significantly reduced shortness of breath. They concluded that, *"there was a sustained rise in maximum breathing capacity (MBC), vital capacity (VC), and peak expiratory flow rate (PEFR) with the leaf (plant extract) as compared with the placebo."*

In another study, researchers (Gore *et al.* 1980) gave 11 patients with asthma, along with 18 healthy volunteers, 3-6 leaves of Tylorphora per day. They found that the Tylophora significantly reduced sneezing and nasal obstruction. They also found Tylophora increased breathing capacity that lasted almost 10 days after the treatment.

In this last study, the researchers hypothesized that Tylophora stimulated the adrenal gland to release cortisol, with possibly a muscle-relaxant effect to go along with it.

This possibility of Tylophora stimulating the adrenal gland was confirmed in animal studies over a decade later (Udupa *et al.* 1991).

Boswellia (Frankincense)

The medicinal Boswellia species include *Boswellia serratta*, *Boswellia thurifera*, and *Boswellia spp.* (other species). Boswellia contains a variety of active constituents, including a number of boswellic acids, diterpenes, ocimene, caryophyllene, incensole acetate, limonene and lupeolic acids.

The genus of *Boswellia* includes a group of trees known for their fragrant sap resin that grow in Africa and Asia. Frankincense was extensively used in ancient Egypt, India, Arabia and Mesopotamia thousands of years ago, as an elixir that relaxed and healed the body's aches and pains. The gum from the resin was applied as an ointment for rheumatic ailments, urinary tract disorders, and on the chest for bronchitis and general breathing problems. It is classified in Ayurveda as bitter and pungent.

Over the centuries, boswellia has been used as an internal treatment for a wide variety of ailments, including inflammation, bronchitis, asthma, arthritis, rheumatism, anemia, allergies and a variety of infections. Its properties are described as stimulant, diaphoretic, anti-rheumatic, tonic, analgesic, antiseptic, diuretic, demulcent, astringent, expectorant, and antispasmodic.

Researchers from Germany's Tübingen Institute of Pharmacology (Gupta *et al.* 1998) gave placebo or 300 milligrams of Boswellia gum resin three times a day for six weeks to 80 long-time asthma patients. After the treatment period, 70% of the Boswellia group had significant reductions or a disappearance in asthma symptoms and episodes—compared to 27% among the control group. Forced expiratory flows, volume capacity and peak flows were significantly increased among the Boswellia group. The Boswellia group also displayed a significant reduction in inflammatory eosinophils.

In two studies, boswellic acids extracted from Boswellia were found to have significant anti-inflammatory action. The trials revealed that Boswellia inhibited the inflammation-stimulating LOX enzyme (5-lipoxygenase) and thus significantly reduced the production of inflammatory leukotrienes (Singh *et al.* 2008; Ammon 2006).

Another study (Takada *et al.* 2006) showed that boswellic acids inhibited cytokines and suppressed cell invasion through NF-kappaB inhibition.

In *in vivo* studies by researchers from the University of Maryland's School of Medicine (Fan *et al.* 2005), Boswellia extract exhibited significant anti-inflammatory effects. The report also concluded that, *"these effects may be mediated via the suppression of pro-inflammatory cytokines."*

In an *in vitro* study also from the University of Maryland's School of Medicine (Chevrier *et al.* 2005), boswellia extract proved to modulate the balance between Th1 and Th2 cytokines. This illustrated Boswellia's ability to strengthen the immune system and increase tolerance.

A similar-acting anti-asthmatic Ayurvedic herb is Guggul. Guggul is another gum derived from the resin of a tree—*Commiphora mukul.*

Coleus

Coleus forskohlii has been used in Ayurveda for acute airway conditions for thousands of years. Over the past few decades, several studies have shown that it can directly reduce allergic and asthmatic symptoms. The central mechanism appears to be that Coleus stimulates cyclic AMP production. Deficiencies in cAMP have been observed amongst many with airway hypersensitivities.

The central constituent in Coleus is forskolin. This isolated extract has been more specifically studied with clinical success for subduing asthmatic symptoms. In a study from Manzanillo's Hospital del Instituto Mexicano del Seguro Social (González-Sánchez *et al.* 2006), 40 patients with mild asthma were given either 10 milligrams per day of forskolin capsules or two inhalations of sodium cromoglycate every eight hours for things times a day.

For the six month period, only 40% of the forskolin-treated patients had asthma attacks, versus 85% of the sodium cromoglycate-treated patients. Forced expiratory volumes (FEV1) were similar between the two groups after the treatment period. The researchers concluded: *"We conclude that forskolin is more effective than sodium cromoglycate in preventing asthma attacks in patients with mild persistent or moderate persistent asthma."*

For this reason, forskolin inhalers are often prescribed and utilized by physicians for asthmatics, and prominently so in Europe.

Marica (Black Pepper)

While *Piper nigrum* is considered Ayurvedic, it is probably one of the most common spices used in Western foods. In fact, the world probably owes its use of Black pepper in foods to Ayurveda.

Black pepper is used in a variety of Ayurvedic formulations because of its anti-inflammatory action. Ayurvedic doctors describe Black pepper as a stimulant, expectorant, carminative (expulsing gas), anti-inflammatory and analgesic. It has been used traditionally for allergies, rheumatism, bronchitis, coughs, asthma, sinusitis, gastritis and other histamine-related conditions. It is also thought to stimulate a healthy mucosal membrane among the stomach and intestines.

Black pepper used as a spice to increase taste is certainly not un-healthy, but it takes a significantly greater and consistent dose to produce its anti-inflammatory effects.

A traditional Ayurvedic prescription for gastroesophageal reflux or GERD, for example, is to take Black pepper in a warm glass of water on an empty stomach first thing in the morning over a period of time. This dose of Black pepper, according to Ayurveda, stimulates mucosal secre-tion, and purifies the mucosal membranes of the stomach and intestines.

Researchers from South Korea's Wonkwang University (Bae *et al.* 2010) found that the *Piper nigrum* extract piperine significantly inhibited inflammatory responses, including leukocytes and TNF-alpha.

Pippali (Long Pepper)

The related Ayurvedic herb, *Piper longum,* has similar properties and constituents as Black pepper. It is used to inhibit the inflammation and histamine activity that results in lung and sinus congestion. Like Black pepper, Long pepper is also known to strengthen digestion by stimulating the secretion of the mucosal membranes within the stomach and intes-tines. It is also said to stimulate enzyme activity and bile production. One study by researchers from India's Markandeshwar University (Kumar *et al.* 2009) found that the oil of Long pepper fruit significantly reduced in-flammation.

Sirisha

Sirisha or Shirisha is *Albizia lebbeck.* It has been used in Ayurveda for thousands of years for bronchial conditions—notably asthma—and other issues related to systemic inflammation. It has also been used for convul-sions and infections—as it is said to be an antiseptic. *Albizia lebbeck* is also called the Siris tree, and contains a variety of glycosides, flavonoids, tan-nins and saponins. Some of the more notable constituents are betulinic acid, beta-sitosterol, melacacidin, lcuco-anthracyanidin, lebbecacidin, kaempferol and quercetin. The leaves, seeds and bark are used. The bark is used for asthma and other inflammatory conditions; and the leaves are used for their anti-convulsion properties. The leaves are considered remedies for snake and scorpion bites (Kumar *et al.* 2007).

In a study from Gujarat Ayurved University (Jaiswal *et al.* 2006), Sirisha showed significant anti-asthmatic and anti-histamine activities after being given to 41 asthmatic patients.

Tinospora (Guduchi)

Tinospora's Ayurvedic name is Guduchi, and its botanical name is *Tinospora Cordifolia*. Among Western herbalists, this herb has been referred to as Heartleaf moonseed. This climbing shrub—at home in tropical regions of India and China—has been utilized for thousands of years to modulate immunity and increase tolerance. In other words, it is an adaptogen.

The Guduchi plant contains a number of alkaloids, aliphatic compounds, diterpenoid lactones, glycosides, sesquiterpenes, phenolics, steroids, and various polysaccharides. Ayurvedic physicians report that the medicinal properties of Guduchi are anti-allergic, antispasmodic, anti-arthritic, anti-inflammatory, antioxidant, relaxant and hepato-protective (protects the liver).

Guduchi contains two researched constituents called tinosporide and cordioside. These have been shown to significantly stimulate immune cell activity, including NK cells, B-cells, T-cells. They have also been shown to increase the production of cytokines IL-1Beta, IL-6, IL-12, IL-18 INF-alpha and TNF-alpha (Kapil and Sharma 1997; Nair *et al.* 2004).

Guduchi has been used extensively for asthma, chronic coughs, allergic respiratory conditions and allergic rhinitis. Researchers from India's Indira Gandhi Medical College (Badar *et al.* 2005) gave *T. cordifolia* extract or placebo to 75 allergic rhinitis patients for eight weeks. Of the Guduchi extract-treated group, 83% reported complete relief from sneezing associated with allergies. The Guduchi treatment also produced complete relief of nasal discharges in 69% of the group, and relief of nasal obstruction in 61%. There was no relief in most of the placebo group.

The researchers also found that Guduchi reduced pro-inflammatory eosinophil and neutrophil counts. Inflammatory goblet cells were also reduced to nil in nasal smears among the Guduchi-treated group.

Numerous *in vivo* laboratory studies over recent years have confirmed the immune-modulating, liver-protective, antioxidant and anti-inflammatory effects of Guduchi (Upadhyay *et al.* 2010).

Triphala

Triphala means *"three fruits."* Triphala is a combination of three botanicals: *Terminalia chebula*, *Terminalia bellirica* and *Emblica officinalis*. They are also termed Haritaki, Bihitaki and Amalaki, respectively. This combination has been utilized for thousands of years to rejuvenate the intestines, regulate digestion and create efficiency within the digestive tract.

The 'three fruits' also are said to produce a balance among the three doshas of *vata, pitta* and *kapha*. Each herb, in fact, relates to a particular *dosha:* Haritaki relates to *vata*, Amalaki relates to *pitta* and Bibhitaki relates to *kapha*. The three taken together comprise the most-prescribed herbal formulation given by Ayurvedic doctors for digestive issues.

This use has been justified by preliminary research. For example, in a study by pharmacology researchers from India's Gujarat University (Nariya *et al.* 2003), triphala was found to significantly reverse intestinal damage and intestinal permeability *in vivo.*

The traditional texts and the clinical use of triphala today in Ayurveda have confirmed these types of intestinal effects in humans.

We might want to elaborate a little further on Haritaki in particular. *Terminalia chebula* has been used by Ayurvedic practitioners specifically for conditions related to asthma, coughs, hoarseness, abdominal issues, skin eruptions, itchiness, and inflammation. It is also called He-Zi in traditional Chinese medicine.

Research has found that Haritaki contains a large number of polyphenols, including ellagic acids, which have significant antioxidant and anti-inflammatory properties (Pfundstein *et al.* 2010).

Turmeric

Curcuma longa has been extensively used as a medicinal herb for many centuries, and this predicated its use as a curry food spice—as Ayurveda has long incorporated healing herbs with meals. The roots or rhizomes of Turmeric are used. It is a relative of Ginger in the *Zingiberaceae* family.

Just as we might expect from a medicinal botanical, Turmeric has a large number of active constituents. The most well known of those are the curcuminoids, which include curcumin (diferuloylmethane, demethoxycurcumin, and bisdemethoxycurcumin). Others include volatile oils such as tumerone, atlantone, and zingiberene; as well as polysaccharides and a number of resins.

As stated in a recent review of research from the Cytokine Research Laboratory at the University of Texas (Anand 2008), multiple studies have linked Turmeric with *"suppression of inflammation; angiogenesis; tumor genesis; diabetes; diseases of the cardiovascular, pulmonary, and neurological systems, of skin, and of liver; loss of bone and muscle; depression; chronic fatigue; and neuropathic pain."*

Indeed, Turmeric has been used for centuries for asthma, allergies, arthritis, inflammation, gallbladder problems, diabetes, wound-healing, liver issues, hepatitis, respiratory disease, menstrual pain, anemia, and gout. It is described as alterative, antibacterial, carminative and stimulating. It is also

286

known for its wound-healing, blood-purifying and circulatory powers. Studies have illustrated that curcumin has about 50% of the effectiveness of cortisone, without its damaging side effects (Jurenka 2009).

A number of studies have proved over the past decade that Turmeric and/or its key constituents such as curcumin halt or inhibit both inflammatory COX and LOX enzymes. Curcumin has specifically been shown to inhibit IgE signaling processes, and slow mast cell activation (Aggarwal and Sung 2009; Thampithak *et al.* 2009; Sompamit *et al.* 2009; Kulka 2009).

Researchers from Vandoeuvre lès Nancy School of Medicine (Venkatesan *et al.* 2007) reviewed the research on curcumin with regard to chronic lung diseases. They found that the research demonstrated that curcumin *"attenuates lung injury and fibrosis caused by radiation, chemotherapeutic drugs, and toxicants."*

Western/European Anti-Allergy Herbs

It is very difficult to separate Eastern from Western herbalism. This is because each utilizes herbs that are known to the other, and many medicinal herbs grow all over the world.

Here we will summarize herbs that have been utilized by Western, European and other herbal traditions, excluding herbs already discussed amongst the Chinese and Ayurvedic medicines that are shared by Western herbalist traditions for asthmatic conditions.

Bishop's Weed (Khella)

Trachyspermum ammiis is also called Khella or Khellin among Middle-Eastern herbalists. It is also referred to as Ajwain weed or *Ammi visnaga* among Ayurvedic practitioners and traditional herbalists. Some also refer to it as *Carum copticum*, Spanish toothpick, Toothpick weed, *Daucus visnaga* and Honeyplant. The plant is related to celery and parsley, and blooms with clusters of fragile white flowers. From the flower heads come a fruit and seeds known for their medicinal properties.

Bishop's weed has a long tradition of use in Ayurvedic medicine and Egyptian medicine, especially for asthma, coughs, bronchitis and hypersensitivity. Its use was mentioned in the *Ebers Papyrus*, written more than 3,000 years ago.

Often the fruit and seeds are crushed to produce a brown oil, which is called omam. The oil can also be infused into creams and tinctures. Omam water is also produced from Bishop's weed. To make omam water, the seeds are simply soaked in water.

Bishop's weed has been shown to inhibit histamine release. It also opens the bronchi and is considered spasmolytic (stops spasms), anticholinergic (blocks acetylcholine), and vagolytic (inhibits vagus nerve responses).

Khella's most important constituents include thymol, isothymol, pinene, cymene, cromoglycate, terpinene and limonene. The fruits contain coumarins and furocoumarins. Khellin and visnagin are considered the more active compounds in Bishop's weed.

Bishop's weed is also antimicrobial. Its antispasmodic traits may be due to its ability to dilate the bronchial passages and blood vessels without stimulation. These actions make it useful for allergies and inflammation response.

Khella's traditional uses thus include coughing, asthma, bronchitis, heart pain and muscle spasms. It has also been used for wound healing, headaches and urinary conditions. While side effects are few, Bishop's weed has been said to increase the skin's sensitivity to the sun.

There is little research on Bishop's weed proving its usefulness. However, sodium cromoglycate—one of its more active anti-asthmatic constituents—has been extensively studied and proven effective for both allergies and asthma.

Disodium cromoglycate was developed by Dr. Roger Altounyan, an asthma sufferer, based on Khella's sodium cromoglycate. Dr. Altounyan first isolated sodium cromoglycate from Khella, in other words. Today, disodium cromoglycate is often used in many cases as a drug for asthma and allergy patients as an alternative to steroids. Disodium cromoglycate has undergone extensive clinical drug studies, and is considered one of the more effective anti-asthmatic medications—one of the most prescribed drugs for asthma behind prednisone and prednisolone. Disodium cromoglycate stabilizes mast cells and smooth muscle fibers. This is effected through modulation of calcium and other ions involved in cell membrane permeability. This effect also alters the degranulation process, thus inhibiting histamine [and leukotrienes] (González Alvarez and Arruzazabala 1981).

As discussed previously, Khella has a number of other constituents besides sodium cromoglycate. Sodium cromoglycate is isolated from the constituent called khellin, which also contains benzopyran and dimethylmethylfuro. These and other constituents provide spasmolytic (halts spasms) properties that relax the smooth muscles around the airways.

Khella is a member of the carrot family. (Umbelliferae). It also looks very similar to carrot. Some have called it wild carrots. This is notable because carrots and similar tubers such as turnips and Gingers all support lung health, as we'll discuss further.

Bittersweet

Solanum dulcamara, a creeping shrub that grows along streams and bogs, has been used extensively in traditional Western herbal medicine for all varieties of allergic and inflammatory conditions. It has been used for rheumatism and circulatory problems. The alkaloid solamine and the glucoside dulcamarin have been recognized as its active constituents, but as we'll discuss, solasodine appears to be intricately involved in stimulating corticoid production (See Plant Corticoid section for discussion of the research.)

Perhaps it is for this reason that many traditional herbalists have recommended bittersweet in cases of allergic skin conditions and mucous membrane issues. We should note that another constituent, solanine, can be poisonous in significant amounts. Therefore, as in all herbal products, consultation with a health professional is suggested before use.

Coltsfoot

The leaves and flowers of *Tussilago farfara* combines soothing mucilage will expectorant action. It's constituents include saponins, tannin, alkaloid (senkirkine), zinc, potassium, calcium and of course the mucilage.

Traditional herbalists made syrups from coltsfoot, and also recommended it as a smoking herb. The fresh leaves have also been used as poultices for skin ulcers or sores, because of its soothing actions. Herbalists suggest moderate consumption of this herb.

Coriander/Cilantro/Parsley

Coriandrum sativum has documented throughout traditional medicines as an anti-allergy and antioxidant herb. The seeds are called Coriander, and the leaves are called Cilantro. Cilantro has been popularly used throughout Central America, Italy, and also Asia—where it is sometimes called Chinese parsley. Cilantro is the backbone ingredient—together with tomatoes and garlic—of salsa. It is related to Italian parsley, with many of the same constituents. Coriander is taken as fresh or juiced fresh, and it has been used by Ayurvedic practitioners primarily for allergic skin rashes and hay fever.

Fresh Italian parsley can readily be found in supermarkets and farmers' markets. While often used as a garnish (for looks and/or to clean the breath), a therapeutic quantity of parsley is about a *bunch.* A bunch of parsley is about two ounces or about ten stalks together with their branches and leaves. A *bunch* can be added to a salad or put into a soup. Parsley can be delicious with tomatoes, vinegar and olive oil. And of course, it can also freshen the breath.

Cumin Seed

Cuminum cyminum has a long history of use among European and Asian herbalists. It is described as antispasmodic and carminative, so it tends to soothe inflammatory responses. Like Fennel, Cumin has been used traditionally to ease abdominal cramping and gas.

Cumin seed contains mucilage, gums and resins. Traditional herbalists consider these constituents primarily responsible for Cumin's ability to help strengthen the mucosal membranes. This makes Cumin part of a strategy to rebuild the mucosal membranes of the airways.

Dandelion

Dandelion species include *Taraxum officinale, Taraxum mongolicum,* and *Taraxum spp.* Dandelion has been shown to help reverse the underlying issues of allergic rhinitis, as it tends to purify the blood, restore the liver, and reduce inflammation and hypersensitivity.

Dandelion contains hundreds of active constituents, which include beta-carboline alkaloids, beta-sitosterol, boron, caffeic acid, calcium, coumaric acid, coumarin, four steroids, furulic acid, gallic acid, hesperetin, hesperidin, indole alkaloids, inulin, iron, lupenol, lutein, luteolin, magnesium, mannans, monoterpenoids, myristic acid, palmitic acid, potassium, quercetins, rufescidride, sesquiterpenes, silicon, steroid complexes, stigmasterol, syringic acid, syringin, tannins, taraxacin, taraxacoside, taraxafolide, taraxafolin-B, taraxasterol, taraxasteryl acetate, taraxerol, taraxinic acid beta-glucopyranosyl, benzenoids, triterpenoids, violaxanthin, vitamin A, Bs, C, D, K and zinc among others (Hu and Kitts 2003; Hu and Kitts 2004; Seo *et al.* 2005; Trojanová *et al.* 2004; Leu *et al.* 2005; Kisiel and Michalska 2005; Leu *et al.* 2003; Michalska and Kisiel 2003; Kisiel and Barszcz 2000).

Taraxum is derived from the Greek words *taraxos* meaning 'disorder' and *akos* meaning 'remedy.' Dandelion is a common weed with a characteristic beautiful yellow flower that assumes a globe of seeds to spread its humble yet incredible medicinal virtues. Its hollow stem is full of milky juice, with a long, hardy root; and leaves that taste good in a spring salad. Dandelion has been one of the "go-to" traditional herbs for all sorts of ailments that involve toxicity within the blood, liver, kidneys, lymphatic system and urinary tract. Dandelion has been listed in a variety of herbal formularies around the world for many centuries.

Dandelion's use was expounded by many cultures from the Greeks to the Northern American Indians—who used it for stomach ailments and infections. It is also used for the treatment of viral and bacterial infections as well as cancer.

The latex or milky sap that comes from the stem has a mixture of polysaccharides, proteins, lipids, rubber, and metabolites such as polyphenoloxidase. The latex has been used to heal skin wounds and protect those wounds from infection—also the sap's function when the plant is injured. For this reason, Dandelion can significantly increase mucosal membrane health.

Dandelion is known to stimulate the elimination of toxins and clear obstructions from the blood and liver. This is thought to be why Dandelion helps clear stones and scarring from kidneys, gallbladder and bladder. It has also been used to treat stomach problems, and has been used to reduce blood pressure.

In ancient Chinese medicine, it has been recommended for issues related to the imbalance between liver enzymes and pancreatic enzymes. It has been used in traditional treatments for hypoglycemia, hypertension, urinary tract infection, skin eruptions, breast cancer, appetite loss, flatulence, dyspepsia, constipation, gallstones, circulation problems, skin issues, spleen and liver complaints, hepatitis and anorexia.

Probably the best indication of Dandelion's benefits for airway health is its ability to reduce leukotrienes—the inflammatory mediators that stimulate airway congestion. Laboratory testing has showed that leukotriene production is significantly decreased with an extract of Dandelion (Kashiwada *et al.* 2001).

Dandelion also inhibits other inflammatory mediators. A study by researchers at Canada's University of British Columbia (Hu and Kitts 2004) found that Dandelion extract suppressed the inflammatory mediator prostaglandin E2 (PGE2) without causing cell death. Further tests indicated that COX-2 was inhibited by the luteolin and luteolin-glucosides in Dandelion.

In another study by Hu and Kitts (2005), inflammatory nitric oxide levels were inhibited. Reactive oxygen species—free radicals—were also significantly reduced by Dandelion—attributed to the plant's phenolic acid content. This in turn prevented lipid peroxidation—one of the mechanisms in heightened LDL (bad cholesterol) levels and artery inflammation.

In a 2007 study from researchers at the College of Pharmacy at the Sookmyung Women's University in Korea (Jeon *et al.* 2008), Dandelion was found to reduce inflammation, leukocytes, vascular permeability, abdominal cramping, pain and COX levels among exudates.

Dandelion also supports probiotic survival. Dandelion was found to stimulate fourteen different strains of bifidobacteria—important components of the intestinal immune system (Trojanová *et al.* 2004).

Another study found that Dandelion extract significantly prevented cell death in Hep G2 (liver) cells, while stimulating TNF and IL-1 levels—illustrating its ability to boost immunity and liver health (Koo *et al.* 2004).

291

This was also illustrated in research showing that Dandelion increases the liver's production of superoxide dismutase and catalase, increasing the liver's ability to purify the blood of toxins and allergens (Cho *et al.* 2001).

Other studies have illustrated that Dandelion inhibits both interleukin IL-6 and TNF-alpha—both inflammatory cytokines often involved in allergic asthmatic episodes (Seo *et al.* 2005).

Dandelion has also illustrated the ability to inhibit inflammatory IL-1 cytokines (Kim *et al.* 2000; Takasaki *et al.* 1999), and the ability to stimulate the liver's production of glutathione (GST)—an important antioxidant needed to clear the system of mucous and toxins (Petlevski *et al.* 2003).

Elecampane

The roots and branches of *Inula helenium* have been used for bronchial issues such as asthma, bronchitis and whooping cough for many centuries. It is often the go-to herb to control coughing. It is thus considered antitussive and carminative.

Elecampane contains several sesquiterpene lactones, including alantolactone. However, its soothing effects are likely produced by its relatively high mucilage content—which makes it useful for rebuilding mucous membranes. It also contains 44% inulin, so it is a good prebiotic.

The roots or branches are typically used by traditional healers. Herbalists typically recommend Elecampane use on a moderate basis, as larger doses can be irritating to the digestive system.

Evening Primrose

Another herb known by traditional herbalists to be beneficial for allergic skin responses is Evening primrose, or *Oenothera spp.* The seeds are rich in gamma-linolenic acid (GLA)—a fatty acid known to slow inflammatory responses of prostaglandins, especially those relating to skin hypersensitivity. The oil from Evening primrose can be applied directly onto the skin and/or taken internally. Evening primrose oil has thus been used successfully in cases of allergic eczema, for example.

Fennel

Foeniculum vulgare contains anetholes, caffeoyl quinic acids, carotenoids, vitamin C, iron, B vitamins, and rutins. Ayurvedic and traditional herbalists from many cultures have used Fennel to relieve digestive discomfort, gas, abdominal cramping, bloating and irritable bowels; and to treat hypersensitivities. Fennel stimulates bile production. Bile digests fats and other nutrients, increasing their bioavailability.

One of Fennel's constituents, called anethole, is known to suppress pro-inflammatory tumor necrosis factor alpha (TNF-a). This inhibition slows excessive immune response. The combination of anethole and antioxidant nutrients such as rutin and carotenoids in Fennel also strengthen immune response while increasing tolerance.

Fennel is not appropriate for pregnant moms, because it has been known to promote uterine contractions. As with any herbal supplement, Fennel should be used under the supervision of a health professional. Those with birch allergies should also be aware that they may also be sensitive to Fennel. (The same goes for Cumin, Caraway, Carrot seed and a few others).

Grindelia

Grindelia camporum is a traditional western herb used specifically for allergic intolerance, as well as asthma and bronchitis. Its constituents include resins, saponins such as grindelin, volatile oils, alkaloids, selenium and tannins. The leaves and stems of the plant are used.

Grindelia has been described as antispasmodic, which means that it reduces or eliminates spasms and hypersensitivity. Grindelia more specifically has been documented to relax the smooth muscles around the airways and reduce swelling of the nasal membranes. It is also reputed to help remove mucous from the bronchi and sinuses, lower blood pressure, and slightly reduce the heart rate.

Grindelia has also been used specifically to reduce hay fever. It has also recently become popular as an agent to reduce the skin's hypersensitivity to poison oak and hives from insect bites.

Herbalists recommend that Grindelia can be taken daily, but in small doses, because it can be toxic in large doses.

Job's Tears

Coix lachryma-jobi (L. var. ma-yuen Stapf) is an ancient grass/grain known to grow primarily in Asia. Native to the tropical regions of Southern Asia, it has been increasingly cultivated as an ornamental grass around the world.

Researchers from National Taiwan University (Chen *et al.* 2010) tested the anti-allergic activity of Job's tears in the laboratory. They found that an extract of Job's tears suppressed mast cell degranulation and inhibited histamine release. It also suppressed the release of inflammatory mediators IL-4, IL-6 and TNF-A—known to stimulate leukotrienes. The researchers concluded that Job's tears inhibited the body's physiological allergic response.

Ivy

Hedera helix L., also known as English Ivy or Common Ivy, grows throughout Europe, North America and Western Asia. It is known to climb walls and sides of buildings, and is the basis for the term "ivy league

293

schools," as the aged buildings of some of these universities are covered with Ivy.

Ivy is also known for its expectorant properties. It has this been used to stimulate tearing and loosen phlegm and mucous of the airways.

Ivy has been the subject of a respectable amount of research for allergies and asthma. Pediatric researchers from Germany's Johann Wolfgang Goethe University (Hofmann *et al.* 2003) reviewed five randomized and controlled studies on Ivy, and selected three for analysis. They found that in all three studies, drops of Ivy extract significantly reduced airway resistance and improved respiratory function in children with chronic bronchial asthma. They concluded that: *"extracts from dried ivy leaves are effective in the treatment of chronic airway obstruction in children suffering from bronchial asthma."*

Mallow

Malva silvestris is a close relative of the *Malva verticillata* herb used in the Chinese Ravas Napas remedy mentioned earlier.

Mallow grows throughout Europe and has had an extensive and popular reputation among Western and Middle Eastern traditional medicines as a demulcent herb: It soothes irritated tissues. Mallow contains polysaccharides, asparagine and mucilage—which stimulates a balance among the body's mucosal membranes. The leaves are typically used.

The mucilage is primarily composed by polysaccharides. These include beta-D-galactosyl, beta-D-glucose, and beta-D-galactoses.

Mallow has been used for sore throats, heartburn, dry sinuses, and irritable bowels.

This herb has also been used in decoctions by European herbalists for allergic skin responses and eczema. For this reason, Swiss doctors during the World Wars would apply mallow compresses onto skin rashes with good success.

Mallow's leaves, flowers and roots are all used. It is an emollient and demulcent, rendering the ability to soften and coat, while stimulating healthy mucous among the airways.

Mallow has been documented among traditional medicines to successfully treat GERD, sinusitis and asthma.

Marsh Mallow

Althaea officinalis, has similar properties and constituents as the *Malva verticillata* L (Mallow). It belongs in the same family, Malvaceaea, and has similar constituents.

Marsh mallow has also enjoyed an extensive and popular reputation among traditional medicines around the world. This is because it contains mucilage, which supports and stimulates a healthy mucosal membrane.

For this reason, Marsh mallow is considered a demulcent: it's leaves soothe irritated sore throats, heartburn, dry sinuses, and irritable bowels.

The leaves, flowers and roots are all used in healing. Marsh mallow is known to be emollient, which gives it properties that soften and coat practically any membrane within the body, including the sinuses, throat, stomach, intestines, urinary tract and of course, the airways.

The root of the Marsh mallow will contain up to 35% mucilage. It also contains a variety of long-chain polysaccharides. Extracts use cold water, so they dissolve the mucilage without the starches. For this reason, tea infusions for drinking and gargling using Marsh mallow often use cold water overnight, although it can also be steeped for 15-20 minutes using hot water.

Mullein

The leaves, flowers and herbs of *Verbascum theapsiforme* and *V. philomoides olanum* have been part of the traditional herbalist repertory for thousands of years. It is classified as a demulcent and expectorant, because it is known to soothe irritated airways and help clear thickened mucous.

Mullein's soothing and demulcent properties are due primarily to its mucilage content, which can be as high as 3%. Other constituents include saponins, which are believed to produce the expectorant properties of this herb.

Mullein has thus been used for centuries for hypersensitivity including coughing and bronchialspasm, skin irritations and ear infections. In all these cases, its effects have been considered soothing to epithelial cells.

Pine Bark Extract

Traditional herbalists have used pine bark extracts for respiratory conditions for centuries. The process of extraction is complex, however. Pine bark contains numerous constituents that yield health benefits, but also contains a high-density tannin complex requiring careful purification.

Today's standard for pine bark extracts is an extract of French Maritime Pine (*Pinus pinaster*) called Pycnogenol®. This extract is produced using a process patented by the Swiss company Horphag Research, Ltd. The process renders a number of bioavailable procyanidolic oligomers (PCOs), including catechin and taxifolin, as well as several phenolic acids.

Pycnogenol® has undergone extensive clinical study and laboratory research. Today, Pycnogenol® has been the subject of nearly 100 human clinical studies, testing over 7,000 patients with a variety of conditions. This extract's unique layered proanthocyanidin content has been shown, among other things, to significantly reduce systemic inflammation.

For example, in a German study (Belcaro *et al.* 2008), Pycnogenol® lowered C-reactive protein levels—known to increase during systemic inflammation and allergies—after 156 patients were given 100 milligrams of Pycnogenol® or placebo for three months. The average CRP decrease went from 3.9 to 1.1 following the treatment period. This is a 354% reduction in this important systemic inflammation marker after only three months of use.

Pycnogenol® has also been shown to directly improve asthma symptoms and increase lung function. Researchers from Loma Linda University's School of Medicine (Lau *et al.* 2004) gave 60 asthmatic children from 6 to 18 years old Pycnogenol® or placebo for three months. The Pycnogenol® group experienced a significant reduction of asthma symptoms, and an increase in pulmonary function. Pycnogenol® also allowed the patients to reduce or discontinue the use of inhalers significantly more than the placebo group.

Researchers from the University of Arizona's School of Medicine (Hosseini *et al.* 2001) gave up to 200 milligrams of Pycnogenol® or a placebo to 26 asthma patients for four weeks. Then the researchers crossed over the two groups, and the placebo group took the Pycnogenol® and vice versa, for another four weeks. In both four-week periods, the Pycnogenol® treated groups showed significantly lower levels of leukotrienes as compared with the placebo groups. Forced expiratory volumes (FEV1) also were significantly improved for the Pycnogenol® groups over the placebo groups. The research also resulted in no adverse side effects.

In a study of allergic rhinitis to birch pollen, 39 allergic patients were given Pycnogenol® several weeks before the start of the 2009 birch allergy season. The treatment reduced allergic eye symptoms by 35% and sinus symptoms by 20%, compared to the placebo group. Better results were found among those who took Pycnogenol® seven to eight weeks before the birch pollen season began (Wilson *et al.* 2010).

In a study from the National Research Institute for Food and Nutrition in Rome, Italy (Canali *et al.* 2009), 150 milligrams of Pycnogenol® were given to six healthy adults for five days. After the five days, blood tests showed that Pycnogenol® interrupted the genetic expression of 5-lipoxygenase (5-LOX) and cyclooxygenase-2 (COX-2). It also inhibited phospholipase A2 (PLA2) activity. The Pycnogenol® supplementation program also reduced leukotriene production and altered prostaglandin levels. As discussed earlier, COX-2 and 5-LOX production is tied to inflammation processes, while leukotriene synthesis is tied specifically with airway hypersensitivity.

Pycnogenol® also reduces histamine, another critical systemic inflammatory mediator as we've discussed. Researchers from Ireland's Trinity College (Sharma *et al.* 2003) found that Pycnogenol® inhibited the release of histamine from mast cells. The researchers commented that this effect appeared to be the result of the significant bioflavonoid content of Pycnogenol®.

Pycnogenol® has also been shown to reduce and inhibit NF-kB by an average of 15%. NF-kB is involved in the expression of airway hyperreactive leukotrienes, as well as adhesion molecules. The matrix metalloproteinase 9 (MMP-9) enzymes known as conducive to asthmatic responses, are also reduced by Pycnogenol® (Grimm *et al.* 2006).

The bottom line is that Pycnogenol®, an extract bark of the French maritime pine tree, has been shown not only to reduce systemic inflammation in general through the radical scavenging abilities of procyanidolic oligomers. It has also been shown to directly reduce allergic hypersensitivity and increase airway health by inhibiting inflammatory mediators that stimulate leukotrienes and histamines.

Red Algae

Red algae—from the *Rhodophyta* family—have been used for thousands of years to treat inflammation-oriented conditions, including bronchitis and hypersensitivity.

Researchers from the National Taiwan Ocean University (Kazłowska *et al.* 2010) studied the ability of the red seaweed *Porphyra dentata*, to halt allergic responses. The researchers found that a *Porphyra dentata* phenolic extract suppressed nitric oxide production among macrophages using a NF-kappa-Beta gene transcription process. This modulated the hypersensitivity immune response on a systemic level. The phenolic compounds within the Red algae have been identified as catechol, rutin and hesperidin.

Skunk Cabbage

The root of *Symplocarpus foetidus* has also been used traditionally for asthma, as well as whooping cough and bronchitis. The herb has a funky odor, but it is considered a strong antispasmodic and expectorant. Antispasmodic means, again, that it relaxes the airways and the smooth muscles around the airways. Expectorant means that it helps clear mucous from the lungs.

Skunk cabbage contains silica, iron, manganese, a resin, volatile oil and acrid principle—which causes its odor. It has sedative effects, and therefore is also used as a nervine, to calm nervousness.

Wild Pansy

This herb, botanical name *Viola tricolor*, has been used extensively in Western herbal medicine for skin and mucous membrane issues. Its wonderful colorful flowers are difficult to miss in grasslands across North America and Europe.

Wild pansy is known to be high in saponins, as many other anti-allergic herbs are. Saponins are the glycosides such as triterpenes—active compounds in many of the medicinal plants we've discussed in this chapter. Ginseng is a rich source of saponins, for example.

Wild pansy has a significant reputation in traditional herbal medicine of improving respiratory conditions like asthma and bronchitis. Today's its extracts are used in a number of popular herbal tonics, extracts, antitussives and dermatology medicines (Rimkiene *et al.* 2003).

Wild pansy's saponins are drawn out via simple tea infusion. This can be applied externally onto skin rashes, as well as taken internally.

Mucilage Seeds

A number of seeds are helpful for calming and settling the airways, including seeds such as Flax, Safflower, Rapeseed, Caraway, Anise, Fennel, Licorice seed, Black seed and others. Seeds contain basic compounds that offer mucilage, saponins and other polysaccharides that contribute to the health of the mucous membranes.

Not surprisingly, combinations or single versions of these seeds have been used in traditional medicine for centuries.

Pharmacology researchers from Cairo's Helwan University (Haggag *et al.* 2003) treated allergic asthmatic patients with an herbal blend containing of Anise, Fennel, Caraway, Licorice, Black seed and Chamomile—all known for their anti-asthmatic effects. They found that the water extract significantly decreased cough frequency and intensity. It also increased lung function, with higher FEV1/FVC percentages among the asthmatic patients, as compared to those who consumed a placebo tea.

Herbal Ointments and Inhalants

It is no surprise that oils of these compounds tend to clear the sinuses and airways when they are rubbed on the chest, sinuses and neck. They are nature's decongestants. Herb-derived ointments that are applied to the skin of the neck and chest have been traditional treatments for asthmatics and chest congestion due to colds and bronchitis for thousands of years among traditional medicine cultures. We discussed this potential with Ma Huang and Boswellia.

In the nineteenth and early twentieth centuries, these traditions were developed into commercial products, primarily as ointments containing menthol and camphor. They were eventually applied to vaporizers, chest rubs and in inhalants.

In a study from the hospital researchers from Toronto (Rynard *et al.* 1968), 65 patients with chronic respiratory conditions—20 of which had asthma—were treated with nightly vapor inhalations of a blend that included oils of Camphor, Garlic and Eucalyptus. Most patients experienced *"lasting improvement"* of symptoms after three to five months of treatment, while asthmatics *"felt relief from acute symptoms during the first three weeks,"* according to the researchers.

Of the 34 patients who completed the full treatment period of five months, 28 patients volunteered for follow-ups that extended for another 18 months after the treatment was completed. Of these, 19 patients remained healthy with no symptoms or respiratory episodes during the 18 months. Another three were *"much improved"* and two experienced a bout of pneumonia during the follow-up period but completely recovered. One had an upper respiratory infection but also recovered. In other words, only three previously chronic respiratory patients suffered further respiratory symptoms.

Researchers from New York's Albert Einstein College of Medicine (Reznik *et al.* 2004) studied the use of these commercial camphor-menthol rubbing ointments with 127 adolescent asthmatics. Those asthmatics who used the rubbing ointments had significantly fewer emergency hospitalizations and anaphylactic crises than those using medications alone.

Camphor

Camphor oil is derived from the camphor tree, which is native to Asia and Japan. The tree will grow from 50 to 100 feet tall, and will live for many decades. The oil has been used for thousands of years throughout Asia and the Middle East for anointing, healing and embalming.

Camphor oil is steam-extracted from the tree's wood and roots. Its central constituents include camphene, eugenol, cineole, pinene, phellandrene, limonene, terpinene, cymene, terpinolene, sabinene, furfural, safrole, linalool, terpinen, caryophyllene, borneol, piperitone, geraniol and cinnamaldehyde, among others.

This extensive list of components illustrates the complexity of camphor. It thus has many properties. It is considered anti-inflammatory, antiseptic, analgesic, carminative, diuretic, rubefacient and stimulating.

Camphor has been used traditionally for coughs, bronchial infections, colds, muscle pain and arthritis. It is either rubbed onto the skin, put into a compress or vaporized with steam. It is not consumed internally. Some consumed herbal formulations have utilized camphor oil, but these have only very tiny portions of camphor. Care must be taken by breastfeeding mothers applying camphor on the chest not to allow the baby to consume any.

Camphor research has typically concentrated on ointments formulated with menthol.

Eucalyptus

Eucalyptus is a large fragrant genus of trees that have primarily come from Australia, although they have been migrating to different regions over the past few hundred years. Today, California and many Pacific Rim countries are now home to eucalyptus species, as is the Mediterranean, Africa and many parts of Asia. The tree's bark and leaves are a source of a medicinal sap known for its decongestant and anti-inflammatory properties.

Eucalyptus oil is derived from this sap, and it is the 1.8-cineol called eucalyptol—a monoterpene—that is the key constituent of eucalyptus oil. Eucalyptol has been shown to suppress arachidonic acid metabolism as well as inhibit cytokine release from monocytes.

Researchers from Germany's Bonn University Hospital (Juergens *et al.* 2003) tested eucalyptus extract (eucalyptol) on 32 asthmatics dependent upon steroid medications. The patients were given 200 mg 1.8-cineol (eucalyptol) orally three times daily in capsules or a placebo for twelve weeks. At the same time, the patients' oral steroid medications (prednisolone) were reduced by 2.5 mg increments every 3 weeks as appropriate with symptoms. The eucalyptus extract group was able to maintain a 36% controlled reduction in oral steroids after twelve weeks, compared to just 7% among the placebo group. The researchers concluded that the eucalyptus extract has *"significant steroid-saving effect in steroid-depending asthma."*

Mints and Menthol

The plants of the mint family include Peppermint (*Mentha piperita*), Watermint (*Mentha aquatica*), Spearmint (*Mentha spicata*), Pennyroyal (*Mentha pulegium*) and several others. They have a variety of common constituents, of which menthol is the most applicable to respiratory issues. Other active constituents of many mints will include menthylacetate, menthone, mentofuran, limonene, cineole, isomenthol, neomenthol, azulenes and rosmarinic acid.

Mint is well-known for its ability to settle digestion and ease flatulence. These effects are due to azulene's ability to relax the smooth muscles around the intestines. Azulene also relaxes the smooth muscles around the airways as well. Note that Chamomile also contains azulene.

Menthol is most known for its ability to clear congestion and expand the airways. It is the expectorant property of menthol that produces this effect. Menthol reduced coughing in a study from Britain's Leicester University Hospitals (Kenia *et al.* 2008) of 42 children.

Menthol also increases perceived nasal airflow. A study from researchers from the Tokyo Women's Medical College (Tamaoki *et al.* 1995) tested nebulized menthol on patients with mild asthma. The menthol group suffered less wheezing and used less bronchodilator medication.

A review of research from the UK's University of Wales (Eccles 1994) indicated that menthol's respiratory reflex effects may at least partially come from its ability to modulate calcium ion channels among the smooth muscles and their associated nerves.

Other Herbal Inhalants

These extracts also make for superb inhalant oils. Oils from camphor, menthol, and eucalyptus have been used alone in diffusers or in humidifiers for bronchial congestion of various types in traditional medicines. These also have been combined with other known bronchial inhalants in some traditional formulations, including:

> ➢ Benzoin tincture (a resin extracted from the bark of the Benzoin tree of the genus *Styrax*)
> ➢ Pine needle oil
> ➢ Canadian balsam extract from the Fir tree
> ➢ Mullein

Plant Derived Corticoids

Corticosteroids systemically reduce allergic symptoms by blocking histamine release and curbing inflammation. For this reason, prednisone and similar cortisone drugs are the most-prescribed drugs for allergies. Prednisone and methylprednisone mimic the actions of cortisol produced by the adrenal gland. The central mechanism of cortisol and cortisone is to slow or shunt the inflammatory response and suppress the immune system by interfering interleukin cytokines. Thus, it is used for a wide range of inflammatory conditions.

However, because prednisone acts like a hormone, it significantly alters moods. This may begin with mild frustration or annoyance over trivial things. With consistent use, this can turn into rage, depression, mania, personality changes and psychotic behavior. Other side effects include weight gain, high blood pressure, sodium retention, headaches, ulcers, cataracts, irregular menstruation, elevated blood sugar, growth retarding, osteoporosis, wound healing moon face (puffiness of the face), glaucoma, bruising, buffalo hump (rounded upper back), and thinning of the skin.

In addition, over time, prednisone dosing can reduce the body's own production of cortisol. Furthermore, increased doses are usually required to maintain the same suppression of symptoms. This can result in an inflammatory and immunosuppressed situation should the prednisone dosing be reduced or withdrawn (Todd *et al.* 2002).

The body produces cortisol and other corticoids using a complex adrenal process that begins with the body's production of a type of cholesterol made from plant-based phytosterols. The body uses these plant-derived cholesterols to produce the steroidal compounds that stimulate cortisone production through the adrenal glands. In other words, the best raw materials for cortisone production come from a healthy plant-based diet of phytosterols. Let's discuss some of the plants that provide these natural raw materials.

For many years, the pharmaceutical industry utilized Wild yam (*Dioscorea floribunda* and *D. floribunda*) to produce the raw corticoid ingredient diosgenin. Diosgenin was utilized to produce progesterone and other steroid drugs. In the human body, the diosgenin in Wild yam is a steroid, and is converted into progesterone and DHEA. Remember also that *Dioscorea opposite* or Chinese yam, is part of a successful Chinese anti-hypersensitivity formula discussed earlier.

As Wild yam production could not keep pace with pharmaceutical steroid demand, stigmasterols and sitosetrols from soy and solasodine from *Solanum dulcamara* became the preferred source of corticoid precursors for the pharmaceutical industry.

Illustrating the anti-inflammatory nature of Solanum, researchers from the Institute of Internal Medicine and Madras Medical College (Govindan *et al.* 2004) gave 300 mg of *Solanum xanthocarpum* and *Solanum trilobatum* for three days to 60 adult asthmatic patients and compared their effects with conventional bronchodilator drugs. The herb groups found that cough, forced expiratory levels (FEV1), peak expiratory flows, breathlessness and sputum were all significantly improved two hours after taking the herbs. FEV1 levels increased by 65% from *Solanum xanthocarpum* and 67% from the *Solanum trilobatum*. Symptom relief lasted from 6-8 hours among the herbal group. The herbs also produced no adverse side effects.

Anti-inflammatory Herbal Spices

A number of other herbs also contain anti-inflammatory properties. These work in different ways, and while they may or may not specifically modulate food sensitivities, they can help strengthen the immune system, and thus reduce the inflammatory process that provokes hypersensitivity. Thus, they can contribute to the modulation of the immune system, allowing us to begin tolerating foods that were not previously tolerated. Here is a quick overview of some of the most well-known (and most available) of these anti-inflammatory herbs:

Basil (*Osimum basilicum*) contains ursolic acid and oleanolic acid, both shown in laboratory studies to inhibit inflammatory COX-2 enzymes.

Garlic (*Allium sativum*) probably deserves a larger section, but that information could easily encompass a book in itself—as was well documented by Paul Bergner: *The Healing Power of Garlic* (1996). Garlic is an ancient medicinal plant with a wealth of characteristics and constituents that stimulate the immune system, protect the liver, purify the bloodstream, reduce oxidative species, reduce LDL lipid peroxidation, reduce inflammation, and stimulate detoxification systems throughout the body. This is supported by a substantial amount of rigorous scientific research.

Garlic is also one of the most powerful antimicrobial plants known. A fresh garlic bulb has at least five different constituents known to inhibit bacteria, fungi and viruses. Much of this antimicrobial capability, however, is destroyed by heat and oxygen. Therefore, eating freshly peeled bulbs are the most assured way to retain these antimicrobial potencies.

Cooked, aged or dehydrated garlic powder also has a variety of powerful antioxidants, but little of its raw antibiotic abilities. Garlic is also a tremendous sulfur donor as well. The combination of garlic's antibiotic, antioxidant, anti-inflammatory and immune-building characteristics make it a *must* spice-herb-food for any inflammatory condition.

Oregano (*Origanum vulgare*) contains at least thirty-one anti-inflammatory constituents, twenty-eight antioxidants, and four significant COX-2 inhibitors (apigenin, kaempferol, ursolic acid and oleanolic acid).

Rosemary (*Rosmarinus officinalis*) contains ursolic acid, oleanolic acid and apigenin—a few of the many constituents in this important botanical—shown to inhibit inflammatory enzymes in laboratory studies. Research has also shown that rosemary's volatile oils can halt airway constriction by inhibiting mast cell degranulation.

Other Anti-Allergy Herbs

The list does not end here. Still other herbs have been used among traditional medicines throughout the world to reverse the hypersensitive metabolism. Many of these are supportive in that they serve to purify the blood, strengthen the liver, strengthen the adrenals, strengthen the immune system and inhibit inflammation.

Comfrey, Aloe and **Slippery elm,** for example, aid the health of the mucosal membranes with their high mucilage and mucopolysaccharide content—while **Cayenne, Nutmeg** and **Goldenseal** stimulate the body's detoxification processes to clear catarrh.

In addition to these airway herbs, there are herbs that relax the muscles and support the nervous system in general. This is a common formulation strategy used by herbalists. These types of herbs are called nervines, and they include **Chamomile, Tulsi, Hops, Wild lettuce** and **Skullcap.**

Polynesian herbalism is also rich with anti-allergy herbs. In fact, the traditional Hawaiians utilized at least 58 different herbs for airway conditions. These included *Piper methysticum* **(Kava),** *Solanum americanum, Aleurites molucana,* and *Sophora chrysophylla,* which have all showed airway-clearing effects in research and clinical application.

South Pacific islanders (Fiji, Tonga, New Guinea) also used Kava, as well as *Cananga odorata, Epipremnum pinnatum, Scaevola taccada, Artocarpus altilis, Syzygium malccanse, Stachytarpheta urticifolia* and *Fagraea berteriana* for airway conditions.

Each has its special benefit, depending upon the specific weakness that is producing the hypersensitivity symptoms; and each has shown clinical benefits among traditional medicines to help reverse the underlying conditions involved in allergic rhinitis:

- Aloe (*Aloe vera*)
- Anise (*Pimpinella anisum*)
- Black sage (*Cordia curassavica*)
- Borage (*Borago officinalis*)
- Cayenne (*Capsicum* spp.)
- Chamomile (*Matricaria chamomilla*)
- Comfrey (*Symphytum officinale*)
- Duckweed (*Stellaria media*)
- Echinacea (*Echinacea purpurea*)
- Goldenseal (*Hydrastis canadensis*)
- Green Tea (*Camellia sinensis*)
- Guggul (*Commiphora mukul*)
- Lemongrass (*Cymbopogon citratus*)
- Nutmeg (*Myristica fragrans*)
- Shadon beni (*Eryngium foetidium*)
- Shandileer (*Leonotis nepetifolia*)
- Slippery elm (*Ulmus fulva*)
- Spurge (*Euphorbia hirta* L.)
- Stinging Nettle (*Urtica dioica*)
- Thyme (*Thymus serphyllum*)
- Tulsi (*Ocimum gratissimum*)
- Wild onion (*Hymenocallis tubiflora*)

Herbal Techniques

This chapter contains a long list of herbs and herbal formulations that have been shown in research and clinical use among traditional medicines to have anti-allergy, anti-congestion, anti-inflammatory and anti-asthma effects. Choosing the right herb and/or formula for a particular case can thus be a little tricky. For this reason, a seasoned expert in herbal formulations should offer specific suggestions that directly relate to ones constitution and precise level of sensitivities should be considered.

That said, one of the strategies many traditional physicians have utilized is to select those herbs that directly target the underlying condition related to each symptom of the patient. With each underlying condition often comes yet another underlying condition. These are targeted one by one with either a formulation, or a series of herbs or formulas. While an herb's primary constituents might be effective for particular symptoms, the rest of the herb's constituents will typically work on the underlying condition. This *"from the outside in"* strategy is known to produce a deeper correction of the systemic immunity issues typically at the root of allergic hypersensitivity.

For example, high liver enzymes (or other liver weakness symptoms such as heavy bags under the eyes) together with hyperreactivity may indicate to the herbalist the use of Dandelion along with other anti-inflammatory herbs—because Dandelion is specifically helpful to the liver. Another example might be that Marsh mallow, Mallow and Mullein might be recommended in a case of GERD along with asthmatic symptoms, because GERD illustrates a weakness in the mucosal membranes. Or perhaps, for issues where sinusitis presents along with allergic rhinitis, the herbalist may first recommend the use of ventilation or ointment of camphor, menthol and eucalyptus along with anti-allergy herbs to clear the sinus passageways, speed the removal of mucous from the nasal region, and exert some antimicrobial effects that these bring.

While ones specific condition may be unique, these examples illustrate the herbalist's strategy of healing underlying conditions from the *outside-in* as well as *inside-out* using the herbs we've discussed in this section.

Dosages and Methods

We have not detailed precise dosages in this section because there are many considerations when determining dosages. These include age, physical health, constitution, unique weaknesses, diet, lifestyle and other factors. Herbs should also be carefully matched, and some herbs and formulations have been known to interact with certain medications.

Therefore, it is suggested that herbs are chosen, formulated and dosed by an experienced herbalist. If there are any medications being used, the prescribing physician should be consulted.

This said, most of the herbs mentioned above, with the exception of essential oils, are safest when used as *infusions*. An infusion is simply the steeping of the fresh or dried root, bark, leaf, seed, stem or fruit in water.

In the case of most herb leaves and stems, the water is brought to a boil, and the herb can be steeped for 5-10 minutes using a strainer or tea-ball. In the case of most roots, seeds and barks, the root can be steeped a little longer, for 10-20 minutes, depending on the herb. In some cases a seed, root or bark is better when it is soaked overnight in room temperature water. A teaspoon of course ground herb or formula per cup of water is a good general rule of thumb to consider.

Another strategy is to simply ingest a capsule or pressed tablet of a powdered version of the herb or herbal formulation. Liquid extracts are also available from many reputable herbal suppliers. In these cases, the literature accompanying these products should be closely examined for dosages and possible interactions.

Indeed, many of the formulations (or their derivatives) mentioned in this section are available as encapsulated, pressed tablets or liquid extracts, together with dosage suggestions. Before using this strategy, care should be taken to assure that the herbal formulation has been ultimately de-signed by a reputable herbalist. Most of the popular commercial brands of herbal formulations employ trained herbalists to design their formula-tions and write out their dosage instructions. Many will also name the herbalist on the marketing material or label of the product. These should be considered more trustworthy formulations.

Essential oils of herbs can also be rubbed into the skin of the chest or sinus region. We discussed this earlier in the case of camphor, menthol and eucalyptus rubs. Care should be taken not to ingest these; or rub these into the eyes, ears, nostrils or onto the breasts before or during breastfeeding. There are several reputable formulations of mentholated rubs with camphor on the market today.

By far the best approach is to have an herbalist formulate and rec-ommend herbs specific to ones constitution, allergy severity, medication use and lifestyle. In the alternative, a commercial formula (such as ones discussed in this chapter) that has been blended or overseen by a reputa-ble herbalist—together with instructions on the packaging—can provide a level of expertise in the formulation, dose and packaging. Remember, again, anyone taking medications should consult with the prescribing physician to avoid possible interactions. Also, very small doses, gradually building up to the suggested dose, are typically recommended at the out-set to test ones tolerance to the herb or formulation.

Homeopathy and Flower Remedies

While homeopathy has been used with some success for allergies, the current research data on homeopathy use for allergies has been disap-pointing. For example, a Cochrane review by researchers from Britain's

Imperial College (McCarney *et al.* 2004) analyzed six studies of homeo-pathic treatments for allergies and asthma, and found the results conflict-ing and without significant positive effects.

On the other hand, in a non-placebo controlled audit study (Sevar 2005) of 455 patients of various diseases including allergies, 77% of 195 patients who had eczema, anxiety, depression, osteoarthritis, asthma, back pain, chronic cough, chronic fatigue, headaches or hypertension reported improvement in their respective conditions. While this effort illustrates homeopathy's potential in a number of disorders, it pointed to homeo-pathic practitioners' prescriptives rather than generalized remedies.

We thus cannot, from the research data, qualify certainty about ho-meopathic remedies and allergies. Homeopathy in its current form does not have the historical clinical application of traditional herbal medicines (although it does have over two centuries of clinical use). This means that we are limited in saying whether or to what extent homeopathy may be helpful.

Moreover, the choosing of the classic homeopathy remedy is highly individualistic. Using diluted doses requires the practitioner to ferret out precise causal issues in the patient that relate specifically to remedy prov-ings—and there are over 2,000 possible homeopathic remedies. This di-agnostic process can be exhaustive, and very successful. Yet it is nonethe-less a complex process that is difficult to conduct without a well-trained classical homeopath.

It would be more accurate to say that the application of homeopathy should not focus on particular remedies, but rather be subject to the skill level of the classical homeopathic practitioner and a willing patient.

Noting these points, this text will not list any specific homeopathic remedies, even those commonly listed for allergies in some alternative texts. We will simply suggest that should a person find no success in the many strategies and herbal remedies available for allergies, a classical ho-meopathic practitioner may be worth considering.

We might add that there is some logic to the concept that an allergy might be mitigated by taking the homeopathic remedy that is a dilution of the allergen itself. This, however, has not always proven out to work, and may also come with complications.

Flower Essences

This said, another approach worth considering is Flower Essences. This is especially true for someone dealing with stress and anxiety.

Flower essences are also diluted doses (less diluted than most homeo-pathic remedies, however) of flower volatiles. Because of their medium dilution, they are seen by most practitioners as extremely safe, even for self-dosing. Dr. Edward Bach, an English medical doctor at the turn of the twentieth century, created his flower formulary with the goal of allow-ing people to self-dose, using his descriptions for the properties of each. Many of these properties pertain to emotional and nervous conditions—which as we've mentioned, can help stimulate allergic hypersensitivity. Otherwise, many practitioners have considered flower remedies especially useful for pollen allergies.

Here are a few of the conditions and specific flower essences that pertain to anxiety and stress:

Anxiousness: **Agrimony** for hidden restlessness); mimulus for known worries; **Red chestnut** for worry about others; **Aspen** for un-known worries; and **White chestnut** for general worrying thoughts.

Apprehension: **Aspen, Mimulus, Rock rose** for fear for oneself; **Red chestnut** for fear for others; **Gentian** for doubt and despondency, and larch for worry over possible failure.

Depression: **Gentian** for known reason, or after set-back; **Mustard** for unknown cause; gorse and gentian for hopelessness; **Sweet chestnut** for utter dejection; and **Mustard** for sudden dark descent.

Fear: **Aspen** for unknown or general fear; **Mimulus** for fear of dark-ness; **Rock rose** for fear of death; **Larch** for fear of failure; and **Chicory** and **Heather** for fear of losing friends.

Fixation: **Vervain** for fixations on project or injustices; **Heather** and **Crab apple** for fixations upon oneself or upon details.

Grief: **Star of Bethlehem** for sudden, shocking loss; **Water violet** for silently grieving; **Sweet chestnut** for heartache and chronic grieving; **Honeysuckle** for longing for the past; **Pine** for guilt and self-blame; and **Crab apple** for self-condemnation.

It is interesting that in Dr. Bach's research, he often found that aller-gies to certain plant pollens often related to a particular anxious deficiency that could be calmed by the flower essences of that particular plant. This of course, ties into immunotherapy and developing tolerance, but on a more subtle, nervous system level.

For those who prefer a general formulation, the **Rescue Remedy** might be an option. It contains many of the core nervousness and stress essences. The Rescue remedy is a mix of five essences: Rock rose, Impa-tiens, Clematis, Star of Bethlehem and Cherry Plum.

Chapter Seven

Rebuilding the Mucosal Membranes

There are numerous herbs that have been utilized in traditional medicine for modifying hypersensitivity. While each herb works in a unique manner, many of these herbs have similar constituents.

As we've illustrated in this text, allergic rhinitis for most people involves a breakdown of the mucosal membranes that line the airways. This produces a hypersensitivity response because:

> ➤ Toxins and microorganisms come into closer contact with airway epithelia that have damaged mucosal membrane layers.
> ➤ The cilia within the airways do not have the right basement fluid to operate effectively. Either they are overwhelmed by too much mucous or don't have enough basement membrane to effectively 'sweep' out toxins, cell parts and mucous.
> ➤ The airways become more sensitive to changes in temperature or increased exercise due to the lack of these membranes.
> ➤ Defects in the mucosal membranes stimulate inflammation due to the decreased protection they offer those parts of the body they normally protect.

Things that Deplete Our Mucosal Membranes

The foods and beverages that deplete our mucosal membranes, not surprisingly, are some of the same ones that increase the risk of allergies in the research. These also increase systemic inflammation because they contribute free radicals and toxins, stimulating inflammation.

These include:

> ➤ Alcohol
> ➤ Foods/beverages high in refined sugars
> ➤ Highly processed foods/beverages
> ➤ Foods/beverages high in refined salt
> ➤ Foods high in saturated fats
> ➤ Fried foods and fast foods
> ➤ Foods that are burnt or overcooked
> ➤ Foods containing chemical additives

These foods and beverages serve to irritate the mucous membranes. This is because they either change the pH of mucous as they make contact with the mucosal membranes, or they directly contribute free radicals.

Other Things that Deplete Our Mucosal Membranes

A number of activities also reduce our mucosal health. These include:

➤ Stress
➤ Anxiety
➤ Anger
➤ Pharmaceuticals
➤ Illicit drugs
➤ Tobacco smoke (primary and secondary)
➤ Air pollution
➤ Lack of sunshine
➤ Infections (fungal, bacterial, viral)
➤ Lack of hydration

As for anger and stress, when our body is stressed, our body switches to fight-or-flight metabolic mechanisms that pull energy away from the processes of the sub-mucosal glands and gastric glands—which produce our mucosal membrane fluids. This is why a person who is nervous or anxious will also often have dry mouth and an upset stomach. They are not producing enough mucosal secretions to protect those epithelial cells.

The others on the list are either toxins that directly alter the pH of our mucosal membranes, or simply infect them.

A lack of sunshine robs the body of vitamin D and key pineal/pituitary master hormones. As for hydration, we'll discuss this again shortly.

Many pharmaceuticals are toxic to the mucosal membranes. This is why a significant side effect of most medications is dry mouth and an upset stomach. These chemicals can deplete our mucosal membranes and/or block mucosal secretions by virtue of inhibiting the COX-2 process. This also goes for other drugs, chemicals, pollutants, and so on.

The Mucosal Membrane Nutrient

Nature also provides nutrients from whole foods that can help rebuild our mucosal membranes. One of the more productive whole foods applicable to rebuilding our body's mucosal membranes is cabbage. Cabbage contains a unique constituent, s-methylmethionine, also referred to as vitamin U. Through a pathway utilizing one of the body's natural enzymes, called Bhmt2, s-methylmethionine is converted to methionine and then to glutathione in several steps.

In this form, glutathione has been shown to stimulate the repair of the mucosal membranes within the stomach, intestines and airways. Glutathione has also been shown to increase the health and productivity of the liver.

Raw cabbage or cabbage juice has been used as a healing agent for ulcers and intestinal issues for thousands of years among traditional medicines, including those of Egyptian, Ayurvedic and Greek systems. The

Western world became aware of raw cabbage juice in the 1950s, when Garnett Cheney, M.D. conducted several studies showing that methylme-thionine-rich cabbage juice concentrate was able to reduce the pain and bleeding associated with ulcers.

In one of Dr. Cheney's studies, 37 ulcer patients were treated with ei-ther cabbage juice concentrate or a placebo. Of the 26-patient cabbage juice group, 24 patients were considered "successes"—achieving an as-tounding 92% success rate.

Medical researchers from Iraq's University Department of Surgery (Salim 1993) conducted a double-blind study of 172 patients who suffered from gastric bleeding caused by nonsteroidal anti-inflammatory drugs (NSAIDs). They gave the patients either cysteine, methylmethionine sul-fonium chloride (MMSC) or a placebo. Those receiving either the cysteine or the MMSC stopped bleeding. Their conditions became *"stable"* as com-pared with many in the control group, who continued to bleed.

Plants use s-methylmethionine to help heal cell membrane damage among their leaves and stems. This is reminiscent of antioxidants: Plants produce antioxidants to help to protect them from damage from the sun, insects and diseases. In other words, the very same biochemicals that pro-tect plants also help heal our bodies.

Note that MMSC or cabbage juice does not inhibit the flow of gastric juices in the stomach to produce these effects as do acid blocking medica-tions. Rather, they stimulate the body's natural production of mucous, which serves to protect the stomach's cells from the effects of acids.

Herbs that Stimulate Mucosal Health

In addition, a number of the herbs we discussed in the herbal medi-cine section of this book have been used for allergies specifically because they help revitalize the mucous membranes. Some of these, such as Aloe, Slippery elm, Marsh mallow and Mallow, specifically contribute muco-polysaccharides in the form of mucilage. These constituents supplement the mucosal membranes, providing protection. At the same time, they contain nutrients that stimulate submucosal gland secretions, which in-clude the glycoproteins and mucopolysaccharides that form the founda-tion for our mucous membranes.

Most will also exert antioxidant effects and, in the case of aloe, will exert an antimicrobial effect upon the mucosal membranes. This of course, helps remove infective microorganisms, which in turn helps lighten the burden on our immune system.

Here is a concise list of those herbs known by traditional herbalists and/or seen amongst the research to stimulate mucosal membrane health:

- Ban Xia - Pinella root (*Pinellia Ternata*)
- Triphala (*Terminalia chebula, Terminalia bellirica* and *Emblica officinalis*)
- Marica - Black Pepper (*Piper nigrum*)
- Pippali - Long Pepper (*Piper longum*)
- Mallow (*Malva sylvestris*)
- Marsh Mallow (*Althaea officinalis*)
- Cumin Seed (*Cuminum cyminum*)
- Coltsfoot (*Tussilago farfara*)
- Aloe (*Aloe vera*)
- Comfrey (*Symphytum officinale*)
- Chamomile (*Matricaria chamomilla*)
- Slippery elm (*Ulmus fulva*)
- Flaxseed (*Linum usitatissimum*)

All of these contain multiple constituents that either stimulate sub-mucosal glands and/or balance the pH of the membrane fluids.

There are several ways to incorporate these herbs into our daily regimen. We can add more freshly ground Black pepper to our foods. We can add a teaspoon of Aloe to a smoothie or juice. We can spice our foods with fresh Cumin seed (also a spice used in many curries). We can make teas (infusions) from one of the Mallows, some Comfrey, Chamomile and Coltsfoot. Flaxseed may also be steeped into tea, eaten raw, baked into breads, or sprinkled directly on foods.

We can also take a teaspoon of Triphala in a glass of warm water each day or every few days. Reputable Triphala formulations are available at health food stores and online.

Isolated nutrients known to help the mucosal membranes include vitamin A, glutamine and folic acid. N-acetylcysteine (NAC) can also nourish mucosal membranes. NAC is made in the cells, using the amino acid cysteine, which can be derived from nuts, seeds and other plant-based foods. NAC is also sold as a supplement, but large dosages come with warnings.

Mucosal (Oral) Probiotics

Research documented in the last chapter shows that our probiotics are critical elements in the health of our mucosal membranes. This is because they inhabit and police our mucosal membranes. They are defenders and facilitators for the recycling of mucous, and they help break down toxins and pathogens.

They also secrete very important biochemicals—which contribute to the ionic and nutrient makeup of the mucosal membranes. Without healthy probiotic colonies, our mucosal membranes are subject to pathogen attack and inflammatory alteration.

312

For the health of our airway mucosal membranes, we can take oral probiotics. These are particular species of probiotic bacteria, such as *Lactobacillus reuteri* and *L. salivarius,* which (among others) line the mucosal membranes of our mouths, sinuses, pharynx, larynx and bronchial airways. Research has illustrated—as we showed earlier—that oral probiotics help clean, prevent infection and maintain the strength and flexibility of our mucosal passages.

Hydration for Mucosal Membranes

As Dr. Jethro Kloss pointed out decades ago (1939), the average person loses about 550 cubic centimeters of water through the skin, 440 cc through the lungs, 1550 cc through the urine, and another 150 cc through the stool. This adds up to 2650 cc per day, equivalent to a little over 2-½ quarts (about 85 fluid ounces).

Meanwhile many have suggested drinking eight 8-oz glasses per day. Actually, 64 ounces will result in a state of dehydration for most adults. In 2004, the National Academy of Sciences released a study indicating that women typically meet their hydration needs with approximately 91 ounces of water per day, while men meet their needs with about 125 ounces per day. This study also indicated that approximately 80% of water intake comes from water/beverages and 20% comes from food. Therefore, we can assume a minimum of 73 ounces of fresh water for the average adult woman and 100 ounces of fresh water for the average adult man should cover our hydration needs. That is significantly more water than the standard eight glasses per day—especially for men.

The data suggests that 50-75% of Americans have chronic dehydration. Fereydoon Batmanghelidj, M.D., probably the world's foremost researcher on water, suggests a ½ ounce of water per pound of body weight. Drinking an additional 16-32 ounces for each 45 minutes to an hour of strenuous activity is also a good idea, with some before and some after exercising. More water should accompany temperature and elevation extremes, and extra sweating or fevers. Note also that alcohol is dehydrating.

A glass of room-temperature water first thing in the morning on an empty stomach can significantly help our mucosal membranes. Then we should be drinking water throughout the day. Our evening should accompany reduced water consumption, so our sleep is not disrupted by urination.

There are easy ways to tell whether we are dehydrated. A sensation of being thirsty indicates that we are already dehydrated. A person with allergic hypersensitivity should thus be drinking enough water to not ever feel

313

thirsty. Dark yellow urine also indicates dehydration. Our urine color should be either clear, or bright yellow if after taking multivitamins.

Drinking just any water is not advised. Municipal water and even bottled water can contain many contaminants that can burden the immune system, and trigger or aggravate hypersensitivity. Care must be taken to drink water that has been filtered of most toxins yet is naturally mineralized. Research has confirmed that distilled water and soft water are not advisable. Natural mineral water is best. Please refer to the author's book, *Pure Water* for more information on water content, filters and water treatment options.

Chapter Eight

Other Strategies to Rebuild the Immune System

As we've discussed at length, allergic rhinitis is a symptom of systemic inflammation combined with weakened airway mucous membranes. Therefore, whatever we can do to remove or avoid consuming toxins will help unburden the immune system. This can help take the immune system off of the alert mode—which will reduce hypersensitivity and help the body rebuild its mucosal membranes.

Furthermore, when the body's normal detoxification systems are not operating at effective levels, the body will be forced to increase detoxification through the mucosal membranes. This means that toxin parts, dead cells and pathogens will be sent out through the mucosal membranes of the lungs and nasal cavities. This in turn thickens those mucous membranes as a result—swamping the cilia and preventing normal mucous activity.

Detoxification Techniques

First let's review some of the toxins (and their sources) that can accumulate in our bodies—especially among our fat cells:

Source	Toxins
Air pollutants	Lead, mercury, carbon monoxide, sulfur, arsenic, nitrogen dioxide, ozone…
Animals	Dried skin, bacteria, waste excreted from animal (dander)
Carpets, rugs	Molds, dander, lice, PC-4, latex
Cigarette/Cigar/Pipe Smoke	Carbon monoxide, nicotine, aldehydes, ketones, soot, formaldehyde, others
Cosmetics	Aluminum, phosphates and chemicals
Spray cans	Propellants, other chemicals
Food Additives	Food colors, preservatives, trans fats, pesticides, arachidonic acids, acrylamide, phytanic acid, artificial flavors
House	Radon, formaldehyde, pesticides, cleaning products, asbestos, lead, paint
Household chemicals	Cleaners, pesticides, herbicides, paints
Insects	Endotoxins from mites, cockroaches and other insects
Laundry soaps	Fragrances, detergents, surfactants

Microorganisms	Mold, bacteria, viruses
Mattresses/pillows	Endotoxins, molds, formaldehyde
Paints	Lead, arsenic, VOCs, adhesives
Pets	Dander, up to 240 infectious diseases & parasites (65 from dogs/39 from cats)
Pharmaceuticals	Numerous
Water	Chorine byproducts, pesticides, pharmaceuticals, many others
Pools and spas	Chlorine byproducts such as trihalomethanes (THMs), various carbonates
Soaps and Shampoos	Fragrances, detergents, surfactants
Stoves, Fireplaces	Carbon monoxide, NO_2, arsenic, soot
Work and school environments	SBS, practically all of the above

Sweating

The adult body has about 2.6 million sweat glands located throughout the body's skin cells. This makes the skin the body's greatest outlet for the elimination of toxins. As exposure to chemicals has increased, our need for regular sweat is even greater. Our ancestors worked and sweated daily in order to survive. Today, many of us sit in our temperature-controlled environments all day without ever breaking a sweat. This trend has suspiciously increased with the prevalence of allergies, asthma, and many other conditions. University of Alberta researchers (2010) concluded in a study published in the *Archives of Environmental Contamination and Toxicology* that, *"induced sweating appears to be a potential method for elimination of many toxic elements from the human body."*

Typical methods of sweating include exercise, saunas and steam rooms. However, most people overlook the fact that outdoor work, walking and manual labor can produce a healthy sweat. Most people crank on the air conditioning at the slightest sign of heat. Sweating to cool off is a better strategy, as this will stimulate the turnover of toxins that burden our immune system.

Sweating outdoors in the summer heat also makes our body more heat tolerant, which allows us to live in warmer conditions in general. This means we can use the air conditioner less, which is better for our lungs and sinuses in the long run.

A good sweat is healthiest when the skin is free of chemicals. Sweating with chemical-based sunscreens, antiperspirants or skin softeners will simply provide a greater conduit for those chemicals to access and poison our tissues.

316

Fasting

Fasting can quickly reduce our toxic burden and systemic inflammation, because it allows the body's liver, kidneys and immune system to clear waste with a lower dietary workload.

However, fasting must be done cautiously. Fasting too aggressively may stimulate too much detoxification too quickly. This can overload the bloodstream with toxin byproducts as the tissues clear waste. For this reason, it may be safer to do short, one-day fasts once or twice a week, or fasting with soups, juices or fruits.

Fasting with healthy but limited food selections also allows the liver, kidneys and immune system to do a deep cleanse, yet renders some energy and nutrients to sustain blood sugar levels.

A systematic approach to fasting is recommended. Here are a few optional approaches to consider:

> ➤ A water fast (drink only water) from morning until dinner time twice a week
> ➤ A water fast for 24 hours.
> ➤ A fast for one or two days per month with lemon juice.
> ➤ A fast for one or two days with only vegetable soups and fresh juices of carrot and celery.

Any of these fasts should be accompanied by the following:

> ➤ Increased water consumption: ¾ ounce per pound of weight (as opposed to ½ counce).
> ➤ Increased relaxation and rest (days off work are suggested).
> ➤ Only light exercise, such as walking or swimming.
> ➤ Peaceful environments (no parties or shouting matches).

These hints can help assure the fast is productive and thoroughly detoxifying.

Colonics and Enemas

The colon of practically every adult on a western diet is significantly putrefied. This means there is a thick crusty layer of putrefied pathogenic bacteria lining our colon. For many such colons, only a small opening allows waste to move out. The rest of the colon is clogged with crusted bacteria and waste products. These release microorganism endotoxins and various other toxic materials that leak back into our bloodstream, including histamines, ketones, ammonia. Research has shown these waste materials directly contribute to systemic inflammation, and produce radical oxygen species (free radicals).

The best strategy for anyone with systemic inflammation and/or allergic hypersensitivity is to periodically cleanse the colon. This can be done with periodic enemas, or more deeply and effectively, with a colonic.

Enemas can be done quite easily in the privacy of ones bathroom:

> The enema bag can be filled with warm water or herbal tea—anti-allergic herbs listed earlier can be used.
> Hang the bag up, with the tubing clamped.
> Insert the tubing nozzle into the rectum about 3-4 inches. A small amount of castor bean oil or vegetable oil can be put on the nozzle to help its entry.
> Unclamp the tubing.
> The water/herbal tea should begin moving up into the colon, slightly extending the lower abdomen. Maintain the filling until the colon begins to feel full.
> Reclamp the tubing and remove from the rectum.
> There will soon be a tremendous urge for a bowel movement. Try to resist this urge for two or three minutes.
> Lightly massage the lower abdomen before bowel movement.
> The bowel movement will flush the water and waste out.

An enema can be done fairly regularly, but it is important not to overdo enemas, because they can lead to undisciplined bowel movements. After doing one per day for two or three days; once a week is probably sufficient. Consultation with a health professional is suggested.

Colonics are performed by professionals who graduate from schools that teach and certify what is called *colon hydrotherapy*. The colonic is typically done with a sanitary machine that flushes water through the colon, while vacuuming out the waste. A colonic is significantly better and cleanses more deeply than an enema—or even many enemas.

Hydrotherapists typically recommend a colonic at least twice a year if not more. For someone with allergic hypersensitivity, three colonics per year is probably minimal. Consult a colon hydrotherapist for more information.

Deep Breathing

Breathing deeper facilitates two detoxification processes at once: It facilitates the consumption of more oxygen, which provides the ability to neutralize radicals. Breathing out deeply effectively eliminates many toxins. As the carbon dioxide/carbonic acid levels in the blood build up, our bloodstream accumulates other acids and toxins. This facilitates more toxins in the blood, and burdens the immune system with efforts to neutralize and eliminate these acids.

We'll discuss specific techniques for deep breathing, but here we should just say that the burden on our immune systems can be immediately lightened, at any moment, by simply breathing deeper. Let's discuss a couple of deep-breathing techniques:

Deep core breathing:

➢ Slowly push out the abdomen around the belly button. As the lungs fill, push out the upper abdomen. If lying down, a book or hand may be placed on the abdomen to feel and see it rise.

➢ Continue pushing out until the lungs are full and the abdomen is fully pushed out.

➢ Top it off by expanding the rib cage to completely fill the lungs.

➢ Hold in position and relax for 3-7 seconds.

➢ Then push the air out by slowly contracting the upper abdominal muscles, followed by a contraction of the lower abdomen as the lungs are completely emptied. This last step is called *flooring*.

Deep diaphragm breathing:

➢ Slowly push out at the top of the abdomen, enlarging the diaphragm to its capacity as the lungs fill.

➢ Follow by expanding the rib cage to fill out the lungs. Hold for 2-5 seconds.

➢ Then begin contracting the upper abdominal muscles to contract the diaphragm. This will begin pushing the air out.

➢ Slowly contract the diaphragm completely to force out as much air as possible.

Diaphragm breathing does not as completely fill or empty the lungs as deep core breathing does, but it is often more practical while sitting, walking or exercising. Core breathing can result in sleepiness, so it is best used at home in bed or on a comfortable sofa. Either method, if practiced daily for at least 15 minutes, can significantly increase our lung cavity capacity. We may begin to breathe deeper without trying. Placing a hand on the abdomen to feel its rise and fall can also help us center ourselves on our breathing.

In both methods, good breathing posture can be maintained. If sitting, the lower back can be arched slightly with the upper spine fairly straight and relaxed, and the back of the head in line with our lower spine. We can sit on the front of our 'sit bones' at the base of the pelvis, rather than the backside of our sit bones where the lower spine tends to curve outward. When we are sitting on the right part of our sit bones, our lower back will naturally arch.

If lying down on our back, a large pillow can be put under the knees, with the spine straight and a comfortable neck pillow that keeps the crown of the head aligned with the lower spine. Most *hatha-yoga* postures are also conducive to deep breathing exercises.

Green Foods and Super Foods

As discussed earlier, there are a number of foods that promote detoxification. In general, these are plant-based foods, primarily the fruits, vegetables and roots. Especially productive for detoxification are the green vegetables. Practically any green plant-food is equipped with many biochemicals that neutralize toxins. Pure chlorophyll can also help accomplish this, but whole green foods are better because they provide chlorophyll along with many other phytonutrients. Especially good detoxification foods are parsley, cilantro, broccoli, spinach, romaine lettuce, celery, apples, beets, cranberries and so many others. See the antioxidant section.

Soups, Juices and Water

Detoxification can be speeded up by increasing water intake. This increases urination, which pushes more toxins out. Fresh soups and raw juices also have this effect, with the addition of neutralizing free radicals by antioxidants present in the phytonutrients of their ingredients. Great detoxification juices include celery, carrot, beet and tomato. Soups can include these, with the addition of barley and antioxidant spices.

Herbs and Spices

Speaking of spices, earlier we detailed a variety of herbs and spices that stimulate detoxification. Some of the more popular and available include garlic, ginger, cayenne, basil, rosemary, dill, black pepper and nutmeg. Most of these are also anti-inflammatory, as described previously.

Skin Brushing

Brushing the skin with a natural fiber brush can also encourage detoxification by stimulating the lymphatic system and opening skin pores. This also stimulates circulation in general, which increases detoxification.

Timing and Intensity

A detoxification strategy while on vacation can be very useful. Being away from the typical toxins and stressors that circulate through our daily lives can allow us to more thoroughly purge them and lift the burden off of our immune system. This is especially true if the vacation is to a natural environment, such as a camping trip or a trip to the beach.

As mentioned briefly earlier, detoxification intensity should match our age, immune system condition, health in general and other specifics unique to our bodies. Generally, the healthier and younger we are, the easier we will cleanse toxins. As we age, our body retains more toxins, depending upon our exposures. Detoxing too fast can be unsafe, especially for elderly persons—as too many toxins can be released at once. Thus, a gradual, slow process is advisable. The process is best supervised by a health professional trained in detoxification strategies.

There are a number of other approaches to detoxification and lifting the burden on the immune system. Let's go through some of these.

Exercise Strategies

Exercise stimulates the immune system and detoxification processes because it increases metabolism, turns over oxygen and carbon dioxide, increases circulation, increases toxin removal, increases nutrient supply and stimulates the liver. Longer, slower exercise achieves more detoxification because it produces fewer acidic exercise metabolites.

Exercising also involves muscle contraction, which 'pumps' the lymphatic system. This effectively increases lymph circulation, which circulates B-cells and T-cells and other immune factors throughout the body, picking off toxins and pathogens and disposing of their broken down parts. When the lymph is running slow, the body must lean on other detoxification systems, including the mucous membranes.

Many with allergies are afraid of exercise because they've experienced or heard about an episode after a little exercise or physical exertion—regardless of the condition of the person or training regimen. Many of these may well be related to specific instances of exercise-induced asthma. However, exercise has proven beneficial for exercise-induced asthma.

The reality is that an immediate change in exertion levels and breathing might provoke wheezing in the short run for anyone—especially in cold weather conditions. An ongoing exercise routine, on the other hand, is what has proven successful in reducing episodes and symptoms.

This is based on the fact that exercise increases circulation and detoxification, stimulates the immune system, pumps the lymphatic system and increases lung capacity. Exercise is one of the most assured ways to strengthen the immune system and thus increase tolerance. When we exercise, we contract muscles. Again, muscle contraction is what circulates (or pumps) lymph around the body through the lymph vessels. This is because the lymphatic system does not have a heart like the circulatory system has. The lymphatic system relies on muscle contraction for circulation—as we've discussed.

Lymph circulation is critical for systemic inflammation because immune cells circulating through the blood and lymph break down and carry out of the body those broken-down toxins and cell parts.

And of course, exercise also circulates oxygen and nutrients throughout the body. Exercise also stimulates the thymus gland, and speeds up healing of the intestinal cell walls. In all, exercise is one of the best and cheapest therapies available to boost immunity and tolerance.

All of these effects and more are produced by daily exercise and activity.

321

Choosing the Routine

Choosing the right type of exercise depends greatly upon the individual and situation. Good forms of exercise include swimming, walking, running, tennis, golf, baseball, basketball, softball, volleyball, surfing, racquetball and squash. While many say that running can induce more hypersensitive episodes, this greatly depends on the person, their individual health, and weather conditions. In fact, many successful runners have been allergic and asthmatic at times. Same goes for swimmers and other sports. The bottom line is that these individuals were better for their exercise, not worse for it.

Research has concluded that sports involving water and warmer air are easier on the airways. Sports like skiing or wintertime running can stress the mucosal membranes and nasal tissues.

Thus working out in a warmer, slightly humid environment has definite advantages, although exercise in cold weather is better than no exercise at all. We might also consider some accessories. If running or working out outside during the winter, we can wear a ski mask or scarf over the nose and mouth to reduce the cold air, for example. Breathing in through the nose will also help warm the air before it hits the lungs.

The morning also typically contains less air pollutants, so exercising during the morning may prove to cause less hypersensitivity.

Warming up before exercising is also important. A routine of stretching, jumping jacks, push-ups, knee bends and so on will increase circulation and prepare the body for rigorous exercise.

Days with longer exercise activity can alternate with shorter-burst activity. Shorter-burst activity increases lung function and increases tolerance. Longer, slower exercise produces more detoxification because there are fewer waste products being produced. For example, a person might alternate between walking, taking a hike in the woods, or slow swimming on one day, and play some basketball, soccer or do wind sprints the next. This can further be supplemented with abdominal and even weight (or isometric) training—both of which can increase breath control and respiratory health.

The bottom line again that it depends upon the individual. If a person enjoys a particular sport, they ought to pursue that sport. They will be better for it because they will more likely to continue that sport.

Manual Activity

Remember the Pima Indian research on obesity and diabetes discussed previously? While the Mexican Pimas didn't have technical exercise routines, they had plenty of activity. Because they lived a traditional lifestyle, they walked, lifted, chopped, farmed, swept and did other manual labor.

Manual labor is shunned in modern western society, yet it is one of the best means to stay healthy. Manual labor works many muscle groups and stimulates detoxification. For most of us, there is always the choice of doing it ourselves or otherwise. A good example is weeding. While pulling weeds by hand or using the hoe to remove them requires virtually no expense or special skill, most westerners elect to spray the weeds with toxic chemicals. The election to spray not only eliminates the potential for exercise: It also exposes us to chemicals that add to our body's toxin load.

Active choices can also be as easy as taking the stairs instead of the elevator; walking to the next store rather than driving the car to the next parking lot; biking to work instead of driving; raking the leaves instead of using a leaf-blower—and so many other choices.

At the same time, the person with allergic hypersensitivity should not feel that we can just work out daily and not do anything else to improve our health. No. We still will need to eat the right foods, and partake in at least some of the other strategies we've outlined in this chapter and throughout this text. Using this information, we can increase our chances of achieving greater tolerance and increased immunity.

Bursting

In addition to manual labor, both capacity and efficiency can be quickly increased with a particular type of cardiovascular exercise we'll call bursting. Bursting is exercising with periodic bursts of speed and/or intensity. Practically every form of exercise can include bursting.

However, the burst can stop once we reach oxygen debt (evidenced by not being able to catch our breath). When we reach that point, we can slow down to our aerobic pace. Going too far beyond our aerobic state does little to increase lung capacity. It merely causes more acidosis. The key is to burst quickly, get to the upper limit, and then ease back down quickly. The next burst can immediately follow the return to aerobic breathing. Spinning, hill running, basketball, squash and other court sports are great ways to burst.

Note that breath holding, especially under water, does little to increase our lung capacity. It will only hasten the cells' switching over to anaerobic respiration, which again leads to acidosis. The combination of acidosis and the pressure under water can result in brain damage and unconsciousness: Not a good idea.

Clearing the Nasal Passages

This brings us to the logical conclusion that we need to keep the nasal passages clear. Obviously, keeping the sinuses and nasal passages clear is the key to breathing comfortably for someone with sinus and nasal congestion. When these regions are clogged, our mucous membranes are not draining properly. Mucous needs to be swept out, and if the mucous is too thick or crustified with waste matter, our airways will be narrowed.

So how do we accomplish clearing the nasal passages? Well, besides the other detoxification measures we discuss in this chapter, we might consider periodic nasal irrigation.

Nasal lavage is the first consideration. This can utilize a special Ayurvedic lavage device called the neti pot. Neti has been in practice for thousands of years. The pot is simply filled with warm weakly-salty water, and poured through each nostril. A small teapot can also be used.

- The technique is to first mix about a quarter-teaspoon of non-iodized, refined salt to about a cup of lukewarm water. A pinch of baking soda may also be added, especially if the salt is iodized or otherwise burns in any way.

- Lean forward, over the sink. With the chin level with the nose, turn the head sideways so the nose on a plane parallel with the ground as much as possible.

- The water is lightly poured into one nostril, traveling around the septum and out the other nostril. There is no force or pressure involved. There is no snuffing in or pulling in. The solution is simply poured into one nostril, and out through the other. Just hold the head still while it pours out.

Nasal Irrigation: This can also be accomplished by gently pushing warm saline (water and salt) into each nostril using a soft squeeze bottle. Soft squeeze bottles designed for cleaning the nasal region are often available at most drug stores. After using the saline in the bottle, the bottle can be refilled. Care must be taken not to forcefully squirt the water through, which can get water into the upper sinuses.

Another technique is to simply sniff water up the nose and back down through to the pharynx and throat, where it is spit out. This can provide a more complete cleansing of the pharynx and sinuses, but should not be overdone, and only if the sinuses are at least partially clear.

Nasal irrigation has been proven in research to aid in allergic conditions and sinusitis. For example, researchers from Taiwan's Chung Shan Medical University Hospital (Wang *et al.* 2009) gave nasal irrigation or not to 69 children with acute sinusitis. The saline irrigation group improved significantly better than the other group with regard to symptoms and quality of life.

Nasal irrigation was also effective in reducing sinus congestion, rhinorrhea, sneezing and nasal itching in a study by medical researchers from Italy's University of Milano (Garavello *et al.* 2010). In this study, 23 pregnant women with seasonal allergic rhinitis underwent either nasal irrigation or not for six weeks.

In another study, presented at the 50th Scientific Assembly of the American Academy of Family Physicians, Dr. Richard Ravizza and Dr. John Fornadley of Pennsylvania State University divided 294 students into three groups, one of which did nasal irrigation with salt water and the other two groups either took a placebo pill or did nothing. The nasal irrigation group experienced fewer colds during the treatment period compared to the other two groups.

To be fair, some have questioned whether daily regular nasal irrigation for long periods is necessarily good. In a study presented at the American College of Allergy, Asthma and Immunology (Nsouli 2009), researchers tested 68 patients with a history of sinusitis, who had been using nasal irrigation daily. Of the total, 44 patients discontinued the irrigation while 24 continued the daily treatment. After a year, those who had discontinued the irrigation had 62% less sinusitis infections than the group who continued to use nasal irrigation daily. Dr. Tamal Nsouli commented that daily irrigation may deplete healthy mucous from the sinuses. As we've discussed, healthy mucous membranes also cover the sinuses, helping protect us from infection. Dr. Nsouli also commented that he is not opposed to irrigation for three or four times a week, but suggested avoiding daily irrigation for long periods.

We should note that the study details and protocol have yet to be published, and was only presented in abstract form at the conference. Diane Heatley, M.D., a Professor at University of Wisconsin's School of Medicine, questioned the report, stating, *"nasal irrigation has previously been proven safe and effective for treatment of sinus symptoms in both adults and children in a number of studies already published in peer-reviewed journals."*

An appropriate conclusion here is that regular nasal irrigation should still include some moderation. Using it during periods of congestion and sensitivity is certainly appropriate. Use after or during environmental conditions where there is an increased level of pollution and/or infectious agents is also appropriate. But we can remember that our mucous membranes also house important immune cells and probiotics, which help protect us. We don't want to flush those away needlessly.

Air Pollution

This leads to the topic of avoiding indoor and outdoor air pollution—a major source of toxins that can overload our immune systems.

Natural Air Sanitation

We can restrict the level of indoor pollutants by choosing to use household products with natural ingredients free as possible from chemicals and VOCs. This means using natural flooring and furniture, natural fragrance-free soaps and cosmetics, and cotton clothing. This also means buying fewer plastic household goods and more natural fiber goods. Should we change our purchasing behavior, we may also alter the behavior of those companies manufacturing these items.

When it comes to freshening up stale indoor air, pressurized aerosol air fresheners are not the way to go. They may contain various synthetic fragrances, benzyl ethanols, naphthalene, and formaldehydes among other undesirables. Various micro-particles are also created by these aerosols.

As mentioned, many aerosols and pump sprays contain noxious propellants—many of which are also volatile organic compounds (VOCs). These include butane and propane. Despite their demand in the marketplace, aerosols are not required for survival: Humankind did just fine without them for thousands of years. An effective disbursing method is a simple spray bottle. An active natural essence—say lemon juice—can be diluted with water and lightly sprayed through a room to freshen it up nicely. There are, of course, many other uses for such a common spray bottle—effectively replacing propellant aerosols.

Beware of perfumes and colognes that may reside in the bathroom or on family members. And be careful of fashion magazines and men's magazines that insert fragrances into their pages and advertisements. These perfumes might smell nice, but they can also contain toxins that can burden the immune system in addition to triggering an allergic episode.

Candles may smell nice, but they are often made with synthetic fragrances, hydrocarbon-based paraffin waxes, and lead or other heavy metal wicks. The combination often releases unhealthy black soot into our air. Beeswax candles with essential oils can provide good alternatives for the candle-loving household, combined, of course, with fresh air.

Healthy alternatives to toxic household cleaners include lemon, vinegar, borax and/or baking soda. Borax is a great scrubbing detergent for heavy household and yard cleaning jobs. Olive oil, lemon oil or beeswax make for good natural furniture polishes.

Cleaning surfaces with these will also significantly freshen indoor air as well. Rotting food and unclean surfaces create mildew and bacteria quite quickly. Fresh air is quite easy to achieve with clean surfaces. Dusting and wiping down flooring and walls with vinegar can be a good strategy. A small cup of vinegar or a box of baking soda placed in a corner can also absorb odors and airborne toxins. Septic unfriendly chlorine bleach or rubbing alcohol can be used sparingly to remove mold or other microorganisms.

As far as pesticides, there are also natural alternatives. These include clove oil, mints, orange oil, borax and others. Many pest control companies will now apply these alternatives upon request.

326

House Plants

A house full of indoor plants will do wonders for improving our indoor air quality. Placing between two and five plants in a hundred square foot room—depending upon the outside air—can significantly remove carbon and raise oxygen levels. Research from the *Mississippi Stennis Space Center* concluded that indoor plants absorbed and broke down formaldehydes, trichloroethylenes, benzenes and zylenes.

Better performing plants included the lady palm, the rubber plant, English ivy, and the areca palm plants. Toxin removal rates can range from 1,000 to 1,800 micrograms per hour. One study done in Norway (Fjeld *et al.* 1998) found 23% fewer complaints of fatigue and sinus congestion among workers working around plants.

Studies performed in Texas and at Washington State University found that cognition response and problem-solving were also significantly higher among people working around plants (Wolverton 1997).

It should be noted that potting soils of indoor plants can also harbor microorganisms such as molds, so care can be taken to dry out the soil between waterings, and keep some sunlight on the soil surface.

We can also create forests around our homes. This means planting, maintaining indigenous trees that provide oxygen, shade, and soil health: Soils without good plant life and rooting systems become loose and dusty. Nearby outdoor plants can significantly decrease the carbon and toxins in our immediate circulating environment. This also means instead of tearing out trees and paving our courtyards, we can leave the trees or replant them. Living in a space surrounded by trees can also render more privacy, allowing us to keep our windows open more often.

Pros and Cons of Air Conditioning

Air conditioning offers benefits and downsides. On the benefit side, a good one can filter out pollens, soot, insect endotoxins and other potential allergy triggers. This of course depends on the filter inside the air conditioner—and how often it is cleaned.

Filters not cleaned frequently can build up with fungi and bacteria that can significantly infect our airspace.

Most air conditioners reduce humidity as well. The problem with this massive reduction in humidity is that it can dry out the mucosal membranes in our airways. This, along with the cold air provided by many air conditioners, can lead to or worsen hypersensitivity.

Swamp coolers provide filtering and cooling, but add humidity. This can keep the airways more moist. However, swamp coolers can easily get infected with molds and bacteria: So they have to be cleaned periodically, perhaps every few weeks in the summer time, and definitely before using after the winter.

327

Practically every air conditioner creates condensation, which results in small droplets of water dripping around the unit or inside the unit. This can encourage fungi and bacteria growth around the walls and ventilation ducts of the system.

Air conditioning artificially cools down body temperature and airways. While this might be considered a good thing when it is hot outside, artificially cooling the body also stresses the body and the airways. The body must work harder to heat and humidify the air before it hits the lungs. This can stress the turbinates, the airway mucosal membranes, and the immune system. Remember the research we laid out earlier that confirms colder, dryer air can increase hypersensitivity.

Also note that car air conditioning systems typically intake air from around the car—full of traffic exhaust. The air can also contain exhaust from the car itself, or combustion byproducts from the engine. While screened through a filter, this air still contains toxins. We can periodically refresh the car's indoor air by stopping and rolling down the car windows.

Air filters in car air conditions can also become filled with fungi and bacteria, so they can be periodically cleaned. Generally, people do not clean their car air filters. So it is safe to say that any older car has a significant build up of mold and other toxins within its air conditioner system and filters.

Noting these issues, it is probably more sustainable to simply minimize air conditioning and utilize fans when possible. Opening the car windows while driving also provides a fan of sorts. Fanned air on the skin helps cool the skin down without chilling the air. Remember that circulated air is typically cleaner than the same type of air when stagnant.

A fan strategy also allows our bodies to better acclimate to the outdoor temperatures. This is healthier for the body. Our bodies have cooling mechanisms that include sweating and relaxing. Both of these are healthy strategies. Sweating removes waste and toxins from the body, and relaxing takes pressure off the adrenal glands.

Natural Materials

Using nature's materials for floors, walls and furniture is also a good strategy. This means using stone, ceramic, wood, wool, cotton and so on. Practically every synthetic piece of furniture, wall covering or floor covering contains a host of chemicals, including formaldehyde, VOCs, insecticides, asbestos and fire retardants. While retarding fires is certainly commendable, these can also make us sick in the worst case, and add to our toxin load in the best case. Besides, stone can be a great fire retardant.

Stone, ceramic tile or wooden floors can also be easily cleaned with vinegar and baking soda to safely eliminate dust and allergens. Wood can also be polished and cleaned with olive oil. Nowadays, most walls are sheet rock, which often contains chalks and asbestos that can slowly build up in the airways. Covering these well with a good paint is a good idea.

Outgassing

Outgassing (or offgassing) any new materials we buy is a good idea, regardless. To outgas a material, we can simply set it in the sun for a day before using it. This is a good idea for any new piece of furniture, wall covering, and anything else that may have been coated in VOCs or form-aldehydes during manufacturing. Plastics may also be outgassed, but out-gassing plastic in direct sunlight can also release additional monomer plas-ticizers.

Outgassing a new car might also be considered. That "new car smell" is more than just an interesting odor. We can leave the car in the sun for a few days or weeks with the windows open. It is also not a bad idea to always keep any car's windows cracked.

Ventilation

A great remedy for air pollution is to allow natural airflow into all of our indoor environments. While most might assume air is just a gas float-ing around aimlessly, moving air orchestrates various filtering and self-cleaning processes as it circulates. Air flows in channels of temperature, pressure, and radiation currents. Air also carries with it a number of elec-tromagnetic and waveform properties. These include negative and positive ions, as we have discussed, and more.

Airflow also provides filtering. Its mixture of elements enables the breakdown of toxins through vaporization and diffusion. While many molecules such as fluorocarbons damage our atmosphere and trap warm air, the combined elements in air work together to break down these ele-ments, gradually eliminating and dispersing their toxic effects. So we need to keep our indoor air moving.

Air works much as water does, as it uses electrostatic forces to remove toxins. This means that our freshest air will be the air that flows through our environment. Stagnated air is polluted air. Moving air is typically cleaner and provides the best means to minimize toxicity. Circulating air also has the greatest tendency of maintaining normal atmospheric com-position, humidity and pressure values.

Therefore, if possible, we might consider keeping our windows open at all times, even in the wintertime. When it is cold outside, we can crack the window barely—just enough to allow for some airflow. Environ-mental filters are also great, because they bring in airflow while filtering pollutants. Fans can do the rest.

Work and School Strategies

Work and school environments are toxin and allergen traps. Why? Because they bring people and limited ventilation systems together under the same roof. They also host a number of toxins among building materials, carpets, desks, chairs, cleaning agents, pesticides, and whatever anyone brings in to work or school. This of course includes animal dander, dust mites, microorganisms and mold attached to people's clothing, hair and skin as they venture into the building.

This was illustrated in the New Zealand research discussed in Chapter Three, where cat allergens were found throughout schools, workplaces, theaters and airplanes.

While there is no way to eliminate these potential allergens, we can certainly take measures to lower our exposure, since as a whole, toxins from the workplace and school do contribute to our overall toxic load and burden upon our immune system. Furthermore, exposure to workplace toxicity in the form of manufacturing wastes, cleaners, gases and other chemical toxins can single-handedly make a person downright sick.

There are a number of policies and strategies among workplaces and schools that can reduce our exposures or toxic loads:

Hazardous Materials: Workplaces and schools typically utilize various chemicals and cleaning materials. Some workplaces use hazardous materials on a daily basis. These should be handled with care, to make sure that exposures are minimized.

According to United States Occupational Safety Code, *Manufacturer's Safety Data Sheets* (MSDS) are required for every chemical used by consumers, workers or cleaning professionals. These should be carefully read over to make sure that the material is being used in accordance with the MSDS. This means that enough ventilation is supplied. For most hazardous materials, this is the greatest risk: Hazardous materials are frequently used without the proper ventilation. These are toxins that can also cause illness and death, depending upon the chemical and exposure level.

HVAC: Our school and workplace should have a heating, ventilating and air conditioning system (also called HVAC) that is adequate for the population, space and environmental conditions. The more people, space and toxins present, the better the HVAC system needs to be. In the United States, these are typically determined by local, state or county building codes. When a building is designed, its HVAC must comply with the building code in place.

The standard codes are determined by The *American Society of Heating, Refrigerating and Air Conditions Engineers* (ASHRAE), who have developed the standards that most municipalities abide by. For example, the 1989 standards (6.2-1989) called for 15-20 cubic feet of fresh air to be brought in per minute (CFM) and per person occupying an indoor space. This means, for example, that an office with 10 people must have a system that pumps in 150-200 cubic feet of fresh filtered air per minute.

This same calculation can be done for any school or other space.

In addition, building codes have changed over the years with respect to insulation. This means that if the building has been built in the past few decades, the building codes are tighter, and there will be likely less ventilation in general. This puts an extra strain on the HVAC system.

Windows are certainly a form of ventilation, but they should not be included in this calculation, because during cold or hot weather, the windows are often closed (though they should not be).

Any building needs to be checked with current code to make sure that the HVAC system matches the use and occupancy of the building. The building specifications designed by the architect before the building was built can easily be different from the building's current use. There may be many more workers or children in the building than originally specified for example. Or if the HVAC was designed for office space, but the building is now used as manufacturing space, for example, the HVAC requirements will be different—depending upon the manufacturing facility and the municipality. So the company owners or school administrators must be reminded to assure their workers or parents that the workplace's/school's HVAC systems are compliant with current codes. This should also be reviewed for any apartment or condominium.

HVAC systems also should also be periodically cleaned. This includes the drip pans and ducting. These can build up with molds and other microorganisms, and infect their occupants. As we discussed earlier, cases have shown that extreme weather changes (from cold to warm or wet) can dramatically affect the HVAC system ducting in terms of mold and microorganisms—significantly infecting the building's occupants.

Flooring: Carpeting in workplaces and schools is particularly problematic. This is because they attract bacteria, molds, dander, allergens and other toxins quickly. Cleaning carpets is typically expensive and difficult. Wood, stone or concrete floors clean easier and can be disinfected more easily, as we've discussed.

Furniture: Chairs and sofas in the work place are susceptible to mold, toxin and allergen build-up as they age, and formaldehydes when newer. Therefore, they need to be periodically cleaned or replaced. Wooden furniture or furniture with cleanable surfaces and moisture barriers are preferred.

Windows: From an individual perspective, sitting or working close to an openable window is suggested in any workplace or school classroom. Any time there is an offensive odor or concern about indoor air quality, the window should be opened and left open until the risk has subsided. Hotel rooms can also be checked for openable windows before they are reserved. A closed-in room with a dirty HVAC system can practically produce a hypersensitive episode in itself.

Fans: Fans are a valuable and inexpensive addition to any room. These can help blow offensive air out the door or window, for example. Fans, in fact, are better strategies than air conditioning, because they do not artificially cool the body down—as we've discussed. In the opinion of this author, every workplace and school should be equipped with fans.

Air purifiers: Small air purifiers can significant help a person working in a workplace with questionable air. There are several purifiers that can be placed on the desk. These can significantly help remove particulates, mold and allergens from our immediate breathing airspace.

Regular Cleaning: This is a requisite for any workplace, school or apartment building. Common areas should be cleaned at least weekly. Floors and walls should be sanitized. Good natural cleaners include vinegar, lemon, borax and baking soda. Chlorine or rubbing alcohol can be used sparingly to disinfect. Furniture requires regular dusting and sanitization, and HVAC systems and ducts require regular cleaning.

Outdoor Air Pollution Strategies

This naturally brings us to strategies to combat air pollution. There is certainly good reason to develop strategies to avoid air pollution. But how practical can these strategies be? Are we to wear a gas mask all day?

The best recommendation we find in most hay fever/allergy texts is simply to shut all the windows as much as possible. Is this really a solution? As we illustrated earlier, research has confirmed that indoor pollution is generally worse than outdoor pollution. What are we to do, then?

As we've discussed, ozone, particulate matter (soot) and carbon monoxide can contribute to and worsen allergy episodes. There is no doubt that allergies are linked to an overloading of the airways with toxins in the form of air pollution.

We might remember that fewer people living in the more pollen-heavy rural areas have less allergic rhinitis than those in cities. This really says a lot when it comes to the strategy of closing the windows.

Country Air

There is little doubt that city living increases allergy and asthma risk. For example, a study done by the Arizona Health Care Cost Containment System (Smith *et al.* 2010) found that among 3,013 people, urban residents had a 55% greater likelihood of asthma and hay fever than did rural residents.

Living around or at least visiting a natural setting such as a forest or beach has many advantages. For example, researchers from Japan's Chiba University (Park *et al.* 2010) conducted 24 field experiments using 280 subjects among 24 forests throughout Japan. In each of the tests, six subjects walked through a forest, while another six walked through a city. The next day the six that walked the city would walk the forest and vice versa. The research concluded that forest environments reduce stress-related cortisol levels, lower heart rate, reduce blood pressure, lower anxiety and increase reaction time. The researchers concluded that: *"These results will contribute to the development of a research field dedicated to forest medicine, which may be used as a strategy for preventive medicine."*

Other studies have confirmed these results. One study found that people living in natural environments had lower levels of stress than those living in urban environments (Ulrich *et al.* 1991). Another, from Emory University, found that natural environments improve health conditions (Frumkin 2001).

Research has also found that even looking at natural environments, even in photos or through windows, enhances positive moods (Blood *et al.* 1999; Kaplan 2001).

All of these improvements, including lower stress levels, positive moods, lower blood pressure and reduced heart rate are all linked to less inflammation and hypersensitivity. Thus, we can conclude that living in a natural setting or spending some significant time in natural settings would be an important strategy to consider for reducing hypersensitivity—for reasons beyond simply reducing air pollution intake.

City Strategies

As much as we may want to, not everyone can pick up and move away from the city. In this case, focus can turn towards reducing immediate air pollutant exposure. We can make logical choices to reduce our exposure. This doesn't mean staying inside and closing all the windows either. It is important that we get enough sunshine and "fresh" air, and this requires us to go outside. We can simply use some common sense. For example, we can *avoid* the following:

> ➤ Running, walking or biking next to a freeway where soot and carbon monoxide levels are greatest.
> ➤ Hanging out downwind of a smoke-stack of an industrial plant known to throw toxins into the air.
> ➤ Sitting or standing downwind, or next to, an outdoor fire or gas stove for an extended period.
> ➤ Standing, sitting or walking next to someone spraying pesticides, herbicides or other chemicals.
> ➤ Frequenting tobacco-filled bars or other smoky places.

> Avoiding dusty areas such as construction sites, runways, racetracks, rodeos and other events that stir up lots of air-borne particulates.

In addition, there are a number of proactive things we can do to reduce our airborne toxins. As discussed earlier, breathing in through the nose helps to filter out some particulates and other foreigners. This also warms the air. As we discussed, cold air can dry the mucous membranes, and thinned mucous membranes expose our airways to more airborne toxins.

If we live in an urban area with poor air quality we might consider exercising or getting outside during the morning, when the air quality is typically better. As temperatures rise, immediate ozone levels increase. We might also consider exercising near a lake, river, or ocean. Polluted air around water tends to disperse more quickly in the presence of wind, humidity, pressure gradients, and temperature differences.

The wearing of a face mask is typically not practical—although during an extreme situation, it is not a bad idea. More subtle strategies include wearing a scarf during winter months, and covering our mouth and nose with it when outside. In colder climates, a fleece ski mask could also help filter out some particulates.

Acupuncture and Acupressure Strategies

A number of studies have shown that acupuncture can reduce symptoms of allergic rhinitis.

Researchers from Germany's Institute of Social Medicine and Charité University Medical Center in Berlin (Brinkhaus et al. 2008) studied acupuncture and allergic rhinitis among 5,237 patients with allergic rhinitis. The acupuncture group received 15 acupuncture treatments over a three-month period. The control groups received conventional medical treatment and no acupuncture.

After three months, using the Rhinitis Quality of Life Questionnaire (RQLQ), they found that the acupuncture group as a whole had 48% improvement while the control group had a 50% worsening of their symptoms according to their RQLQ scores.

Acupuncturists are now licensed in many states in the U.S., and there are a number of accredited acupuncture schools in Western countries graduating skilled acupuncturists. Acupuncture treatments are also very reasonably priced in comparison to most conventional therapies.

In addition to professional treatment, we can also consider acupressure, which may be self-applied, applied by a friend or mate, or applied by a professional acupressure therapist. Acupressure is very safe. It requires no needles, and does not invade the body in any way.

There is good reason to believe that acupressure works for allergic rhinitis. Researchers from the World Health Organization Collaborating Center for Traditional Medicine at Australia's RMIT University (Zhang *et al.* 2010) identified 92 research papers that studied ear acupressure for allergic rhinitis. They found among these, five studies that, in the aggregate, determined that ear acupressure was more effective than antihistamine medications in the long run, and as good as antihistamines in the short run. We should note that while the studies contained some randomization, they did not have blindedness (actually a bit difficult to accomplish in acupressure).

Both acupuncture and acupressure stimulate key points along our body's *meridians*—energy channels through which flow the body's subtle energy, termed *qi* or *chi*.

While acupuncture applies needles at these points, acupressure requires the application of the fingertips—or better, the tip of the thumb. The acupressure *"point"* along the meridian is deeply pressed with the fingertips or thumb. The ear points can be pressed (or "pinched") with a fingertip or dull matchstick (Kenyon 1988). While the points are deeply pressed, pressing should stop short of any pain—as some of these points may be sensitive.

The diagrams on the next page show acupressure points suggested for hay fever by leading acupressure expert and acupuncturist, Julian Kenyon, M.D. By "TOP" the diagram means to apply the pressure on the top of the foot. By "SIDE" the diagram means the side that has the symptoms, although for most rhinitis sufferers, both sides would probably be appropriate.

These points can be massaged or pressed deeply for 15-30 minutes a day, or several times a day. There is no set time limit or restriction. Easily accessible points can be self-massaged or self-pressed virtually at any time. This technique is safe, and as illustrated in the acupuncture research, has value for anyone with allergic hyperreactivity.

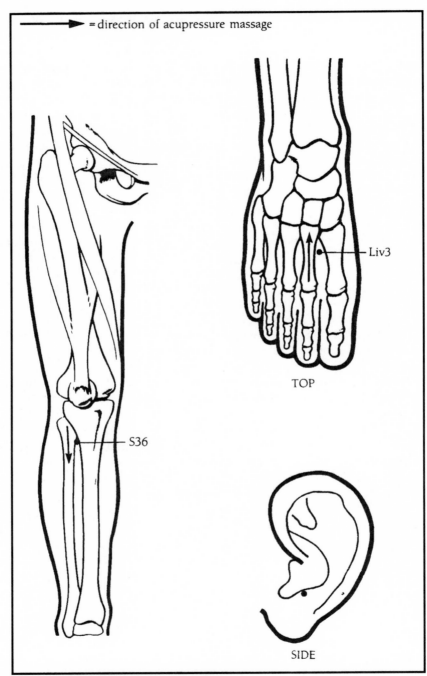

= direction of acupressure massage

Liv3

TOP

S36

SIDE

(Kenyon 1988; Reprinted with permission)

336

Liver Strategies

Throughout this text, we have illustrated that immunosuppression and systemic inflammation is the primary underlying condition in hay fever and allergies—combined with functional weaknesses among airway mucosal membranes. The liver is the primary organ involved in removing toxins that burden the immune system—and contribute to systemic inflammation. In other words, liver health is crucial for inhibiting allergic hypersensitivity.

The liver produces a number of enzymes that help break down toxins and endotoxins (waste material from microorganisms). The liver also filters blood through its hepatocytes to remove toxins, while breaking apart pathogens using its kuppfer cells. We discussed the liver's functionality in more detail in the second chapter. There are several strategies we can consider to strengthen the liver, and we've discussed most of these:

➢ Reducing or eliminating our intake of chemical preservatives, food dyes and synthetic sweeteners. All of these require the liver's resources to break them down.

➢ Reducing or eliminating our exposure to formaldehydes, cleaning chemicals, pesticides, herbicides, benzenes, VOCs and other harsh chemicals that the liver must work hard to break down once absorbed into the skin or lungs.

➢ Drinking enough water. Water nourishes and helps the liver flush and detoxify the blood and lymph.

➢ Eliminating unnecessary pharmaceuticals, as pharmaceuticals are typically rough on the liver—as is alcohol. This requires that we work closely with those doctors who have prescribed our pharmaceuticals, while asking the doctor a clear question: *"Do I really need to continue taking this pharmaceutical?"* Most pharmaceuticals are intended and tested for short-term use. Most were never intended for long-term use, and many studies have shown that long-term use of medications can severely damage the liver. Note also that some pharmaceuticals are worse than others. Acetaminophen is particularly harsh on the liver, for example. For a more complete list of pharmaceuticals that aggravate or cause hypersensitivity, see the list in Chapter Four.

➢ Correcting the fatty acid balance in our diet to comply more closely to that outlined earlier in the dietary strategies section. The liver must work hard to accommodate our fats. High levels of the wrong fats can put a strain on the liver.

➢ Keeping our cholesterol levels in balance through wise dietary choices. Foods that produce high levels of low-density

337

lipoproteins (such as fried foods, saturated fats, grilled meats and so on) will strain the liver as it seeks to balance cholesterol and reduce lipid peroxidation.

➤ Liver strengthening foods include beets, carrots, turnips, radishes, onions, leafy-green vegetables, spirulina, chlorella, squash, celery and other plant-based foods.

➤ Liver restoring herbs include Milk Thistle, Turmeric, Garlic, Dandelion, Goldenseal, Ginger, Bupleurum and Guduchi.

Adrenal Strategies

The adrenal glands respond to stress by way of biochemical signals from the hypothalamus and pituitary gland. These biochemical signals come in the form of adrenocorticotropic hormone (or ACTH). This master hormone signals nerve centers, and stimulates the adrenal glands to produce cortisol and other glucocorticoids. This is called the *hypothalamic-pituitary-adrenal axis stress response.*

Remember that the adrenals are critical to balancing inflammatory responses. During times of stress, we can overload the adrenal gland. Over time, with continued stress, we can exhaust the adrenals.

The adrenal glands produce cortisol, androgens, glucocorticoids and many other hormones that stabilize and balance the body's metabolism. Without a strong and active adrenal complex, the body's hormone and steroid system becomes unbalanced and out of whack. This encourages inflammatory responses to become uncontrolled, producing a number of possible symptoms—including allergic hypersensitivity.

When the adrenals are exhausted, they have problems controlling the inflammatory response as healthy adrenals do. In this state, we are more prone to hyperinflammatory conditions such as allergies.

This is also why relaxation exercises are so productive in reducing allergy symptoms. As the system relaxes more, the adrenal glands are allowed some time to refresh, enabling them to better respond to small inflammatory episodes—before they get out of control.

But what about adrenal glands that are already exhausted? Can we do anything to rebuild and strengthen them? Absolutely.

In fact, many of the strategies we have outlined in this book, including many of the herbs, foods, detoxification and exercises will directly or indirectly strengthen the adrenal glands. This is accomplished because these methods can:

➤ Reduce inflammation—unburdening the adrenal glands.

➤ Stimulate relaxation—allowing the adrenals to recuperate.

➤ Directly stimulate healthy adrenal activity.

> ➤ Supply adrenals with the raw materials to produce corticoids and androgens.

What are some of the more immediate ways to increase adrenal capacity? Here are a few of the many that either unburden or strengthen the adrenals:

> ➤ Decrease toxin consumption, increase detoxification.
> ➤ Greenfoods, fruits and vegetables that provide antioxidants.
> ➤ Plenty of water, as defined earlier.
> ➤ Relaxation: Letting things roll off the back, so to speak. Not sweating inconsequential things. This is particularly important for those who drive everyday. Driving is highly stressful. It can help, therefore, to listen to soothing music while driving. Or take public transportation.
> ➤ Deep breathing: This is important for relaxation, as we discussed above. Breathing not only nourishes the adrenals with oxygen and alkalinity: It also stimulates the VNO nerves.
> ➤ Visual imagery: Looking at scenes of nature, or imagining natural settings.
> ➤ Higher sounds: Consider what we hear. Are we hearing a lot of chatter about what other people are stressed about? (This includes television.) Hearing stressful language can stimulate our adrenals. In fact, a dramatic movie or TV program has been shown to stimulate the adrenals and increase cortisol levels. This may be okay periodically, but not constantly. For those with already over-stimulated adrenals, being around uplifting sounds and discussions is a better strategy.
> ➤ Foods particularly good for the adrenals include onions, garlic, peppers, papaya, mango, apricots, squash and broccoli.
> ➤ Herbs that help strengthen and revitalize the adrenals include Shizandra, Tylophora, Astragalus, Dandelion, Licorice and Chinese Licorice.

We might add that the Licorice mentioned here should not be deglycyrrhized Licorice, as in the DGL used primarily for stomach ulcers. This is because glycyrrhizin and its triterpenoid, glycyrrhizinic acid, are considered primary adrenal-restorative constituents. This said, a 2003 European Commission suggested that a person should not consume more than 100 milligrams of glycyrrhizinic acid per day. Note, however, that even concentrated extracts of Licorice herb will contain only 4-25% glycyrrhizinic acid. This means that 400-500 mg a day of *raw, unconcentrated* Licorice root will contain far less than the maximum levels documented by the European Commission. Natural Licorice root, in fact, has been used safely by Western and Eastern traditional herbalists for many centuries.

Hydrotherapy Strategies

Water Therapies

The ancient physician Hippocrates was a proponent of hydrotherapy for respiratory conditions, and there have been many treatment successes among the many hydrotherapy treatment centers all over Europe, Asia and the U.S. over the centuries. Early nineteenth century physician Vincent Priessnitz from Austria popularized many types of modern water treatments, as did Father Sebastian Kneipp—a 19th century German monk. These included water compresses, cold-water therapy, contrast baths, hot baths, and warm baths.

Dr. Wilhelm Winternitz, an Austrian neurologist, observed one of Priessnitz's treatment centers and became one of the most celebrated proponents of water treatment in modern times. Dr. Winternitz designed a number of different water treatments and influenced American physicians such as Dr. John Harvey Kellogg, Dr. Jethro Kloss and Dr. Simon Baruch. Dr. Kellogg operated the famous Michigan Battle Creek Health Center for many years until it burnt down in 1902. The center utilized hydrotherapy as a key healing agent. Dr. Kloss ran his own clinic and also worked closely with the Battle Creek Center.

Despite its history of success, opposition to hydrotherapy came from pharmaceutical medicine circles in the decades that followed. Water cures became targeted by the new medical establishment, and many hydrotherapy treatment centers were shut down between 1920 and 1950. Hydrotherapy experienced a resurgence in the U.S. following World War II, when physical therapists found success in whirlpool treatment. Today hydrotherapy is widely used in various modalities, treatments, and physical therapy centers. Many hot springs and wellness spas are unmistakably similar to the hydrotherapy centers of years past. Today these centers draw millions of people seeking therapy and relaxation.

Research has also confirmed that living near or exercising in water significantly lowers the risk and incidence of allergies. A number of studies have confirmed that swimming reduces allergy and asthma occurrence. In two studies investigating hypersensitivities in children, it was determined that swimming significantly reduced asthma and allergy episodes and severity—at levels greater than those offered by other forms of exercise (Inbar *et al.* 1980).

Hot and Cold Water Techniques

Hot and warm water therapy increases circulation, relaxation and detoxification efforts. Let's review some of the techniques recommended:

Cold water showers or a quick cold water rinse off after a warm water shower is invigorating and stimulating to the immune system and nervous system. It also helps balance the body's thermoregulation systems, cool the body in hot weather, as well as heat the body (through muscle contraction) in cold weather.

These actions are produced by our blood vessels' response to cold water. Cold water constricts the blood vessels and leads to involuntary muscle contraction. This type of muscle contraction increases the body's immune function by pumping the lymphatic vessels. In other words, lymph flow is circulated by movement and muscle contraction.

The mechanism works like this: As cold water hits the skin, internal muscles autonomically contract. This effectively pumps or squeezes lymphatic vessels. When the lymph vessels are pumped, the lymphatic fluid speed is increased—much like our heart's pumping increases blood circulation.

Lymph circulation distributes macrophages, T-cells, B-cells and other immune factors throughout the body, enabling them to break down invading bacteria, viruses, and chemical toxins. This effectively speeds up our immune response. As our immune system is responding faster, our toxic load is decreased and our infective burden lightens.

Blood vessel constriction from cold water also stimulates the health of our blood vessels. This serves to increase blood vessel wall elasticity, especially when the cold shower follows a warm or hot shower. Alternating cold water can also help open a blocked nose, as the blood vessels contract, lessening vascular permeability.

German researchers (Goedsche *et al.* 2007) studied the treatments used of Dr. Kneipp on twenty patients with chronic obstructive pulmonary disease. Cold-water hydrotherapy was tested for immunostimulation, maximal expiratory flow, quality of life, and respiratory function. After ten weeks of three cold effusions and two cold washings on the upper body per day, IFN-gamma lymphocytes increased, quality of life increased, lung function improved and the frequency of respiratory infections decreased.

Many traditional healers have used cold water therapy with great success for allergic hypersensitivity. Additional cold water strategies include walking in a few inches to a few feet of cold water by a lake, river or ocean for at least a few minutes, building to up to 30 minutes a day.

Contrast baths reference a therapy of alternating hot water and cold water bathing. This therapy has been used with great success, and can be easily practiced at home by simply following a hot shower with a short cold one before toweling off.

Besides constricting blood vessels and stimulating lymph flow, a cold rinse at the end of a shower causes the skin pores to close. This leaves the body prepared to step out of the shower or bath. A cold rinse also reduces the potential of a basal cell chilling, which can stress the body. In other words, a cold rinse will better prepare the body for the temperature change.

Wet Sock hydrotherapy has been used to rebuild immunity for centuries. The feet are soaked in hot water for 10-30 minutes while a pair of thin socks are soaked in cold, icy water. The feet are taken out of the hot water and the cold socks are wrung out and put on, with a pair of thick wool socks over top. This is followed by lying down or sitting with the feet up for an hour or two while relaxing.

Finnish sauna and plunge system: The Fins are famous for their wooden saunas, often built outside near a cold-water plunge. A vigorous sweat in the sauna immediately followed by the cold plunge stimulates the immune system dramatically. This ritual has also been a part of other cultures, including many North American Indian tribes, who used *sweat lodges* with great success. These cultures are known for their long lives and strengthened immunity. Infrared saunas are great modern devices for this purpose. Infrared saunas have the added benefit of quickly and safely dilating blood vessels.

Hot baths also have a great tradition of success among those with respiratory ailments. Hippocrates, known to western medicine as the father of medicine, stated that the hot bath *"...promotes expectoration, improves the respiration, and allays lassitude; for it soothes the joints and the outer skin, and is diuretic, removes heaviness of the heat and moistens the nose."*

Hot water calms the body and slows the heart rate, as the body's blood vessels relax and dilate in response to thermal radiation. A hot bath will open skin pores, allowing a detoxification and exfoliation of skin cells and their contents. For sore or damaged muscle tissues, the dilation of capillaries and micro-capillaries speeds up the process of cleansing the muscle cells of lactic and carbonic acids—the byproducts of inadequate respiration.

Recovery times from strenuous activity are typically reduced by the use of hot water therapy. Hot water is also *hydrostatic*—it gently massages the dermal layers. Hot water also slows internal organ activity, and relaxes the airways. This provides a soothing effect upon the innervations to these areas. The result is reduced stress and widened airways. This effect is increased when hot water is in motion—for example a hot tub.

Hot baths can also be medicated with a variety of anti-allergic herbs, as listed earlier. Simply make an infusion tea and pour it into the bath.

It should be noted that too much hot water for too long of a period can lead to cardiovascular stress. Hot water can also lead to heat exhaustion. For best results, hot water applications or saunas should be limited to about 10-15 minutes at the hotter levels.

Also, care should be taken to prevent chlorine and chlorine byproduct overload. The byproducts of chlorine breakdown are trihalomethanes (TTHM) and haloacetic acids (TAA5). Over-exposure to these can increase our toxin burden. Today there are healthier alternatives to chlorine, including bromine and salt water blends.

Hot Mineral Springs: From deep within the earth's surface come special waters of a thermal nature. Geothermal heat from volcanic magma creates a rich environment for charging aquifers with high temperatures and a variety of minerals. Many hot springs have a wholesome mixture of bicarbonates, iron, boron, silica, magnesium, copper, lithium, and many trace elements. Some contain exotic elements such as arsenic—believed to help heal skin issues and digestive issues. In other words, not all hot springs are alike.

Due to the earth's sulfur conveyor system, many of these hot spring waters are rich in sulfur in the form of hydrogen sulfide or sulfate. These can loosen phlegm and relax the airways.

Other mineral ions in hot springs have beneficial effects. Magnesium baths have been shown in studies to relax muscles and ease tension. Magnesium also strengthens arteries and relaxes the airway smooth muscles. Iron in hot springs has been associated with strengthening the immune system. Bicarbonates in hot springs—also called "soda springs"—have been associated with easing tension and aiding digestion.

Epson Salt Bath: For those without a nearby hot springs, a simple bath can be easily turned into therapeutic waters. At home, we can duplicate a magnesium and sulfur mineral springs bath by adding natural mineral salts such as Epson salts to our bath water. Epson salts—originally named after the magnesium-rich waters of Epson, England—are primarily magnesium sulfate, which will ionize in the water into magnesium ions and sulfur ions. As mentioned, ionic magnesium is beneficial to body tissues—relaxing the skin, reducing muscle tension, and lowering stress. Sulfur was also discussed above.

The Epson salt bath can be supplemented with the addition of rock salt. Natural rock salt contains upwards of 80 minerals and trace elements, which can make the bath a nourishing soak for the entire body.

A drop or two of an essential oil such as lavender or rose oil into the bath will further support relaxation. Lavender oil in particular can significantly calm the nerves.

The skin is said to be the largest organ of the body and absorbs water quite readily. The skin is similar to a mucous membrane. Ancient seamen understood this fact well. When out to sea and dehydrated, seamen would soak their garments in seawater for survival.

For this same reason, our bath waters should not contain toxic chemical bubble baths, chemical-laden perfumed soaps, or heavily chlorinated water. The skin will readily absorb these toxins, putting an extra burden upon the liver and detoxification systems. Best to use clean water and only natural additives.

Steam baths are especially helpful for allergies, sinus congestion, headaches and asthmatic hypersensitivity. The steam bath can be accomplished with a formal steam room, by the use of a humidifier, or simply with a hot bath in an enclosed room. A cool or coldwater rinse after is helpful for immune stimulation and temperature adjustment. Eucalyptus can be added to increase the expectoration effect. With this and all hot baths, water intake should be increased dramatically, depending upon duration.

Steams can also be done with a pan of boiled water steeped with anti-asthmatic herbs, or boiled potatoes. Just put a towel over the head and over the pan to breathe in the steam.

Humidified Air

As mentioned previously, the air is full of water in the form of vapor. When water is vaporized within our atmosphere, it is called humidity. Humidity levels are typically measured as *relative humidity*. This is the level of moisture the air can contain at a particular temperature. This means that 100% relative humidity indicates that this is the highest amount of moisture the air can contain at that temperature. Warmer temperatures can hold more vapor than colder temperatures, which is why hot humidity is especially uncomfortable.

Humidity levels can range from 100% percent at 100 degrees in the tropics to 25% at the same temperatures in the desert. At zero degrees F, however, 100% relative humidity is equivalent to only 4% humidity at room temperature. So cold temperatures are typically very dry, even at higher relative humidity levels.

As most of us have experienced, higher humidity during warm weather is uncomfortable. Too low of a humidity level will also be uncomfortable, as it will dry our skin and irritate our lungs. Our lungs are full of moisture, and a slightly humid environment is typically better for the lungs.

What this all means is that typical winters are too dry and summers are too humid in most places. This can be exacerbated indoors if we are not careful, creating an unhealthy indoor environment.

The trick is to create healthy indoor humidity levels. This does not mean reducing outdoor air levels, however. It is important that we have a constant flow of oxygen from nature into our indoor environment. Not only does this give us good oxygen content: It also reduces the amount of radon the house will contain. A closed up house attracts more radon than an open-air house because of the pressure gradient.

So how do we create a comfortable indoor humidity? Our bodies are most comfortable at 25% to 60% humidity at room temperature—with the upper range more conducive to better airway function. Indoor humidity can be affected by a house's building materials, ventilation systems, whatever air conditioning or heating units are in place, and human activity. Simply being in the house will increase its humidity. As we breathe, we send out about a cup of water into our environment every four hours—effectively raising the humidity level by 6-8%.

Most furnaces, fireplace fires and forced air heating units will dry the atmosphere. Most refrigerant air conditioners also dry the air as their evaporator coils draw water vapor. Swamp coolers or evaporative coolers increase the indoor humidity (and use less electricity). Also how we cook, take showers and use water in general will determine our indoor humidity levels. A shower will raise the humidity levels about as much as four hours of breathing.

To test humidity levels in the absence of a humidity gauge (advisable), we can watch the moisture levels on the surface of a glass of ice water. If little or no moisture forms immediately on the outside surface of the glass, our house is too dry. If we see moisture build up or mold on the ceilings, our house is likely too humid.

Changing our humidity is quite easy if it is too dry. A shower, humidifier or a room full of people will increase the humidity quite quickly. If the air is too moist, opening up all the windows (assuming it is dryer outside) is the simplest method. In a humid outside environment, we can reduce indoor plants, cook under an oven fan, and in general keep rotating the moist air out. Dehumidifiers are now available for extreme environments, but better to create our own dehumidifier by ventilating our home with fans and keeping windows open to move the moist air out.

Nasal congestion, lung infections and sinusitis will often respond well to moderately humid environments. Humid air will allow the lungs and nasal tissues to detoxify more efficiently. For this reason, humidifiers and steam rooms can be extremely helpful for infections and congestion. Eucalyptus oil, peppermint oil and/or camphor can be put in the water or steam tray to increase mucous clearance. Be aware, however, that too much humidity can also breed mold.

Anxiety and Stress Strategies

As we discussed, allergic disorders often directly relate to emotional stress and anxiety. Fortunately, there are several techniques that can have proven to reduce our stress, and also bring about a more centered, balanced mind:

Hatha Yoga and Meditation

A number of studies have shown that the practice of *hatha-yoga* can significantly benefit respiratory health. Furthermore, *hatha-yoga* has been shown to reduce airway hyperreactivity.

Researchers from the New Delhi's All India Institute of Medical Sciences (Vempati *et al.* 2009) assigned 57 asthmatic adults to either a *hatha-yoga* group or a control group. The control group was given conventional medication, while the *hatha-yoga* group was given conventional medication plus daily *hatha-yoga* training. The *hatha-yoga* training was supervised for the first two weeks, and then done at home for six weeks.

After the eight weeks, the *hatha-yoga* group had significantly more improvement in forced expiratory volume (FEV1) and peak expiratory flow rates (PEFR). The *hatha-yoga* group also had a significant reduction in exercise-induced asthmatic episodes as compared to the control group.

Remember that oxidative stress is directly associated with degenerative allergic conditions. Indian Researchers (Yadav *et al.* 2005) also determined that psychological stress directly produces increased levels of oxidative radicals. This was determined by measuring the relative concentrations of oxidative byproducts called thiobarbituric acid reactive substances (TBARS) in the bloodstream. We discussed TBARS in the diagnostic and inflammatory section.

The researchers tested 104 men and women with a nine-day educational course on the theory and practice of *hatha-yoga*. These included trainings on postures (*asanas*) and breathing exercises (*pranayama*), together with lectures on stress management, meditation, relaxation (*shavasana*) and nutrition. Blood samples collected before and after the training showed that TBARS concentrations decreased significantly over the 12 day test period.

Mental Imagery

Mental imagery is just about what it sounds like. We can imagine in our minds, a place where we find peace and solace from the stresses of our world. For some, this might be an empty beach on a tropical island. For others, this might be a quiet lake, a dense forest, or a rushing waterfall high in the mountains. It may also be taking oneself back to a place and time where they experienced a peaceful or tranquil feeling.

Research and clinical mental imagery typically uses one or a choice of these images to achieve a state of relaxation. Studies have illustrated that mental imagery can significantly reduce stress and anxiety; and in turn reduce allergic hypersensitivity.

The process of mental imagery takes a person through an exercise that brings the chosen image into the forefront of the mind. This means to focus upon it. The process can be one of picturing, in detail, the various aspects of the image: The color of the sky and clouds; the shape of the mountains; the length of the beach; the color of the ocean, for example. As we begin to picture and even describe these details, our stress levels decrease as we are distracted from our worries. Other techniques, such as looking at a picture, listening to sounds of waves or a stream or even describing our reaction and feeling to these details. This interjects our emotions into the imagery, distracting us further from our worries.

As we imagine the details of our escape, we can see and feel ourselves in the environment. For example, we can see ourselves floating down a river in a raft. We can feel the eddies swirling us as we stare up at the clouds drifting overhead. Practically any relaxing experience can be relived using mental imagery. The more real the experience, the more relaxed we will be—assuming the experience was relaxing.

While doing this, we can also visualize the airways widening and filling with more air and efficiency—by visualizing expanding pipes or hoses.

Researchers from New York's Mount Sinai Medical Center (Epstein *et al.* 2004) tested mental imagery on 68 adults with asthma for seventeen weeks. The study took place at New York's Lenox Hill Hospital. The imagery group volunteers were given a choice of seven imagery exercises to practice three times every day. The practiced for 15 minutes a day.

Of the imagery group, 47% discontinued or reduced their asthma control medications, while only 19% of the control reduced medication use (no one in the control group discontinued medication). Lung function also improved among the mental imagery group. The researchers concluded: *"The study also demonstrated that imagery is inexpensive, safe and, with training, can be used as an adjunct therapy by patients themselves."*

Massage

Massage—whether it is performed by a professional, our mate or friend, or even ourselves (self-massage), can provide a combination of relaxation, stress-relief and increased circulation. All of these can benefit a person with hypersensitivity. And the research supports this.

Researchers from the University of Miami School of Medicine (Field *et al.* 1998) tested 32 asthmatic children with either massage therapy or relaxation therapy. The therapy was applied by the children's parents, who were taught the therapy for 20 minutes prior to bedtime every night for a month. Younger children receiving the massage therapy had immediate decreases in anxiety and cortisol levels after their massages. Over the month, attitudes improved. Peak respiratory flows, along with other lung functions, also improved. Older children who were massaged also reported similar benefits.

Laughter

Laughing is a great stress releaser, and anyone with any type of stress or anxiety can direct themselves towards humor for releasing stress. Laughter in particular is good for hypersensitivity because it also exercises the airways, sinuses and nasal membranes. Experts have compared laughing to exercise: The physiological effects are practically identical. Laughing also stimulates the production of feel-good hormone dopamine into a the pleasure center of the brain. It also reduces levels of stress-related hormones, and increases levels of immunoglobulin A—which in turn increases mucosal membrane immunity.

Illustrating these effects, a series of human clinical studies from Japan's Ujitakeda Hospital and Osaka Prefecture research institute (Kimata 2004; 2004; 2009; 2007; 2010) found that laughter decreased allergies, reduced allergen-specific IgE levels, lowered allergic hypersensitivity, and reduced asthma among groups of patients.

In one these studies, this one using twenty allergic patients, an 87-minute movie of Charlie Chaplin increased levels of dermcidin-derived peptide (DCD) from sweat glands. DCD is an antimicrobial substance that tends to decrease levels of eczema in allergic individuals.

In another study, watching a funny video decreased pollen-specific immunoglobulin E (IgE) and IgG4 levels and increased IgA levels in patients with allergic conjunctivitis.

In another (2004), laughter by mothers reduced allergies among their children.

In yet another, watching Rowan Atkinson's "Mr. Bean" reduced allergen skin wheal responses and reduced levels of neurotrophin-3—a nerve growth factor involved in allergic responses.

In the study that takes the cake (2010), 24 healthy subjects and 24 allergic dermatitis patients were monitored during seven days of watching a humorous movie each day. The comedy resulted in heightened colonization of probiotic lactobacilli and bifidobacterium populations, and decreased levels of infective *Staphylococcus aureus* and enterobacteria. In other words, it seems our (anti-allergic) probiotics also enjoy a good laugh!

Well, maybe not that directly. But certainly, our probiotics respond positively to our body's physiological response to laughter.

There are many ways to bring on genuine laughter, including comedians and humorous theatrical performances. Laughing with friends—and laughing at ourselves and the weird things we do—can also be very therapeutic.

Letting It Out/Letting It Go

Many people with allergies often internalize the issues they have with others. In fact, some research has indicated that some people express themselves (or cry out to others) *through* their allergic episodes—possibly as a result of not adequately expressing themselves otherwise.

This tendency to hold things in can be mitigated by (nicely) letting the people around us know how we are feeling. If we are feeling upset about something someone else did, we can sensitively explain this to them. Assuming that we are not accusatory, often they will simply apologize for their actions, explaining that they did not mean to have that effect. This is because most people do things that affect others without realizing it. They are simply focused elsewhere, and not aware that their actions may be affecting someone adversely. Should we sensitively inform them, most people are prepared to accommodate or make changes.

With regard to children, parents can encourage honesty and directness in their communications.

Having a deeper, spiritual direction in life can also significantly reduce our stresses and anxieties, especially as they pertain to survival issues.

Strategies to Keep Track

The biggest pitfall in any condition is ignorance. Many epidemiological studies performed on allergies have underscored a similar problem: Many people assume they are allergic or intolerant to a particular trigger when they may not be. For this reason, it is important that we approach this issue carefully, and recognize what our specific sensitivities are.

It is one thing to have a negative reaction after exposure to a potential trigger. But it is quite another to have a severe response following multiple potential triggers, yet not be clear on which caused that severe response. In this case, awareness could save a lot of time and energy.

The key to self-awareness is keeping a good diary. A diary simply allows for jotting down what exposures are followed by allergic responses. A sample episode diary format is given on the following page.

This dairy records the date, time and length of an episode, the possible triggers, and the severity of the allergy episode. *"Episode Severity"* is gauged on a one to ten basis, with ten being the worst imaginable, and one being a very slight episode. *"Episode time"* is the length of the allergy symptoms from beginning to end.

HAY FEVER AND ALLERGIES

Episode Diary

Episode Date & Time	Possible Allergens/ Triggers	Episode Length	Episode Description	Episode Severity (1-10)

Conclusion: Putting it All Together

We have proven, through the application and review of hundreds of scientific studies and rigorous clinical applications, that allergic rhinitis is not a disease: Allergic rhinitis/hay fever is a symptom of an underlying deficiency of the immune system and systemic inflammation; combined with functional weaknesses among the nasal mucosal membranes, nerve plexus, sinuses and/or airways in general. We have also showed that the most prominent underlying issue in allergic rhinitis—the linchpin if you will—is systemic inflammation.

This text has offered an extensive review on the range of causes of hypersensitivity, together with the scientific evidence. We have also offered a range of allergens and rhinitis triggers in detail, and the role those triggers play in hypersensitivity. We also discussed in detail the physiology of allergic rhinitis: illustrating the mechanisms involving systemic inflammation, hypersensitivity, and the immune system's inflammatory functions.

These last chapters have laid out an extensive array of strategies to resolve the underlying conditions that produce allergic rhinitis. Some are designed to reverse the underlying causes, while others are targeted for stimulating the body's own healing processes. These have included:

➤ Reducing toxins to lighten our immune system burden.

➤ Immunotherapy to increase tolerance to allergens.

➤ Herbal formulations and individual herbs shown to strengthen the immune system, help the body expel toxins, increase tolerance, neutralize and balance the bloodstream, supply nutrients, strengthen underlying weaknesses among the airways, restore mucosal membrane health, produce hormone and steroid balance, encourage relaxation, remove infections, and many others. We laid out the research illustrating that these traditional herbal formulations can be effective—using the protocols of modern research. We also showed the successful application of these herbs in thousands of years of clinical herbalism.

➤ Diet concepts, foods and recipes shown to help eliminate or ameliorate the underlying causes of hypersensitivity.

➤ Natural nutritional supplements shown to provide extensive antioxidant and adaptogenic properties.

➤ Early diet practices shown to help decrease the risk of allergies among infants.

➤ Techniques to rebuild and revitalize the body's mucosal membranes—shown to decrease hypersensitivity.

➢ Methods to increase our probiotic populations: Shown to stimulate tolerance and maintain a stronger immune system.

➢ Strategies to increase body fluids: Shown to reduce inflammation and hyperresponsiveness.

➢ Ways to increase detoxification in order to lighten the load on our immune systems.

➢ Increasing our deep sleep in order to help strengthen our immunity and increase detoxification.

➢ Acupuncture and self-applied acupressure techniques shown to ease allergic hypersensitivity.

➢ Exercise strategies to lighten our toxic burden, improve circulation, stimulate immunity and increase relaxation.

➢ Nasal- and sinus-clearing techniques to decrease congestion and open the airways.

➢ Steps to reduce consumption of outdoor pollutants: Shown to reduce inflammation and lighten our toxin load.

➢ Techniques to improve and filter our indoor air in order to reduce allergens and triggers during periods of immune system boosting.

➢ Approaches to improve our work and school environments in order to avoid sick building syndrome and hypersensitivity among children and employees.

➢ Programs to strengthen our liver: Shown to increase the elimination of toxins that produce systemic inflammation.

➢ Methods to revitalize our adrenal glands: Shown to increase our natural hormone and steroid balance, and inhibit inflammation and hypersensitivity.

➢ Ways to reduce stress and anxiety, in order to produce increased tolerance, improve our probiotic populations and decrease hypersensitivity.

➢ Tools to track our triggers, episodes, and allergens: To increase our allergy awareness and gauge our improvement as we apply these strategies.

As shown in numerous studies, clinical application and practical evidence, each strategy above can significantly reduce or even reverse hypersensitivity, allergy symptoms, and the underlying causes of allergies.

What does this mean? Does this mean a total curing of our allergies? Well, since allergic rhinitis is not a disease, we cannot cure it. What we can do is remove its underlying conditions, which removes the potential for those symptoms.

One of the beautiful things about modern research is that a properly conducted study will attempt to eliminate all the other possible factors that could be at play. This, in effect, isolates the particular strategy and its chance for success. In the studies used in this text, this isolation of each strategy means that if we were to apply many of these strategies at the same time, our chances for completely removing the underlying causes becomes exponentially greater than the successes resulting from utilizing only one particular strategy.

Remember that a significant result must typically be greater than the placebo effect, which is considered to be under 32%. So let's say that each strategy reduced allergic and asthmatic symptoms (removed underlying causes) in only 33% of the cases. (in most of the research, the improvement was significantly better). This would mean that at the worst, statistically and hypothetically, we would expect a complete elimination of underlying causes if three or more of these scientifically verified strategies were applied concurrently.

While we have segregated the possible strategies into about two dozen categories, we have actually laid out *hundreds* of specific strategies in this book. Therefore, should a person seriously incorporate these strategies—or even a handful—the chance of removing the underlying causes of allergic hypersensitivity becomes exponentially greater.

The word *"seriously"* is used because we are not talking about making some half-hearted lifestyle changes for a few weeks and then stopping. We are talking about making a *commitment* to long-term change: Making lasting and disciplined changes that last for years.

We must remember that the underlying causes of most allergic hypersensitivity have developed over a long period of time: Years, and possibly decades, of a combination of diet, environment and other lifestyle factors. Thus we simply cannot expect results overnight.

What we can expect, assuming that we institute a good number of these strategies, is renewed vigor, strengthened immunity, increased tolerance, better breathing, more relaxation and among others, a greater quality of life.

Depending upon the severity of the allergy, this process should be partnered with one's health professional. For severe symptoms, the lifestyle changes detailed in this book should be made with consultation and supervision of someone skilled in allergic hypersensitivity and aware of the person's particular constitution.

Regardless of how temporary relief is employed, the only way we can remove the potential for allergic symptoms is to remove the underlying causes. This text focuses there. While discipline and determination are necessary, the long-term health rewards and improvements to quality of life provided by these strategies will undoubtedly far outweigh the effort required.

References and Bibliography

Abdureyim S, Amat N, Umar A, Upur H, Berke B, Moore N. Anti-inflammatory, immunomodulatory, and heme oxygenase-1 inhibitory activities of ravan napas, a formulation of uighur traditional medicine, in a rat model of allergic asthma. Erid Based Complement Alternat Med. 2011;2011. pii: 725926.

Aberg N, Hesselmar B, Aberg B, Eriksson B. Increase of asthma, allergic rhinitis and eczema in Swedish schoolchildren between 1979 and 1991. Clin Exp Allergy. 1995;25:815-819.

Adel-Patient K, Ah-Leung S, Creminon C, Nouaille S, Chatel JM, Langella P, Wal JM. Oral administration of recombinant Lactococcus lactis expressing bovine beta-lactoglobulin partially prevents mice from sensitization. Clin Exp Allergy. 2005 Apr;35(4):539-46.

Agache I, Ciobanu C. Risk factors and asthma phenotypes in children and adults with seasonal allergic rhinitis. Phys Sportsmed. 2010 Dec;38(4):81-6.

Agarwal SK, Singh SS, Verma S. Antifungal principle of sesquiterpene lactones from Anamirta cocculus. Indian Drugs. 1999;36:754-5.

Aggarwal BB, Harikumar KB. Potential therapeutic effects of curcumin, the anti-inflammatory agent, against neurodegenerative, cardiovascular, pulmonary, metabolic, autoimmune and neoplastic diseases. Int J Biochem Cell Biol. 2009 Jan;41(1):40-59.

Aggarwal BB, Sung B. Pharmacological basis for the role of curcumin in chronic diseases: an age-old spice with modern targets. Trends Pharmacol Sci. 2009 Feb;30(2):85-94.

Agostoni C, Fiocchi A, Riva E, Terracciano L, Sarratud T, Martelli A, Lodi F, D'Auria E, Zuccotti G, Giovannini M. Growth of infants with IgE-mediated cow's milk allergy fed different formulas in the complementary feeding period. Pediatr Allergy Immunol. 2007 Nov;18(7):599-606.

Aho K, Koskenvuo M, Tuominen J, Kaprio J. Occurrence of rheumatoid arthritis in a nationwide series of twins. J Rheumatol. 1986 Oct;13(5):899-902.

Akinbami LJ, Moorman JE, Garbe PL, Sondik EJ. Status of childhood asthma in the United States, 1980-2007. Pediatrics. 2009;123:S131-45.

Aldinucci C, Bellussi L, Monciatti G, Passàli GC, Salerni L, Passàli D, Bocci V. Effects of dietary yoghurt on immunological and clinical parameters of rhinopathic patients. Eur J Clin Nutr. 2002 Dec;56(12):1155-61.

Alemán A, Sastre J, Quirce S, de las Heras M, Carnés J, Fernández-Caldas E, Pastor C, Blázquez AB, Vivanco F, Cuesta-Herranz J. Allergy to kiwi: a double-blind, placebo-controlled food challenge study in patients from a birch-free area. J Allergy Clin Immunol. 2004 Mar;113(3):543-50.

Alexander DD, Cabana MD. Partially hydrolyzed 100% whey protein infant formula and reduced risk of atopic dermatitis: a meta-analysis. J Pediatr Gastroenterol Nutr. 2010 Apr;50(4):422-30.

Alexandrakis M, Letourneau R, Kempuraj D, Kandere-Grzybowska K, Huang M, Christodoulou S, Boucher W, Seretakis D, Theoharides TC. Flavones inhibit proliferation and increase mediator content in human leukemic mast cells (HMC-1). Eur J Haematol. 2003 Dec;71(6):448-54.

Alfvén T, Braun-Fahrländer C, Brunekreef B, von Mutius E, Riedler J, Scheynius A, van Hage M, Wickman M, Benz MR, Budde J, Michels KB, Schram D, Ublagger E, Waser M, Pershagen G; PARSIFAL study group. Allergic diseases and atopic sensitization in children related to farming and anthroposophic lifestyle—the PARSIFAL study. Allergy. 2006 Apr;61(4):414-21. PubMed PMID: 16512802.

Al-Harrasi A, Al-Saidi S. Phytochemical analysis of the essential oil from botanically certified oleogum resin of Boswellia sacra (Omani Luban). Molecules. 2008 Sep 16;13(9):2181-9.

Almqvist C, Garden F, Xuan W, Mihrshahi S, Leeder SR, Oddy W, Webb K, Marks GB; CAPS team. Omega-3 and omega-6 fatty acid exposure from early life does not affect atopy and asthma at age 5 years. J Allergy Clin Immunol. 2007 Jun;119(6):1438-44.

Amato R, Pinelli M, Monticelli A, Miele G, Cocozza S. Schizophrenia and Vitamin D Related Genes Could Have Been Subject to Latitude-driven Adaptation. BMC Evol Biol. 2010 Nov 11;10(1):351.

American Conference of Governmental Industrial Hygienists. Threshold limit values for chemical substances and physical agents in the work environment. Cincinnati, OH: ACGIH, 1986.

American Dietetic Association; Dietitians of Canada. Position of the American Dietetic Association and Dietitians of Canada: vegetarian diets. Can J Diet Pract Res. 2003 Summer;64(2):62-81.

Ammon HP. Boswellic acids (components of frankincense) as the active principle in treatment of chronic inflammatory diseases. Wien Med Wochenschr. 2002;152(15-16):373-8.

Ammon HP. Boswellic acids in chronic inflammatory diseases. Planta Med. 2006 Oct;72(12):1100-16.

Anand P, Thomas SG, Kunnumakkara AB, Sundaram C, Harikumar KB, Sung B, Tharakan ST, Misra K, Priyadarsini IK, Rajasekharan KN, Aggarwal BB. Biological activities of curcumin and its analogues (Congeners) made by man and Mother Nature. Biochem Pharmacol. 2008 Dec 1;76(11):1590-611.

Anderson JL, May HT, Horne BD, Bair TL, Hall NL, Carlquist JF, Lappé DL, Muhlestein JB; Intermountain Heart Collaborative (IHC) Study Group. Relation of vitamin D deficiency to cardiovascular risk factors, disease status, and incident events in a general healthcare population. Am J Cardiol. 2010 Oct 1;106(7):963-8.

Anderson M., Grissom C. Increasing the Heavy Atom Effect of Xenon by Adsorption to Zeolites: Photolysis of 2,3-Diazabicyclo[2.2.2]oct-2-ene. *J. Am. Chem. Soc.* 1996;118:9552-9556.

Anderson RC, Anderson JH. Acute respiratory effects of diaper emissions. *Arch Environ Health.* 1999 Sep-Oct;54(5):353-8.

Anderson RC, Anderson JH. Acute toxic effects of fragrance products. *Arch Environ Health.* 1998 Mar-Apr;53(2):138-46.

Anderson RC, Anderson JH. Respiratory toxicity in mice exposed to mattress covers. *Arch Environ Health.* 1999 May-Jun;54(3):202-9.

Anderson RC, Anderson JH. Respiratory toxicity of fabric softener emissions. *J Toxicol Environ Health.* 2000 May 26;60(2):121-36.

Anderson RC, Anderson JH. Respiratory toxicity of mattress emissions in mice. *Arch Environ Health.* 2000 Jan-Feb;55(1):38-43.

Anderson RC, Anderson JH. Sensory irritation and multiple chemical sensitivity. *Toxicol Ind Health.* 1999 Apr-Jun;15(3-4):339-45.

Anderson RC, Anderson JH. Toxic effects of air freshener emissions. *Arch Environ Health.* 1997 Nov-Dec;52(6):433-41.

Anderson SD, Charlton B, Weiler JM, Nichols S, Spector SL, Pearlman DS; A305 Study Group. Comparison of mannitol and methacholine to predict exercise-induced bronchoconstriction and a clinical diagnosis of asthma. *Respir Res.* 2009 Jan 23;10:4.

Andoh T, Zhang Q, Yamamoto T, Tayama M, Hattori M, Tanaka K, Kuraishi Y. Inhibitory Effects of the Methanol Extract of Ganoderma lucidum on Mosquito Allergy-Induced Itch-Associated Responses in Mice. *J Pharmacol Sci.* 2010 Oct 8.

André C, André F, Colin L. Effect of allergen ingestion challenge with and without cromoglycate cover on intestinal permeability in atopic dermatitis, urticaria and other symptoms of food allergy. *Allergy.* 1989;44 Suppl 9:47-51.

André C. Food allergy. Objective diagnosis and test of therapeutic efficacy by measuring intestinal permeability. *Presse Med.* 1986 Jan 25;15(3):105-8.

Andre F, Andre C, Feknous M, Colin L, Cavagna S. Digestive permeability to different-sized molecules and to sodium cromoglycate in food allergy. *Allergy Proc.* 1991 Sep-Oct;12(5):293-8.

Anim-Nyame N, Sooranna SR, Johnson MR, Gamble J, Steer PJ. Garlic supplementation increases peripheral blood flow: a role for interleukin-6? *J Nutr Biochem.* 2004 Jan;15(1):30-6.

Annweiler C, Schott AM, Berrut G, Chauviré V, Le Gall D, Inzitari M, Beauchet O. Vitamin D and ageing: neurological issues. *Neuropsychobiology.* 2010 Aug;62(3):139-50.

Antczak A, Nowak D, Shariati B, Król M, Piasecka G, Kurmanowska Z. Increased hydrogen peroxide and thiobarbituric acid-reactive products in expired breath condensate of asthmatic patients. *Eur Respir J.* 1997 Jun;10(6):1235-41.

Aoki T, Usuda Y, Miyakoshi H, Tamura K, Herberman RB. Low natural killer syndrome: clinical and immunologic features. *Nat Immun Cell Growth Regul.* 1987;6(3):116-28.

Apáti P, Houghton PJ, Kite G, Steventon GB, Kéry A. In-vitro effect of flavonoids from Solidago canadensis extract on glutathione S-transferase. *J Pharm Pharmacol.* 2006 Feb;58(2):251-6.

APHA (American Public Health Association). Opposition to the Use of Hormone Growth Promoters in Beef and Dairy Cattle Production. Policy Date: 11/10/2009. Policy Number: 20098. http://www.apha.org/advocacy/policy/id=1379. Accessed Nov. 24, 2010.

Araki K, Shinozaki T, Irie Y, Miyazawa Y. Trial of oral administration of Bifidobacterium breve for the prevention of rotavirus infections. *Kansenshogaku Zasshi.* 1999 Apr;73(4):305-10.

Araujo AC, Aprile LR, Dantas RO, Terra-Filho J, Vianna EO. Bronchial responsiveness during esophageal acid infusion. Lung. 2008 Mar-Apr;186(2):123-8. 2008 Feb 23.

Arbes SJ Jr, Gergen PJ, Vaughn B, Zeldin DC. Asthma cases attributable to atopy: results from the Third National Health and Nutrition Examination Survey. *J Allergy Clin Immunol.* 2007 Nov;120(5):1139-45. 2007 Sep 24.

Argento A, Tiraferri E, Marzaloni M. Oral anticoagulants and medicinal plants. An emerging interaction. *Ann Ital Med Int.* 2000 Apr-Jun;15(2):139-43.

Arif AA, Delclos GL, Colmer-Hamood J. Association between asthma, asthma symptoms and C-reactive protein in US adults: data from the National Health and Nutrition Examination Survey, 1999-2002. *Respirology.* 2007 Sep;12(5):675-82. .

Arif AA, Shah SM. Association between personal exposure to volatile organic compounds and asthma among US adult population. *Int Arch Occup Environ Health.* 2007 Aug;80(8):711-9.

Arshad SH, Bateman B, Sadeghnejad A, Gant C, Matthews SM. Prevention of allergic disease during childhood by allergen avoidance: the Isle of Wight prevention study. *J Allergy Clin Immunol.* 2007 Feb;119(2):307-13.

REFERENCES

Arshad SH, Bateman B, Sadeghnejad A, Gant C, Matthews SM. Prevention of allergic disease during childhood by allergen avoidance: the Isle of Wight prevention study. *J Allergy Clin Immunol.* 2007 Feb;119(2):307-13.

Arslanoglu S, Moro GE, Schmitt J, Tandoi L, Rizzardi S, Boehm G. Early dietary intervention with a mixture of prebiotic oligosaccharides reduces the incidence of allergic manifestations and infections during the first two years of life. *J Nutr.* 2008 Jun;138(6):1091-5.

Arslanoglu S, Moro GE, Schmitt J, Tandoi L, Rizzardi S, Boehm G. Early dietary intervention with a mixture of prebiotic oligosaccharides reduces the incidence of allergic manifestations and infections during the first two years of life. *J Nutr.* 2008 Jun;138(6):1091-5.

Arterburn LM, Oken HA, Bailey Hall E, Hamersley J, Kuratko CN, Hoffman JP. Algal-oil capsules and cooked salmon: nutritionally equivalent sources of docosahexaenoic acid. *J Am Diet Assoc.* 2008 Jul;108(7):1204-9.

Arterburn LM, Oken HA, Hoffman JP, Bailey-Hall E, Chung G, Rom D, Hamersley J, McCarthy D. Bioequivalence of Docosahexaenoic acid from different algal oils in capsules and in a DHA-fortified food. *Lipids.* 2007 Nov;42(11):1011-24.

Arvaniti F, Priftis KN, Panagiotakos DB. Dietary habits and asthma: a review. *Allergy Asthma Proc.* 2010 Mar;31(2):e1-10.

Asero R, Antonicelli L, Arena A, Bommarito L, Caruso B, Colombo G, Crivellaro M, De Carli M, Della Torre E, Della Torre F, Heffler E, Lodi Rizzini F, Longo R, Manzotti G, Marcotulli M, Melchiorre A, Minale P, Morandi P, Moreni B, Moschella A, Murzilli F, Nebiolo F, Poppa M, Randazzo S, Rossi G, Senna GE. Causes of food-induced anaphylaxis in Italian adults: a multi-centre study. *Int Arch Allergy Immunol.* 2009;150(3):271-7.

Asero R, Mistrello G, Roncarolo D, Amato S, Caldironi G, Barocci F, van Ree R. Immunological crossreactivity between lipid transfer proteins from botanically unrelated plant-derived foods: a clinical study. *Allergy.* 2002 Oct;57(10):900-6.

Ashrafi K, Chang FY, Watts JL, Fraser AG, Kamath RS, Ahringer J, Ruvkun G. Genome-wide RNAi analysis of Caenorhabditis elegans fat regulatory genes. *Nature.* 2003 Jan 16;421(6920):268-72.

Atkinson W, Harris J, Mills P, Moffat S, White C, Lynch O, Jones M, Cullinan P, Newman Taylor AJ. Domestic aeroallergen exposures among infants in an English town. *Eur Respir J.* 1999 Mar;13(3):583-9.

Atsumi T, Tonosaki K. Smelling lavender and rosemary increases free radical scavenging activity and decreases cortisol level in saliva. *Psychiatry Res.* 2007 Feb 28;150(1):89-96.

Bacopoulou F, Veltsista A, Vassi I, Gika A, Lekea V, Priftis K, Bakoula C. Can we be optimistic about asthma in childhood? A Greek cohort study. *J Asthma.* 2009 Mar;46(2):171-4.

Badar VA, Thawani VR, Wakode PT, Shrivastava MP, Gharpure KJ, Hingorani LL, Khiyani RM. Efficacy of Tinospora cordifolia in allergic rhinitis. *J Ethnopharmacol.* 2005 Jan 15;96(3):445-9.

Bae GS, Kim MS, Jung WS, Seo SW, Yun SW, Kim SG, Park RK, Kim EC, Song HJ, Park SJ. Inhibition of lipopolysaccharide-induced inflammatory responses by piperine. *Eur J Pharmacol.* 2010 Sep 10;642(1-3):154-62.

Bafadhel M, Singapuri A, Terry S, Hargadon B, Monteiro W, Green RH, Bradding PH, Wardlaw AJ, Pavord ID, Brightling CE. Body mass and fat mass in refractory asthma: an observational 1 year follow-up study. *J Allergy.* 2010;2010:251758. 2010 Dec 1.

Baker SM. *Detoxification and Healing.* Chicago: Contemporary Books, 2004.

Bakkeheim E, Mowinckel P, Carlsen KH, Håland G, Carlsen KC. Paracetamol in early infancy: the risk of childhood allergy and asthma. *Acta Paediatr.* 2011 Jan;100(1):90-6.

Balch P, Balch J. *Prescription for Nutritional Healing.* New York: Avery, 2000.

Ballentine R. *Diet & Nutrition: A holistic approach.* Honesdale, PA: Himalayan Int., 1978.

Ballentine R. *Radical Healing.* New York: Harmony Books, 1999.

Ballmer-Weber BK, Holzhauser T, Scibilia J, Mittag D, Zisa G, Ortolani C, Oesterballe M, Poulsen LK, Vieths S, Bindslev-Jensen C. Clinical characteristics of soybean allergy in Europe: a double-blind, placebo-controlled food challenge study. *J Allergy Clin Immunol.* 2007 Jun;119(6):1489-96.

Ballmer-Weber BK, Vieths S, Lüttkopf D, Heuschmann P, Wüthrich B. Celery allergy confirmed by doubleblind, placebo-controlled food challenge: a clinical study in 32 subjects with a history of adverse reactions to celery root. *J Allergy Clin Immunol.* 2000 Aug;106(2):373-8.

Banno N, Akihisa T, Yasukawa K, Tokuda H, Tabata K, Nakamura Y, Nishimura R, Kimura Y, Suzuki T. Anti-inflammatory activities of the triterpene acids from the resin of Boswellia carteri. *J Ethnopharmacol.* 2006 Sep 19;107(2):249-53.

Bant A, Kruszewski J. Increased sensitization prevalence to common inhalant and food allergens in young adult Polish males. *Ann Agric Environ Med.* 2008 Jun;15(1):21-7.

Barnes M, Cullinan P, Athanasaki P, MacNeill S, Hole AM, Harris J, Kalogeraki S, Chatzinikolaou M, Drakonakis N, Bibaki-Liakou V, Newman Taylor AJ, Bibakis I. Crete: does farming explain urban and rural differences in atopy? *Clin Exp Allergy.* 2001 Dec;31(12):1822-8.

Barnetson RS, Drummond H, Ferguson A. Precipitins to dietary proteins in atopic eczema. *Br J Dermatol.* 1983 Dec;109(6):653-5.

Barnett AG, Williams GM, Schwartz J, Neller AH, Best TL, Petroeschevsky AL, Simpson RW. Air pollution and child respiratory health: a case-crossover study in Australia and New Zealand. *Am J Respir Crit Care Med.* 2005 Jun 1;171(11):1272-8.

Barrager E, Veltmann JR Jr, Schauss AG, Schiller RN. A multicentered, open-label trial on the safety and efficacy of methylsulfonylmethane in the treatment of seasonal allergic rhinitis. *J Altern Complement Med.* 2002 Apr;8(2):167-73.

Barros R, Moreira A, Fonseca J, de Oliveira JF, Delgado L, Castel-Branco MG, Haahtela T, Lopes C, Moreira P. Adherence to the Mediterranean diet and fresh fruit intake are associated with improved asthma control. *Allergy.* 2008 Jul;63(7):917-23.

Basu A, Devaraj S, Jialal I. Dietary factors that promote or retard inflammation. *Arterioscler Thromb Vasc Biol.* 2006 May;26(5):995-1001.

Bateman B, Warner JO, Hutchinson E, Dean T, Rowlandson P, Gant C, Grundy J, Fitzgerald C, Stevenson J. The effects of a double blind, placebo controlled, artificial food colourings and benzoate preservative challenge on hyperactivity in a general population sample of preschool children. *Arch Dis Child.* 2004 Jun;89(6):506-11.

Bates DW, Cullen DJ, Laird N, Petersen LA, Small SD, Servi D, Laffel G, Sweitzer BJ, Shea BF, Hallisey R, et al. Incidence of adverse drug events and potential adverse drug events. Implications for prevention. ADE Prevention Study Group. *JAMA.* 1995 Jul 5;274(1):29-34.

Batista R, Martins I, Jeno P, Ricardo CP, Oliveira MM. A proteomic study to identify soya allergens—the human response to transgenic versus non-transgenic soya samples. *Int Arch Allergy Immunol.* 2007;144(1):29-38.

Batmanghelidj F. Neurotransmitter histamine: an alternative view point, *Science in Medicine Simplified.* Falls Church, VA: Foundation for the Simple in Medicine, 1990.

Batmanghelidj F. Pain: a need for paradigm change. *Anticancer Res.* 1987 Sep-Oct;7(5B):971-89.

Batmanghelidj F. *Your Body's Many Cries for Water.* 2nd Ed. Vienna, VA: Global Health, 1997.

Beasley R, Clayton T, Crane J, von Mutius E, Lai CK, Montefort S, Stewart A; ISAAC Phase Three Study Group. Association between paracetamol use in infancy and childhood, and risk of asthma, rhinoconjunctivitis, and eczema in children aged 6-7 years: analysis from Phase Three of the ISAAC programme. *Lancet.* 2008 Sep. 20;372(9643):1039-48.

Beaulieu A, Fessele K. Agent Orange: management of patients exposed in Vietnam. *Clin J Oncol Nurs.* 2003 May-Jun;7(3):320-3.

Becker KG, Simon RM, Bailey-Wilson JE, Freidlin B, Biddison WE, McFarland HF, Trent JM. Clustering of non-major histocompatibility complex susceptibility candidate loci in human autoimmune diseases. *Proc Natl Acad Sci U S A.* 1998 Aug 18;95(17):9979-84.

Beddoe AF. *Biologic Ionization as Applied to Human Nutrition.* Warsaw: Wendell Whitman, 2002.

Beecher GR. Phytonutrients' role in metabolism: effects on resistance to degenerative processes. *Nutr Rev.* 1999 Sep;57(9 Pt 2):S3-6.

Belcaro G, Cesarone MR, Errichi S, Zulli C, Errichi BM, Vinciguerra G, Ledda A, Di Renzo A, Stuard S, Dugall M, Pellegrini L, Gizzi G, Ippolito E, Ricci A, Cacchio M, Cipollone G, Ruffini I, Fano F, Hosoi M, Rohdewald P. Variations in C-reactive protein, plasma free radicals and fibrinogen values in patients with osteoarthritis treated with Pycnogenol. *Redox Rep.* 2008;13(6):271-6.

Bell IR, Baldwin CM, Schwartz GE. Illness from low levels of environmental chemicals: relevance to chronic fatigue syndrome and fibromyalgia. *Am J Med.* 1998;105 (suppl 3A).:74-82. S.

Bell SJ, Potter PC. Milk whey-specific immune complexes in allergic and non-allergic subjects. *Allergy.* 1988 Oct;43(7):497-503.

Ben, X.M., Zhou, X.Y., Zhao, W.H., Yu, W.L., Pan, W., Zhang, W.L., Wu, S.M., Van Beusekom, C.M., Schaafsma, A. (2004) Supplementation of milk formula with galactooligosaccharides improves intestinal micro-flora and fermentation in term infants. *Chin Med J.* 117(6):927-931, 2004.

Benard A, Desreumeaux P, Huglo D, Hoorelbeke A, Tonnel AB, Wallaert B. Increased intestinal permeability in bronchial asthma. *J Allergy Clin Immunol.* 1996 Jun;97(6):1173-8.

Bengmark S. Curcumin, an atoxic antioxidant and natural NFkappaB, cyclooxygenase-2, lipooxygenase, and inducible nitric oxide synthase inhibitor: a shield against acute and chronic diseases. *JPEN J Parenter Enteral Nutr.* 2006 Jan-Feb;30(1):45-51.

Bengmark S. Immunonutrition: role of biosurfactants, fiber, and probiotic bacteria. *Nutrition.* 1998 Jul-Aug;14(7-8):585-94.

Benlounes N, Dupont C, Candalh C, Blaton MA, Darmon N, Desjeux JF, Heyman M. The threshold for immune cell reactivity to milk antigens decreases in cow's milk allergy with intestinal symptoms. *J Allergy Clin Immunol.* 1996 Oct;98(4):781-9.

Bennett WD, Zeman KL, Jarabek AM. Nasal contribution to breathing and fine particle deposition in children versus adults. *J Toxicol Environ Health A.* 2008;71(3):227-37.

REFERENCES

Ben-Shoshan M, Harrington DW, Soller L, Fragapane J, Joseph L, St Pierre Y, Godefroy SB, Elliot SJ, Clarke AE. A population-based study on peanut, tree nut, fish, shellfish, and sesame allergy prevalence in Canada. *J Allergy Clin Immunol.* 2010 Jun;125(6):1327-35.

Ben-Shoshan M, Kagan R, Primeau MN, Alizadehfar R, Turnbull E, Harada L, Dufresne C, Allen M, Joseph L, St Pierre Y, Clarke A. Establishing the diagnosis of peanut allergy in children never exposed to peanut or with an uncertain history: a cross-Canada study. *Pediatr Allergy Immunol.* 2010 Sep;21(6):920-6.

Bensky D, Gable A, Kaptchuk T (transl.). *Chinese Herbal Medicine Materia Medica.* Seattle: Eastland Press, 1986.

Bergner P. *The Healing Power of Garlic.* Prima Publishing, Rocklin CA 1996.

Berin MC, Yang PC, Ciok L, Waserman S, Perdue MH. Role for IL-4 in macromolecular transport across human intestinal epithelium. *Am J Physiol.* 1999 May;276(5 Pt 1):C1046-52.

Berkow R., (Ed.) *The Merck Manual of Diagnosis and Therapy.* 16th Edition. Rahway, N.J.: Merck Research Labs, 1992.

Bernstein DI, Epstein T, Murphy-Berendts K, Liss GM. Surveillance of systemic reactions to subcutaneous immunotherapy injections: year 1 outcomes of the ACAAI and AAAAI collaborative study. *Ann Allergy Asthma Immunol.* 2010 Jun;104(6):530-5. .

Berseth CL, Mitmesser SH, Ziegler EE, Marunycz JD, Vanderhoof J. Tolerance of a standard intact protein formula versus a partially hydrolyzed formula in healthy, term infants. *Nutr J.* 2009 Jun 19;8:27.

Berteau O and Mulloy B. 2003. Sulfated fucans, fresh perspectives: structures, functions, and biological properties of sulfated fucans and an overview of enzymes active toward this class of polysaccharide. *Glycobiology.* Jun;13(6):29R-40R.

Beyer K, Morrow E, Li XM, Bardina L, Bannon GA, Burks AW, Sampson HA. Effects of cooking methods on peanut allergenicity. *J Allergy Clin Immunol.* 2001;107:1077-81.

Bielory BP, Perez VL, Bielory L. Treatment of seasonal allergic conjunctivitis with ophthalmic corticosteroids: in search of the perfect ocular corticosteroids in the treatment of allergic conjunctivitis. *Curr Opin Allergy Clin Immunol.* 2010 Oct;10(5):469-77.

Bielory L, Lupoli K. Herbal interventions in asthma and allergy. *J Asthma.* 1999;36:1-65.

Bielory L, Russin J, Zuckerman GB. Clinical efficacy, mechanisms of action, and adverse effects of complementary and alternative medicine therapies for asthma. *Allergy Asthma Proc.* 2004;25:283-91.

Bielory L. Complementary and alternative interventions in asthma, allergy, and immunology. *Ann Allergy Asthma Immunol.* 2004 Aug;93(2 Suppl 1):S45-54.

Bindslev-Jensen C, Skov PS, Roggen EL, Hvass P, Brinch DS. Investigation on possible allergenicity of 19 different commercial enzymes used in the food industry. *Food Chem Toxicol.* 2006 Nov;44(11):1909-15.

Birch EE, Khoury JC, Berseth CL, Castañeda YS, Couch JM, Bean J, Tamer R, Harris CL, Mitmesser SH, Scalabrin DM. The impact of early nutrition on incidence of allergic manifestations and common respiratory illnesses in children. *J Pediatr.* 2010 Jun;156(6):902-6, 906.e1. 2010 Mar 15.

Bisgaard H, Loland L, Holst KK, Pipper CB. Prenatal determinants of neonatal lung function in high-risk newborns. *J Allergy Clin Immunol.* 2009 Mar;123(3):651-7, 657.e1-4. 2009 Jan 18.

Bisset N.. *Herbal Drugs and Phytopharmaceuticals.* Stuttgart: CRC, 1994.

Bjarnason I, MacPherson A, Hollander D. Intestinal permeability: an overview. *Gastroenterology.* 1995 May;108(5):1566-81.

Blackhall K, Appleton S, Cates FJ. Ionisers for chronic asthma. *Cochrane Database Syst Rev* 2003;(3):CD002986.

Blackley, CH. *Experimental Researchers on the Causes and Nature of Catarrhus Aestivus (Hay Fever or Hay-Asthma).* London, 1873.

Blood AJ, Zatorre RJ, Bermudez P, Evans AC. Emotional responses to pleasant and unpleasant music correlate with activity in paralimbic brain regions. *Nat Neurosci.* 1999;2:382-7.

Blumenthal M (ed.) *The Complete German Commission E Monographs.* Boston: Amer Botan Council, 1998.

Blumenthal M, Brinckmann J, Goldberg A (eds). *Herbal Medicine: Expanded Commission E Monographs.* Newton, MA: Integrative Med., 2000.

Boccafogli A, Vicentini L, Camerani A, Cogliati P, D'Ambrosi A, Scolozzi R. Adverse food reactions in patients with grass pollen allergic respiratory disease. *Ann Allergy.* 1994 Oct;73(4):301-8.

Bode C, Bode JC. Effect of alcohol consumption on the gut. *Best Pract Res Clin Gastroenterol.* 2003 Aug;17(4):575-92.

Bodinier M, Legoux MA, Pineau F, Triballeau S, Segain JP, Brossard C, Denery-Papini S. Intestinal translocation capabilities of wheat allergens using the Caco-2 cell line. *J Agric Food Chem.* 2007 May 30;55(11):4576-83.

Boehm, G., Lidestri, M., Casetta, P., Jelinek, J., Negretti, F., Stahl, B., Martini, A. (2002) Supplementation of a bovine milk formula with an oligosaccharide mixture increases counts of faecal bifidobacteria in preterm infants. *Arch Dis Child Fetal Neonatal Ed.* 86: F178-F181

Bolhaar ST, Tiemessen MM, Zuidmeer L, van Leeuwen A, Hoffmann-Sommergruber K, Bruijnzeel-Koomen CA, Taams LS, Knol EF, van Hoffen E, van Ree R, Knulst AC. Efficacy of birch-pollen immunotherapy on cross-reactive food allergy confirmed by skin tests and double-blind food challenges. *Clin Exp Allergy.* 2004 May;34(5):761-9.

Bolleddula J, Goldfarb J, Wang R, Sampson H, Li XM. Synergistic Modulation Of Eotaxin And Il-4 Secretion By Constituents Of An Anti-asthma Herbal Formula (ASHMI) In Vitro. *J Allergy Clin Immunol.* 2007;119:S172.

Bonfils P, Halimi P, Malinvaud D. Adrenal suppression and osteoporosis after treatment of nasal polyposis. *Acta Otolaryngol.* 2006 Dec;126(11):1195-200.

Bongaerts GP, Severijnen RS. Preventive and curative effects of probiotics in atopic patients. *Med Hypotheses.* 2005;64(6):1089-92.

Bongartz D, Hesse A. Selective extraction of quercetrin in vegetable drugs and urine by off-line coupling of boronic acid affinity chromatography and high-performance liquid chromatography. *J Chromatogr B Biomed Appl.* 1995 Nov 17;673(2):223-30.

Bonsignore MR, La Grutta S, Cibella F, Scichilone N, Cuttitta G, Interrante A, Marchese M, Veca M, Virzi' M, Bonanno A, Profita M, Morici G. Effects of exercise training and montelukast in children with mild asthma. *Med Sci Sports Exerc.* 2008 Mar;40(3):405-12.

Borchers AT, Hackman RM, Keen CL, Stern JS, Gershwin ME. Complementary medicine: a review of immunomodulatory effects of Chinese herbal medicines. *Am J Clin Nutr.* 1997 Dec;66(6):1303-12.

Borchert VE, Czyborra P, Fetscher C, Goepel M, Michel MC. Extracts from Rhois aromatica and Solidaginis virgaurea inhibit rat and human bladder contraction. *Naunyn Schmiedebergs Arch Pharmacol.* 2004 Mar;369(3):281-6.

Böttcher MF, Jenmalm MC, Voor T, Julge K, Holt PG, Björkstén B. Cytokine responses to allergens during the first 2 years of life in Estonian and Swedish children. *Clin Exp Allergy.* 2006 May;36(5):619-28.

Bottema RW, Kerkhof M, Reijmerink NE, Thijs C, Smit HA, van Schayck CP, Brunekreef B, van Oosterhout AJ, Postma DS, Koppelman GH. Gene-gene interaction in regulatory T-cell function in atopy and asthma development in childhood. *J Allergy Clin Immunol.* 2010 Aug;126(2):338-46, 346.e1-10.

Bouchez-Mahiout I, Pecquet C, Kerre S, Snégaroff J, Raison-Peyron N, Laurière M. High molecular weight entities in industrial wheat protein hydrolysates are immunoreactive with IgE from allergic patients. *J Agric Food Chem.* 2010 Apr 14;58(7):4207-15.

Bougault V, Turmel J, Boulet LP. Bronchial challenges and respiratory symptoms in elite swimmers and winter sport athletes: Airway hyperresponsiveness in asthma: its measurement and clinical significance. *Chest.* 2010 Aug;138(2 Suppl):31S-37S. 2010 Apr 2.

Boyce JA, Assa'ad A, Burks AW, Jones SM, Sampson HA, Wood RA, Plaut M, Cooper SF, Fenton MJ, Arshad SH, Bahna SL, Beck LA, Byrd-Bredbenner C, Camargo CA Jr, Eichenfield L, Furuta GT, Hanifin JM, Jones C, Kraft M, Levy BD, Lieberman P, Luccioli S, McCall KM, Schneider LC, Simon RA, Simons FE, Teach SJ, Yawn BP, Schwaninger JM. Guidelines for the diagnosis and management of food allergy in the United States: report of the NIAID-sponsored expert panel. *J Allergy Clin Immunol.* 2010 Dec;126(6 Suppl):S1-58.

Bräbäck L, Breborowicz A, Julge K, Knutsson A, Riikjärv MA, Vasar M, Björkstén B. Risk factors for respiratory symptoms and atopic sensitisation in the Baltic area. *Arch Dis Child.* 1995 Jun;72(6):487-93.

Bräbäck L, Kjellman NI, Sandin A, Björkstén B. Atopy among schoolchildren in northern and southern Sweden in relation to pet ownership and early life events. *Pediatr Allergy Immunol.* 2001 Feb;12(1):4-10.

Bradette-Hébert ME, Legault J, Lavoie S, Pichette A. A new labdane diterpene from the flowers of Solidago canadensis. *Chem Pharm Bull.* 2008 Jan;56(1):82-4.

Brandtzaeg P. The mucosal immune system and its integration with the mammary glands. *J Pediatr.* 2010 Feb;156(2 Suppl):S8-15.

Braun-Fahrländer C, Gassner M, Grize L, Neu U, Sennhauser FH, Varonier HS, Vuille JC, Wüthrich B. Prevalence of hay fever and allergic sensitization in farmer's children and their peers living in the same rural community. SCARPOL team. Swiss Study on Childhood Allergy and Respiratory Symptoms with Respect to Air Pollution. *Clin Exp Allergy.* 1999 Jan;29(1):28-34.

Brehm JM, Schuemann B, Fuhlbrigge AL, Hollis BW, Strunk RC, Zeiger RS, Weiss ST, Litonjua AA; Childhood Asthma Management Program Research Group. Serum vitamin D levels and severe asthma exacerbations in the Childhood Asthma Management Program study. *J Allergy Clin Immunol.* 2010 Jul;126(1):52-8.e5. 2010 Jun 9.

Brighenti F, Valtueña S, Pellegrini N, Ardigò D, Del Rio D, Salvatore S, Piatti P, Serafini M, Zavaroni I. Total antioxidant capacity of the diet is inversely and independently related to plasma concentration of high-sensitivity C-reactive protein in adult Italian subjects. *Br J Nutr.* 2005 May;93(5):619-25.

Brinkhaus B, Witt CM, Jena S, Liecker B, Wegscheider K, Willich SN. Acupuncture in patients with allergic rhinitis: a pragmatic randomized trial. *Ann Allergy Asthma Immunol.* 2008 Nov;101(5):535-43.

Brisman J, Torén K, Lillienberg L, Karlsson G, Ahlstedt S. Nasal symptoms and indices of nasal inflammation in flour-dust-exposed bakers. *Int Arch Occup Environ Health.* 1998 Nov;71(8):525-32.

Brodtkorb TH, Zetterström O, Tinghög G. Cost-effectiveness of clean air administered to the breathing zone in allergic asthma. *Clin Respir J.* 2010 Apr;4(2):104-10.

REFERENCES

Brody J. *Jane Brody's Nutrition Book*. New York: WW Norton, 1981.

Broekhuizen BD, Sachs AP, Hoes AW, Moons KG, van den Berg JW, Dalinghaus WH, Lammers E, Verheij TJ. Undetected chronic obstructive pulmonary disease and asthma in people over 50 years with persistent cough. *Br J Gen Pract*. 2010 Jul;60(576):489-94.

Brostoff J, Gamlin L, Brostoff J. *Food Allergies and Food Intolerance: The Complete Guide to Their Identification and Treatment*. Rochester, VT: Healing Arts, 2000.

Brownstein D. *Salt: Your Way to Health*. West Bloomfield, MI: Medical Alternatives, 2006.

Brown-Whitehorn TF, Spergel JM. The link between allergies and eosinophilic esophagitis: implications for management strategies. *Expert Rev Clin Immunol*. 2010 Jan;6(1):101-9.

Bruce S, Nyberg F, Melén E, James A, Pulkkinen V, Orsmark-Pietras C, Bergström A, Dahlén B, Wickman M, von Mutius E, Doekes G, Lauener R, Riedler J, Eder W, van Hage M, Pershagen G, Scheynius A, Kere J. The protective effect of farm animal exposure on childhood allergy is modified by NPSR1 polymorphisms. *J Med Genet*. 2009 Mar;46(3):159-67. 2008 Feb 19.

Bruneton J. *Pharmacognosy, Phytochemistry, Medicinal Plants*. Paris: Lavoisier, 1995.

Bruton A, Lewith GT. The Buteyko breathing technique for asthma: a review. *Complement Ther Med*. 2005 Mar;13(1):41-6. 2005 Apr 18.

Bruton A, Thomas M. The role of breathing training in asthma management. *Curr Opin Allergy Clin Immunol*. 2011 Feb;11(1):53-7.

Bryborn M, Halldén C, Säll T, Cardell LO. CLC- a novel susceptibility gene for allergic rhinitis? *Allergy*. 2010 Feb;65(2):220-8.

Bublin M, Pfister M, Radauer C, Oberhuber C, Bulley S, Dewitt AM, Lidholm J, Reese G, Vieths S, Breiteneder H, Hoffmann-Sommergruber K, Ballmer-Weber BK. Component-resolved diagnosis of kiwifruit allergy with purified natural and recombinant kiwifruit allergens. *J Allergy Clin Immunol*. 2010 Mar;125(3):687-94, 694.e1.

Buchanan TW, Lutz K, Mirzazade S, Specht K, Shah NJ, Zilles K, et al. Recognition of emotional prosody and verbal components of spoken language: an fMRI study. *Cogn Brain Res*. 2000;9:227-38.

Bucher X, Pichler WJ, Dahinden CA, Helbling A. Effect of tree pollen specific, subcutaneous immunotherapy on the oral allergy syndrome to apple and hazelnut. *Allergy*. 2004 Dec;59(12):1272-6.

Budzianowski J. Coumarins, caffeoyltartaric acids and their artifactual methyl esters from Taraxacum officinale leaves. *Planta Med*. 1997 Jun;63(3):288.

Bueso AK, Berntsen S, Mowinckel P, Andersen LF, Lodrup Carlsen KC, Carlsen KH. Dietary intake in adolescents with asthma - potential for improvement. *Pediatr Allergy Immunol*. 2010 Oct 20. doi: 10.1111/j.1399-3038.2010.01013.x.

Bundy R, Walker AF, Middleton RW, Booth J. Turmeric extract may improve irritable bowel syndrome symptomology in otherwise healthy adults: a pilot study. *J Altern Complement Med*. 2004 Dec;10(6):1015-8.

Burdge GC, Jones AE, Wootton SA. Eicosapentaenoic and docosapentaenoic acids are the principal products of alpha-linolenic acid metabolism in young men. *B J Nutr*. 2002 Oct;88(4):355-63.

Buret AG. How stress induces intestinal hypersensitivity. *Am J Pathol*. 2006 Jan;168(1):3-5.

Burgess CD, Bremner P, Thomson CD, Crane J, Siebers RW, Beasley R. Nebulized beta 2-adrenoceptor agonists do not affect plasma selenium or glutathione peroxidase activity in patients with asthma. *Int J Clin Pharmacol Ther*. 1994 Jun;32(6):290-2.

Burks W, Jones SM, Berseth CL, Harris C, Sampson HA, Scalabrin DM. Hypoallergenicity and effects on growth and tolerance of a new amino acid-based formula with docosahexaenoic acid and arachidonic acid. *J Pediatr*. 2008 Aug;153(2):266-71.

Burney PG, Luczynska C, Chinn S, Jarvis D. The European Community Respiratory Health Survey. *Eur Respir J*. 1994;7: 954-960.

Burr ML, Butland BK, King S, Vaughan-Williams E. Changes in asthma prevalence: two surveys 15 years apart. *Arch Dis Child*. 1989;64:1452-1456.

Busse PJ, Wen MC, Huang CK, Srivastava K, Zhang TF, Schofield B, Sampson HA, Li XM. Therapeutic effects of the Chinese herbal formula, MSSM-03d, on persistent airway hyperreactivity and airway remodeling. *J Allergy Clin Immunol*. 2004;113:S220.

Byrne AM, Malka-Rais J, Burks AW, Fleischer DM. How do we know when peanut and tree nut allergy have resolved, and how do we keep it resolved? *Clin Exp Allergy*. 2010 Sep;40(9):1303-11.

Cabanillas B, Pedrosa MM, Rodríguez J, González A, Muzquiz M, Cuadrado C, Crespo JF, Burbano C. Effects of enzymatic hydrolysis on lentil allergenicity. *Mol Nutr Food Res*. 2010 Mar 19.

Caglar E, Kavaloglu SC, Kuscu OO, Sandalli N, Holgerson PL, Twetman S. Effect of chewing gums containing xylitol or probiotic bacteria on salivary mutans streptococci and lactobacilli. *Clin Oral Investig*. 2007 Dec;11(4):425-9.

Caglar E, Kuscu OO, Cildir SK, Kuvvetli SS, Sandalli N. A probiotic lozenge administered medical device and its effect on salivary mutans streptococci and lactobacilli. *Int J Paediatr Dent*. 2008 Jan;18(1):35-9.

Caglar E, Kuscu OO, Selvi Kuvvetli S, Kavaloglu Cildir S, Sandalli N, Twetman S. Short-term effect of ice-cream containing *Bifidobacterium lactis* Bb-12 on the number of salivary mutans streptococci and lacto-bacilli. *Acta Odontol Scand.* 2008 Jun;66(3):154-8.

Calder PC. Dietary modification of inflammation with lipids. *Proc Nutr Soc.* 2002 Aug;61(3):345-58.

Camargo CA Jr, Ingham T, Wickens K, Thadhani R, Silvers KM, Epton MJ, Town GI, Pattemore PK, Espinola JA, Crane J; New Zealand Asthma and Allergy Cohort Study Group. Cord-blood 25-hydroxyvitamin D levels and risk of respiratory infection, wheezing, and asthma. *Pediatrics.* 2011 Jan;127(1):e180-7.

Caminiti L, Passalacqua G, Barberi S, Vita D, Barberio G, De Luca R, Pajno GB. A new protocol for specific oral tolerance induction in children with IgE-mediated cow's milk allergy. *Allergy Asthma Proc.* 2009 Jul-Aug;30(4):443-8.

Campbell TC, Campbell TM. *The China Study.* Dallas, TX: Benbella Books, 2006.

Canakcioglu S, Tahamiler R, Saritzali G, Alimoglu Y, Isildak H, Guvenc MG, Acar GO, Inci E. Evaluation of nasal cytology in subjects with chronic rhinitis: a 7-year study. *Am J Otolaryngol.* 2009 Sep-Oct;30(5):312-7.

Canali R, Comitato R, Schonlau F, Virgili F. The anti-inflammatory pharmacology of Pycnogenol in humans involves COX-2 and 5-LOX mRNA expression in leukocytes. *Int Immunopharmacol.* 2009 Sep;9(10):1145-9.

Canonica GW, Passalacqua G. Noninjection routes for immunotherapy. *J Allergy Clin Immunol.* 2003 Mar;111(3):437-48; quiz 449.

Cantani A, Micera M. Natural history of cow's milk allergy. An eight-year follow-up study in 115 atopic children. *Eur Rev Med Pharmacol Sci.* 2004 Jul-Aug;8(4):153-64.

Cantani A, Micera M. The prick by prick test is safe and reliable in 58 children with atopic dermatitis and food allergy. *Eur Rev Med Pharmacol Sci.* 2006 May-Jun;10(3):115-20.

Cao G, Alessio HM, Cutler RG. Oxygen-radical absorbance capacity assay for antioxidants. *Free Radic Biol Med.* 1993 Mar;14(3):303-11.

Cao G, Shukitt-Hale B, Bickford PC, Joseph JA, McEwen J, Prior RL. Hyperoxia-induced changes in antioxidant capacity and the effect of dietary antioxidants. *J Appl Physiol.* 1999 Jun;86(6):1817-22.

Caramia G. The essential fatty acids omega-6 and omega-3: from their discovery to their use in therapy. *Minerva Pediatr.* 2008 Apr;60(2):219-33.

Carey DG, Aase KA, Pliego GJ. The acute effect of cold air exercise in determination of exercise-induced bronchospasm in apparently healthy athletes. J Strength Cond Res. 2010 Aug;24(8):2172-8.

Carroccio A, Cavataio F, Montalto G, D'Amico D, Alabrese L, Iacono G. Intolerance to hydrolysed cow's milk proteins in infants: clinical characteristics and dietary treatment. *Clin Exp Allergy.* 2000 Nov;30(11):1597-603.

Carroll D. *The Complete Book of Natural Medicines.* New York: Summit, 1980.

Caruso M, Frasca G, Di Giuseppe PL, Pennisi A, Tringali G, Bonina FP. Effects of a new nutraceutical ingredient on allergen-induced sulphidoleukotrienes production and CD63 expression in allergic subjects. *Int Immunopharmacol.* 2008 Dec 20;8(13-14):1781-6.

Casale TB, Amin BV. Allergic rhinitis/asthma interrelationship. *Clin Rev Allergy Immunol.* 2001;21:27-49.

Cats A, Kuipers EJ, Bosschaert MA, Pot RG, Vandenbroucke-Grauls CM, Kusters JG. Effect of frequent consumption of a Lactobacillus casei-containing milk drink in Helicobacter pylori-colonized subjects. *Aliment Pharmacol Ther.* 2003 Feb;17(3):429-35.

Caughey AB, Nicholson JM, Cheng YW, Lyell DJ, Washington AE. Induction of labor and Cesarean delivery by gestational age. *Am J Obstet Gynecol.* 2006 Sep;195(3):700-5.

Celakovská J, Vaněčková J, Ettlerová K, Ettler K, Bukac J. The role of atopy patch test in diagnosis of food allergy in atopic eczema/dermatitis syndrom in patients over 14 years of age. *Acta Medica (Hradec Kralove).* 2010;53(2):101-8.

Celikel S, Karakaya G, Yurtsever N, Sorkun K, Kalyoncu AF. Bee and bee products allergy in Turkish beekeepers: determination of risk factors for systemic reactions. *Allergol Immunopathol (Madr).* 2006 Sep-Oct;34(5):180-4.

Centers for Disease Control and Prevention (CDC). Obesity prevalence among low-income, preschool-aged children - United States, 1998-2008. *MMWR Morb Mortal Wkly Rep.* 2009 Jul 24;58(28):769-73.

Centers for Disease Control and Prevention (CDC). Vital signs: nonsmokers' exposure to secondhand smoke - United States, 1999-2008. *MMWR Morb Mortal Wkly Rep.* 2010 Sep 10;59(35):1141-6.

Centre for Molecular, Environmental, Genetic and Analytic Epidemiology, School of Population Health, The UniverGumowski P, Lech B, Chaves I, Girard JP. Chronic asthma and rhinitis due to Candida albicans, epidermophyton, and trichophyton. *Ann Allergy.* 1987 Jul;59(1):48-51.

Cereijido M, Contreras RG, Flores-Benítez D, Flores-Maldonado C, Larre I, Ruiz A, Shoshani L. New diseases derived or associated with the tight junction. *Arch Med Res.* 2007 Jul;38(5):465-78.

REFERENCES

Chafen JJ, Newberry SJ, Riedl MA, Bravata DM, Maglione M, Suttorp MJ, Sundaram V, Paige NM, Towfigh A, Hulley BJ, Shekelle PG. Diagnosing and managing common food allergies: a systematic review. *JAMA.* 2010 May 12;303(18):1848-56.

Chahine BG, Bahna SL. The role of the gut mucosal immunity in the development of tolerance versus development of allergy to food. *Curr Opin Allergy Clin Immunol.* 2010 Aug;10(4):394-9.

Chaitow L, Trenev N. *Probiotics.* New York: Thorsons, 1990.

Chaitow L. *Conquer Pain the Natural Way.* San Francisco: Chronicle Books, 2002.

Chakŭrski I, Matev M, Koĭchev A, Angelova I, Stefanov G. Treatment of chronic colitis with an herbal combination of Taraxacum officinale, Hipericum perforatum, Melissa officinaliss, Calendula officinalis and Foeniculum vulgare. *Vutr Boles.* 1981;20(6):51-4.

Chan CK, Kuo ML, Shen JJ, See LC, Chang HH, Huang JL. Ding Chuan Tang, a Chinese herb decoction, could improve airway hyper-responsiveness in stabilized asthmatic children: a randomized, double-blind clinical trial. *Pediatr Allergy Immunol.* 2006;17:316-22.

Chandra RK. Prospective studies of the effect of breast feeding on incidence of infection and allergy. *Acta Paediatr Scand.* 1979 Sep;68(5):691-4.

Chaney M, Ross M. *Nutrition.* New York: Houghton Mifflin, 1971.

Chang HT, Tseng LJ, Hung TJ, Kao BT, Lin WY, Fan TC, Chang MD, Pai TW. Inhibition of the interactions between eosinophil cationic protein and airway epithelial cells by traditional Chinese herbs. *BMC Syst Biol.* 2010 Sep 13;4 Suppl 2:S8.

Chang TT, Huang CC, Hsu CH. Clinical evaluation of the Chinese herbal medicine formula STA-1 in the treatment of allergic asthma. *Phytother Res.* 2006;20:342-7.

Chang TT, Huang CC, Hsu CH. Inhibition of mite-induced immunoglobulin E synthesis, airway inflammation, and hyperreactivity by herbal medicine STA-1. *Immunopharmacol Immunotoxicol.* 2006;28:683-95.

Chao A, Thun MJ, Connell CJ, McCullough ML, Jacobs EJ, Flanders WD, Rodriguez C, Sinha R, Calle EE. Meat consumption and risk of colorectal cancer. *JAMA.* 2005 Jan 12;293(2):172-82.

Characterization and quantitation of Antioxidant Constituents of Sweet Pepper (Capsicum annuum - Cayenne). *J Agric Food Chem.* 2004 Jun 16;52(12):3861-9.

Chatzi L, Apostolaki G, Bibakis I, Skypala I, Bibaki-Liakou V, Tzanakis N, Kogevinas M, Cullinan P. Protective effect of fruits, vegetables and the Mediterranean diet on asthma and allergies among children in Crete. *Thorax.* 2007 Aug;62(8):677-83.

Chatzi L, Torrent M, Romieu I, Garcia-Esteban R, Ferrer C, Vioque J, Kogevinas M, Sunyer J. Mediterranean diet in pregnancy is protective for wheeze and atopy in childhood. *Thorax.* 2008 Jun;63(6):507-13.

Chaves TC, de Andrade e Silva TS, Monteiro SA, Watanabe PC, Oliveira AS, Grossi DB. Craniocervical posture and hyoid bone position in children with mild and moderate asthma and mouth breathing. *Int J Pediatr Otorhinolaryngol.* 2010 Sep;74(9):1021-7.

Chawes BL, Bonnelykke K, Kreiner-Moller E, Bisgaard H. Children with allergic and nonallergic rhinitis have a similar risk of asthma. *J Allergy Clin Immunol.* 2010 Sep;126(3):567-73.e1-8.

Chawes BL, Kreiner-Moller E, Bisgaard H. Objective assessments of allergic and nonallergic rhinitis in young children. *Allergy.* 2009 Oct;64(10):1547-53.

Chehade M, Aceves SS. Food allergy and eosinophilic esophagitis. *Curr Opin Allergy Clin Immunol.* 2010 Jun;10(3):231-7.

Chellini E, Talassi F, Corbo G, Berti G, De Sario M, Rusconi F, Piffer S, Caranci N, Petronio MG, Sestini P, Dell'Orco V, Bonci E, Armenio L, La Grutta S; Gruppo Collaborativo SIDRIA-2. Environmental, social and demographic characteristics of children and adolescents, resident in different Italian areas. *Epidemiol Prev.* 2005 Mar-Apr;29(2 Suppl):14-23.

Chen HJ, Shih CK, Hsu HY, Chiang W. Mast cell-dependent allergic responses are inhibited by ethanolic extract of adlay (Coix lachryma-jobi L. var. ma-yuen Stapf) testa. *J Agric Food Chem.* 2010 Feb 24;58(4):2596-601.

Chen JX, Ji B, Lu ZL, Hu LS. Effects of chai hu (radix burpleuri) containing formulation on plasma beta-endorphin, epinephrine and dopamine on patients. *Am J Chin Med.* 2005;33(5):737-45.

Chen Y, Blaser MJ. Helicobacter pylori colonization is inversely associated with childhood asthma. *J Infect Dis.* 2008 Aug 15;198(4):553-60.

Chen Y, Blaser MJ. Inverse associations of Helicobacter pylori with asthma and allergy. *Arch Intern Med.* 2007 Apr 23;167(8):821-7.

Cheney G, Waxler SH, Miller IJ. Vitamin U therapy of peptic ulcer; experience at San Quentin Prison. *Calif Med.* 1956 Jan;84(1):39-42.

Chevallier A. *Encyclopedia of Medicinal Plants.* New York, NY: DK Publishing; 1996.

Chevrier MR, Ryan AE, Lee DY, Zhongze M, Wu-Yan Z, Via CS. Boswellia carterii extract inhibits TH1 cytokines and promotes TH2 cytokines in vitro. *Clin Diagn Lab Immunol.* 2005 May;12(5):575-80.

Chilton FH, Rudel LL, Parks JS, Arm JP, Seeds MC. Mechanisms by which botanical lipids affect inflammatory disorders. *Am J Clin Nutr.* 2008 Feb;87(2):498S-503S.

Chilton FH, Tucker L. *Win the War Within.* New York: Rodale, 2006.

Chin A Paw MJ, de Jong N, Pallast EG, Kloek GC, Schouten EG, Kok FJ. Immunity in frail elderly: a randomized controlled trial of exercise and enriched foods. *Med Sci Sports Exerc.* 2000 Dec;32(12):2005-11.

Choi BW, Yoo KH, Jeong JW, Yoon HJ, Kim SH, Park YM, Kim WK, Oh JW, Rha YH, Pyun BY, Chang SI, Moon HB, Kim YY, Cho SH. Easy diagnosis of asthma: computer-assisted, symptom-based diagnosis. *J Korean Med Sci.* 2007 Oct;22(5):832-8.

Choi SY, Sohn JH, Lee YW, Lee EK, Hong CS, Park JW. Characterization of buckwheat 19-kD allergen and its application for diagnosing clinical reactivity. *Int Arch Allergy Immunol.* 2007;144(4):267-74.

Choi SZ, Choi SU, Lee KR. Phytochemical constituents of the aerial parts from Solidago virga-aurea var. gigantea. *Arch Pharm Res.* 2004 Feb;27(2):164-8.

Chong Neto HJ, Rosário NA; Grupo EISL Curitiba (Estudio Internacional de Sibilancias en Lactantes). Risk factors for wheezing in the first year of life. *J Pediatr.* 2008 Nov-Dec;84(6):495-502.

Chopra RN, Nayar SL, Chopra IC, eds. *Glossary of Indian Medicinal plants.* New Delhi: CSIR, 1956.

Choudhry S, Seibold MA, Borrell LN, Tang H, Serebrisky D, Chapela R, Rodriguez-Santana JR, Avila PC, Ziv E, Rodriguez-Cintron W, Risch NJ, Burchard EG. Dissecting complex diseases in complex populations: asthma in latino americans. *Proc Am Thorac Soc.* 2007 Jul;4(3):226-33.

Christopher JR. *School of Natural Healing.* Springville UT: Christopher Publ, 1976.

Chu YF, Liu RH. Cranberries inhibit LDL oxidation and induce LDL receptor expression in hepatocytes. *Life Sci.* 2005;77(15):1892-1901. 27.

Chung SY, Butts CL, Maleki SJ, Champagne ET. Linking peanut allergenicity to the processes of maturation, curing, and roasting. *J Agric Food Chem.* 2003;51: 4273-4277.

Cibella F, Cuttitta G. Nocturnal asthma and gastroesophageal reflux. *Am J Med.* 2001 Dec 3;111 Suppl 8A:31S-36S.

Cingi C, Demirbas D, Songu M. Allergic rhinitis caused by food allergies. *Eur Arch Otorhinolaryngol.* 2010 Sep;267(9):1327-35.

Ciprandi G, De Amici M, Negrini S, Marseglia G, Tosca MA. TGF-beta and IL-17 serum levels and specific immunotherapy. *Int Immunopharmacol.* 2009 Sep;9(10):1247-9.

Cisneros C, García-Río F, Romera D, Villasante C, Girón R, Ancochea J. Bronchial reactivity indices are determinants of health-related quality of life in patients with stable asthma. *Thorax.* 2010 Sep;65(9):795-800.

Clark S, Bock SA, Gaeta TJ, Brenner BE, Cydulka RK, Camargo CA; Multicenter Airway Research Collaboration-8 Investigators. Multicenter study of emergency department visits for food allergies. *J Allergy Clin Immunol.* 2004 Feb;113(2):347-52.

Clement YN, Williams AF, Aranda D, Chase R, Watson N, Mohammed R, Stubbs O, Williamson D. Medicinal herb use among asthmatic patients attending a specialty care facility in Trinidad. *BMC Complement Altern Med.* 2005 Feb 15;5:3.

Cobo Sanz JM, Mateos JA, Muñoz Conejo A. Effect of *Lactobacillus casei* on the incidence of infectious conditions in children. *Nutr Hosp.* 2006 Jul-Aug;21(4):547-51.

Codispoti CD, Levin L, LeMasters GK, Ryan P, Reponen T, Villareal M, Burkle J, Stanforth S, Lockey JE, Khurana Hershey GK, Bernstein DI. Breast-feeding, aeroallergen sensitization, and environmental exposures during infancy are determinants of childhood allergic rhinitis. *J Allergy Clin Immunol.* 2010 May;125(5):1054-1060.e1.

Cohen A, Goldberg M, Levy B, Leshno M, Katz Y. Sesame food allergy and sensitization in children: the natural history and long-term follow-up. *Pediatr Allergy Immunol.* 2007 May;18(3):217-23.

Cohen RT, Raby BA, Van Steen K, Fuhlbrigge AL, Celedón JC, Rosner BA, Strunk RC, Zeiger RS, Weiss ST; Childhood Asthma Management Program Research Group. In utero smoke exposure and impaired response to inhaled corticosteroids in children with asthma. *J Allergy Clin Immunol.* 2010 Sep;126(3):491-7. 2010 Jul 31. ; .

Collipp PJ, Goldzier S 3rd, Weiss N, Soleymani Y, Snyder R. Pyridoxine treatment of childhood bronchial asthma. *Ann Allergy.* 1975 Aug;35(2):93-7.

Conquer JA, Holub BJ. Dietary docosahexaenoic acid as a source of eicosapentaenoic acid in vegetarians and omnivores. *Lipids.* 1997 Mar;32(3):341-5.

Cooper GS, Miller FW, Germolec DR: Occupational exposures and autoimmune diseases. *Int Immunopharm* 2002, 2:303-313.

Cooper K. *The Aerobics Program for Total Well-Being.* New York: Evans, 1980.

Corbe C, Boissin JP, Siou A. Light vision and chorioretinal circulation. Study of the effect of procyanidolic oligomers (Endotelon). *J Fr Ophtalmol.* 1988;11(5):453-60.

Corbo GM, Forastiere F, De Sario M, Brunetti L, Bonci E, Bugiani M, Chellini E, La Grutta S, Migliore E, Pistelli R, Rusconi F, Russo A, Simoni M, Talassi F, Galassi C; Sidria-2 Collaborative Group. Wheeze and asthma in children: associations with body mass index, sports, television viewing, and diet. *Epidemiology.* 2008 Sep;19(5):747-55.

REFERENCES

Cory S, Ussery-Hall A, Griffin-Blake S, Easton A, Vigeant J, Balluz L, Garvin W, Greenlund K; Centers for Disease Control and Prevention (CDC). Prevalence of selected risk behaviors and chronic diseases and conditions-steps communities, United States, 2006-2007. *MMWR Surveill Summ.* 2010 Sep 24;59(8):1-37.

Courtney R, Cohen M. Investigating the claims of Konstantin Buteyko, M.D., Ph.D.: the relationship of breath holding time to end tidal CO_2 and other proposed measures of dysfunctional breathing. *J Altern Complement Med.* 2008 Mar;14(2):115-23.

Couzy F, Kastenmayer P, Vigo M, Clough J, Munoz-Box R, Barclay DV. Calcium bioavailability from a calcium- and sulfate-rich mineral water, compared with milk, in young adult women. *Am J Clin Nutr.* 1995 Dec;62(6):1239-44.

Covar R, Gleason M, Macomber B, Stewart L, Szefler P, Engelhardt K, Murphy J, Liu A, Wood S, DeMichele S, Gelfand EW, Szefler SJ. Impact of a novel nutritional formula on asthma control and biomarkers of allergic airway inflammation in children. *Clin Exp Allergy.* 2010 Aug;40(8):1163-74. 2010 Jun 7.

Crane J, Ellis I, Siebers R, Grimmet D, Lewis S, Fitzharris P. A pilot study of the effect of mechanical ventilation and heat exchange on house-dust mites and Der p 1 in New Zealand homes. *Allergy.* 1998 Aug;53(8):755-62.

Crescente M, Jessen G, Momi S, Höltje HD, Gresele P, Cerletti C, de Gaetano G. Interactions of gallic acid, resveratrol, quercetin and aspirin at the platelet cyclooxygenase-1 level. Functional and modelling studies. *Thromb Haemost.* 2009 Aug;102(2):336-46.

Crinnion WJ. Toxic effects of the easily avoidable phthalates and parabens. *Altern Med Rev.* 2010 Sep;15(3):190-6.

Cserhati E. Current view on the etiology of childhood bronchial asthma. *Orv Hetil.* 2000;141:759-760.

Cuesta-Herranz J, Barber D, Blanco C, Cistero-Bahíma A, Crespo JF, Fernández-Rivas M, Fernández-Sánchez J, Florido JF, Ibáñez MD, Rodríguez R, Salcedo G, Garcia BE, Lombardero M, Quiralte J, Rodriguez J, Sánchez-Monge R, Vereda A, Villalba M, Alonso Díaz de Durana MD, Basagaña M, Carrillo T, Fernández-Nieto M, Tabar AI. Differences among Pollen-Allergic Patients with and without Plant Food Allergy. *Int Arch Allergy Immunol.* 2010 Apr 23;153(2):182-192.

Cummings M. *Human Heredity: Principles and Issues.* St. Paul, MN: West, 1988.

Custovic A, Simpson BM, Simpson A, Kissen P, Woodcock A; NAC Manchester Asthma and Allergy Study Group. Effect of environmental manipulation in pregnancy and early life on respiratory symptoms and atopy during first year of life: a randomised trial. *Lancet.* 2001 Jul 21;358(9277):188-93.

D'Anneo RW, Bruno ME, Falagiani P. Sublingual allergoid immunotherapy: a new 4-day induction phase in patients allergic to house dust mites. *Int J Immunopathol Pharmacol.* 2010 Apr-Jun;23(2):553-60.

D'Auria E, Sala M, Lodi F, Radaelli G, Riva E, Giovannini M. Nutritional value of a rice-hydrolysate formula in infants with cows' milk protein allergy: a randomized pilot study. *J Int Med Res.* 2003 May-Jun;31(3):215-22.

D'Orazio N, Ficoneri C, Riccioni G, Conti P, Theoharides TC, Bollea MR. Conjugated linoleic acid: a functional food? *Int J Immunopathol Pharmacol.* 2003 Sep-Dec;16(3):215-20.

D'Urbano LE, Pellegrino K, Artesani MC, Donnanno S, Luciano R, Riccardi C, Tozzi AE, Ravà L, De Benedetti F, Cavagni G. Performance of a component-based allergen-microarray in the diagnosis of cow's milk and hen's egg allergy. *Clin Exp Allergy.* 2010 Jul 13.

Dallinga JW, Robroeks CM, van Berkel JJ, Moonen EJ, Godschalk RW, Jöbsis Q, Dompeling E, Wouters EF, van Schooten FJ. Volatile organic compounds in exhaled breath as a diagnostic tool for asthma in children. Clin Exp Allergy. 2010 Jan;40(1):68-76.

Davidson T. *Rhinology: The Collected Writings of Maurice H. Cottle, M.D.* San Diego, CA: American Rhinologic Society, 1987.

Davies G. *Timetables of Medicine.* New York: Black Dog & Leventhal, 2000.

Davin JC, Forget P, Mahieu PR. Increased intestinal permeability to (51 Cr) EDTA is correlated with IgA immune complex-plasma levels in children with IgA-associated nephropathies. *Acta Paediatr Scand.* 1988 Jan;77(1):118-24.

de Boissieu D, Dupont C, Badoual J. Allergy to nondairy proteins in mother's milk as assessed by intestinal permeability tests. *Allergy.* 1994 Dec;49(10):882-4.

de Boissieu D, Matarazzo P, Rocchiccioli F, Dupont C. Multiple food allergy: a possible diagnosis in breast-fed infants. *Acta Paediatr.* 1997 Oct;86(10):1042-6.

De Lucca AJ, Bland JM, Vigo CB, Cushion M, Selitrennikoff CP, Peter J, Walsh TJ. CAY-I, a fungicidal saponin from Capsicum sp. fruit. *Med Mycol.* 2002 Apr;40(2):131-7.

de Martino M, Novembre E, Galli L, de Marco A, Botarelli P, Marano E, Vierucci A. Allergy to different fish species in cod-allergic children: in vivo and in vitro studies. *J Allergy Clin Immunol.* 1990;86:909-914.

De Smet PA. Herbal remedies. *N Engl J Med.* 2002;347:2046-2056.

Dean C. *Death by Modern Medicine.* Belleville, ON: Matrix Verite-Media, 2005.

Debley JS, Carter ER, Redding GJ. Prevalence and impact of gastroesophageal reflux in adolescents with asthma: a population-based study. *Pediatr Pulmonol.* 2006 May;41(5):475-81.

Dehlink E, Yen E, Leichtner AM, Hait EJ, Fiebiger E. First evidence of a possible association between gastric acid suppression during pregnancy and childhood asthma: a population-based register study. *Clin Exp Allergy.* 2009 Feb;39(2):246-53. 2008 Dec 9.

del Giudice MM, Leonardi S, Maiello N, Brunese FP. Food allergy and probiotics in childhood. *J Clin Gastroenterol.* 2010 Sep;44 Suppl 1:S22-5.

Delacourt C. Bronchial changes in untreated asthma. *Arch Pediatr.* 2004 Jun;11 Suppl 2:71s-73s.

Del-Rio-Navarro B, Berber A, Blandón-Vijil V, Ramírez-Aguilar M, Romieu I, Ramírez-Chanona N, Heras-Acevedo S, Serrano-Sierra A, Barraza-Villareal A, Baeza-Bacab M, Sienra-Monge JJ. Identification of asthma risk factors in Mexico City in an International Study of Asthma and Allergy in Childhood survey. *Allergy Asthma Proc.* 2006 Jul-Aug;27(4):325-33.

Dengate S, Ruben A. Controlled trial of cumulative behavioural effects of a common bread preservative. *J Paediatr Child Health.* 2002 Aug;38(4):373-6.

Dente FL, Bacci E, Bartoli ML, Cianchetti S, Costa F, Di Franco A, Malagrinò L, Vagaggini B, Paggiaro P. Effects of oral prednisone on sputum eosinophils and cytokines in patients with severe refractory asthma. *Ann Allergy Asthma Immunol.* 2010 Jun;104(6):464-70.

Derebery MJ, Berliner KI. Allergy and its relation to Meniere's disease. *Otolaryngol Clin North Am.* 2010 Oct;43(5):1047-58.

Desjeux JF, Heyman M. Milk proteins, cytokines and intestinal epithelial functions in children. *Acta Paediatr Jpn.* 1994 Oct;36(5):592-6.

DesRoches A, Infante-Rivard C, Paradis L, Paradis J, Haddad E. Peanut allergy: is maternal transmission of antigens during pregnancy and breastfeeding a risk factor? *J Investig Allergol Clin Immunol.* 2010;20(4):289-94.

Deutsche Gesellschaft für Ernährung. Drink distilled water? *Med. Mo. Pharm.* 1993;16:146.

Devaraj TL. *Speaking of Ayurvedic Remedies for Common Diseases.* New Delhi: Sterling, 1985.

Devirgiliis C, Zalewski PD, Perozzi G, Murgia C. Zinc fluxes and zinc transporter genes in chronic diseases. *Mutat Res.* 2007 Sep 1;622(1-2):84-93. 2007 Feb 17.

Dharmage SC, Erbas B, Jarvis D, Wjst M, Raherison C, Norbäck D, Heinrich J, Sunyer J, Svanes C. Do childhood respiratory infections continue to influence adult respiratory morbidity? *Eur Respir J.* 2009 Feb;33(2):237-44.

Di Gioacchino M, Cavallucci E, Di Stefano F, Paolini F, Ramondo S, Di Sciascio MB, Ciuffreda S, Riccioni G, Della Vecchia R, Romano A, Boscolo P. Effect of natural allergen exposure on non-specific bronchial reactivity in asthmatic farmers. *Sci Total Environ.* 2001 Apr 10;270(1-3):43-8.

Di Gioacchino M, Cavallucci E, Di Stefano F, Verna N, Ramondo S, Ciuffreda S, Riccioni G, Boscolo P. Influence of total IgE and seasonal increase of eosinophil cationic protein on bronchial hyperreactivity in asthmatic grass-sensitized farmers. *Allergy.* 2000 Nov;55(11):1030-4.

Di Marco F, Santus P, Centanni S. Anxiety and depression in asthma. *Curr Opin Pulm Med.* 2011 Jan;17(1):39-44.

Dierksen KP, Moore CJ, Inglis M, Wescombe PA, Tagg JR. The effect of ingestion of milk supplemented with salivaricin A-producing Streptococcus salivarius on the bacteriocin-like inhibitory activity of streptococcal populations on the tongue. *FEMS Microbiol Ecol.* 2007 Mar;59(3):584-91.

Diğrak M, Ilçim A, Hakki Alma M. Antimicrobial activities of several parts of Pinus brutia, Juniperus oxycedrus, Abies cilicia, Cedrus libani and Pinus nigra. *Phytother Res.* 1999 Nov;13(7):584-7.

DiMango E, Holbrook JT, Simpson E, Reibman J, Richter J, Narula S, Prusakowski N, Mastronarde JG, Wise RA; American Lung Association Asthma Clinical Research Centers. Effects of asymptomatic proximal and distal gastroesophageal reflux on asthma severity. *Am J Respir Crit Care Med.* 2009 Nov 1;180(9):809-16. 2009 Aug 6.

Din FV, Theodoratou E, Farrington SM, Tenesa A, Barnetson RA, Cetnarskyj R, Stark L, Porteous ME, Campbell H, Dunlop MG. Effect of aspirin and NSAIDs on risk and survival from colorectal cancer. *Gut.* 2010 Dec;59(12):1670-9.

Diop L, Guillou S, Durand H. Probiotic food supplement reduces stress-induced gastrointestinal symptoms in volunteers: a double-blind, placebo-controlled, randomized trial. *Nutr Res.* 2008 Jan;28(1):1-5.

Dixon AE, Kaminsky DA, Holbrook JT, Wise RA, Shade DM, Irvin CG. Allergic rhinitis and sinusitis in asthma: differential effects on symptoms and pulmonary function. *Chest.* 2006 Aug;130(2):429-35.

Dona A, Arvanitoyannis IS. Health risks of genetically modified foods. *Crit Rev Food Sci Nutr.* 2009 Feb;49(2):164-75.

Donato F, Monarca S, Premi S., and Gelatti, U. Drinking water hardness and chronic degenerative diseases. Part III. Tumors, urolithiasis, fetal malformations, deterioration of the cognitive function in the aged and atopic eczema. *Ann. Ig.* 2003;15:57-70.

Dooley, M.A. and Hogan S.L. Environmental epidemiology and risk factors for autoimmune disease. *Curr Opin Rheum.* 2003;15(2):99-103.

366

REFERENCES

dos Santos LH, Ribeiro IO, Sánchez PG, Hetzel JL, Felicetti JC, Cardoso PF. Evaluation of pantoprazol treatment response of patients with asthma and gastroesophageal reflux: a randomized prospective double-blind placebo-controlled study. *J Bras Pneumol.* 2007 Apr;33(2):119-27.

Dotolo Institute. *The Study of Colon Hydrotherapy.* Pinellas Park, FL: Dotolo, 2003.

Dove MS, Dockery DW, Connolly GN. Smoke-free air laws and asthma prevalence, symptoms, and severity among nonsmoking youth. *Pediatrics.* 2011 Jan;127(1):102-9. 2010 Dec 13.

Dowd JB, Zajacova A, Aiello A. Early origins of health disparities: burden of infection, health, and socio-economic status in U.S. children. *Soc Sci Med.* 2009 Feb;68(4):699-707. 2009 Jan 17.

Ducrotté P. Irritable bowel syndrome: from the gut to the brain-gut. *Gastroenterol Clin Biol.* 2009 Aug-Sep;33(8-9):703-12.

Duke J. *CRC Handbook of Medicinal Herbs.* Boca Raton: CRC; 1989.

Duke J. *The Green Pharmacy.* New York: St. Martins, 1997.

Dunstan JA, Roper J, Mitoulas L, Hartmann PE, Simmer K, Prescott SL. The effect of supplementation with fish oil during pregnancy on breast milk immunoglobulin A, soluble CD14, cytokine levels and fatty acid composition. *Clin Exp Allergy.* 2004 Aug;34(8):1237-42.

Duong M, Subbarao P, Adelroth E, Obminski G, Strinich T, Inman M, Pedersen S, O'Byrne PM. Sputum eosinophils and the response of exercise-induced bronchoconstriction to corticosteroid in asthma. *Chest.* 2008 Feb;133(2):404-11. 2007 Dec 10.

Dupont C, Barau E, Molkhou P, Raynaud F, Barbet JP, Dehennin L. Food-induced alterations of intestinal permeability in children with cow's milk-sensitive enteropathy and atopic dermatitis. *J Pediatr Gastroenterol Nutr.* 1989 May;8(4):459-65.

Dupont C, Barau E, Molkhou P. Intestinal permeability disorders in children. *Allerg Immunol.* 1991 Mar;23(3):95-103.

Dupont C, Soulaines P, Lapillonne A, Donne N, Kalach N, Benhamou P. Atopy patch test for early diagnosis of cow's milk allergy in preterm infants. *J Pediatr Gastroenterol Nutr.* 2010 Apr;50(4):463-4.

Dupuy P, Cassé M, André F, Dhivert-Donnadieu H, Pinton J, Hernandez-Pion C. Low-salt water reduces intestinal permeability in atopic patients. *Dermatology.* 1999;198(2):153-5.

Duran-Tauleria E, Vignati G, Guedan MJ, Petersson CJ. The utility of specific immunoglobulin E measurements in primary care. *Allergy.* 2004 Aug;59 Suppl 78:35-41.

Duwiejua M, Zeitlin IJ, Waterman PG, Chapman J, Mhango GJ, Provan GJ. Anti-inflammatory activity of resins from some species of the plant family Burseraceae. *Planta Med.* 1993 Feb;59(1):12-6.

Dykewicz MS, Lemmon JK, Keaney DL. Comparison of the Multi-Test II and Skintestor Omni allergy skin test devices. *Ann Allergy Asthma Immunol.* 2007 Jun;98(6):559-62.

Eastham EJ, Walker WA. Effect of cow's milk on the gastrointestinal tract: a persistent dilemma for the pediatrician. *Pediatrics.* 1977 Oct;60(4):477-81.

Eaton KK, Howard M, Howard JM. Gut permeability measured by polyethylene glycol absorption in abnormal gut fermentation as compared with food intolerance. *J R Soc Med.* 1995 Feb;88(2):63-6.

Ebers GC, Kukay K, Bulman DE, Sadovnick AD, Rice G, Anderson C, Armstrong H, Cousin K, Bell RB, Hader W, Paty DW, Hashimoto S, Oger J, Duquette P, Warren S, Gray T, O'Connor P, Nath A, Auty A, Metz L, Francis G, Paulseth JE, Murray TJ, Pryse-Phillips W, Nelson R, Freedman M, Brunet D, Bouchard JP, Hinds D, Risch N. A full genome search in multiple sclerosis. *Nat Genet.* 1996 Aug;13(4):472-6.

Eccles R. Menthol and related cooling compounds. *J Pharm Pharmacol.* 1994 Aug;46(8):618-30.

ECRHS (2002) The European Community Respiratory Health Survey II. *Eur Respir J.* 20: 1071-1079.

Edgecombe K, Latter S, Peters S, Roberts G. Health experiences of adolescents with uncontrolled severe asthma. *Arch Dis Child.* 2010 Dec;95(12):985-91. 2010 Jul 30.

Edgell PG. The psychology of asthma. *Can Med Assoc J.* 1952 Aug;67(2):121-5.

Egashira Y, Nagano H. A multicenter clinical trial of TJ-96 in patients with steroid-dependent bronchial asthma. A comparison of groups allocated by the envelope method. *Ann N Y Acad Sci.* 1993 Jun 23;685:580-3.

Ege MJ, Frei R, Bieli C, Schram-Bijkerk D, Waser M, Benz MR, Weiss G, Nyberg F, van Hage M, Pershagen G, Brunekreef B, Riedler J, Lauener R, Braun-Fahrländer C, von Mutius E; PARSIFAL Study team. Not all farming environments protect against the development of asthma and wheeze in children. *J Allergy Clin Immunol.* 2007 May;119(5):1140-7.

Ege MJ, Herzum I, Büchele G, Krauss-Etschmann S, Lauener RP, Roponen M, Hyvärinen A, Vuitton DA, Riedler J, Brunekreef B, Dalphin JC, Braun-Fahrländer C, Pekkanen J, Renz H, von Mutius E; Protection Against Allergy Study in Rural Environments (PASTURE) Study group. Prenatal exposure to a farm environment modifies atopic sensitization at birth. *J Allergy Clin Immunol.* 2008 Aug;122(2):407-12, 412.e1-4.

Eggermont E. Cow's milk protein allergy. *Tijdschr Kindergeneeskd.* 1981 Feb;49(1):16-20.

Ehling S, Hengel M, and Shibamoto T. Formation of acrylamide from lipids. *Adv Exp Med Biol* 2005, 561:223-233.

Ehnert B, Lau-Schadendorf S, Weber A, Buettner P, Schou C, Wahn U. Reducing domestic exposure to dust mite allergen reduces bronchial hyperreactivity in sensitive children with asthma. *J Allergy Clin Immunol.* 1992 Jul;90(1):135-8.

Ehren J, Morón B, Martin E, Bethune MT, Gray GM, Khosla C. A food-grade enzyme preparation with modest gluten detoxification properties. *PLoS One.* 2009 Jul 21;4(7):e6313.

Eijkemans M, Mommers M, de Vries SI, van Buuren S, Stafleu A, Bakker I, Thijs C. Asthmatic symptoms, physical activity, and overweight in young children: a cohort study. *Pediatrics.* 2008 Mar;121(3):e666-72.

Eldridge MW, Peden DB. Allergen provocation augments endotoxin-induced nasal inflammation in subjects with atopic asthma. *J Allergy Clin Immunol.* 2000 Mar;105(3):475-81.

el-Ghazaly M, Khayyal MT, Okpanyi SN, Arens-Corell M. Study of the anti-inflammatory activity of Populus tremula, Solidago virgaurea and Fraxinus excelsior. *Arzneimittelforschung.* 1992 Mar;42(3):333-6.

Ellingwood F. *American Materia Medica, Therapeutics and Pharmacognosy.* Portland: Eclectic Medical Publ., 1983.

Elliott RB, Harris DP, Hill JP, Bibby NJ, Wasmuth HE. Type I (insulin-dependent) diabetes mellitus and cow milk: casein variant consumption. *Diabetologia.* 1999 Mar;42(3):292-6.

Elwood PC. Epidemiology and trace elements. *Clin Endocrinol Metab.* 1985 Aug;14(3):617-28.

Emberlin JC, Lewis RA. Pollen challenge study of a phototherapy device for reducing the symptoms of hay fever. *Curr Med Res Opin.* 2009 Jul;25(7):1635-44.

Emmanouil E, Manios Y, Grammatikaki E, Kondaki K, Oikonomou E, Papadopoulos N, Vassilopoulou E. Association of nutrient intake and wheeze or asthma in a Greek pre-school population. *Pediatr Allergy Immunol.* 2010 Feb;21(1 Pt 1):90-5. 2009 Sep 9.

Engler RJ. Alternative and complementary medicine: a source of improved therapies for asthma? A challenge for redefining the specialty? *J Allergy Clin Immunol.* 2000;106:627-9.

Environmental Working Group. *Human Toxome Project.* 2007. http://www.ewg.org/sites/humantoxome/. Accessed: 2007 Sep.

EPA. *A Brief Guide to Mold, Moisture and Your Home.* Environmental Protection Agency, Office of Air and Radiation/Indoor Environments Division. EPA 2002;402-K-02-003.

Epstein GN, Halper JP, Barrett EA, Birdsall C, McGee M, Baron KP, Lowenstein S. A pilot study of mind-body changes in adults with asthma who practice mental imagery. *Altern Ther Health Med.* 2004 Jul-Aug;10(4):66-71.

Erkkola M, Kaila M, Nwaru BI, Kronberg-Kippilä C, Ahonen S, Nevalainen J, Veijola R, Pekkanen J, Ilonen J, Simell O, Knip M, Virtanen SM. Maternal vitamin D intake during pregnancy is inversely associated with asthma and allergic rhinitis in 5-year-old children. *Clin Exp Allergy.* 2009 Jun;39(6):875-82.

Ernst E. Frankincense: systematic review. *BMJ.* 2008 Dec 17;337:a2813.

Erwin EA, James HR, Gutekunst HM, Russo JM, Kelleher KJ, Platts-Mills TA. Serum IgE measurement and detection of food allergy in pediatric patients with eosinophilic esophagitis. *Ann Allergy Asthma Immunol.* 2010 Jun;104(6):496-502.

EuroPrevall. *WP 1.1 Birth Cohort Update.* 1st Quarter 2006. Berlin, Germany: Charité University Medical Centre.

Evans P, Forte D, Jacobs C, Fredhoi C, Aitchison E, Hucklebridge F, Clow A. Cortisol secretory activity in older people in relation to positive and negative well-being. *Psychoneuroendocrinology.* 2007 Aug 7

Everhart JE. *Digestive Diseases in the United States.* Darby, PA: Diane Pub, 1994.

FAAN. *Public Comment on 2005 Food Safety Survey: Docket No. 2004N-0516 (2005 FSS).* Fairfax, VA: Food Allergy & Anaphylaxis Network.

Fairchild SS, Shannon K, Kwan E, Mishell RI. T cell-derived glucosteroid response-modifying factor (GRMF): a unique lymphokine made by normal T lymphocytes and a T cell hybridoma. *J Immunol.* 1984 Feb;132(2):821-7.

Fajac I, Frossard N. Neuropeptides of the nasal innervation and allergic rhinitis. *Rev Mal Respir.* 1994;11(4):357-67.

Fajac I, Frossard N. Neuropeptides of the nasal innervation and allergic rhinitis. *Rev Mal Respir.* 1994;11(4):357-67.

Fälth-Magnusson K, Kjellman NI, Magnusson KE, Sundqvist T. Intestinal permeability in healthy and allergic children before and after sodium-cromoglycate treatment assessed with different-sized polyethyleneglycols (PEG 400 and PEG 1000). *Clin Allergy.* 1984 May;14(3):277-86.

Fälth-Magnusson K, Kjellman NI, Odelram H, Sundqvist T, Magnusson KE. Gastrointestinal permeability in children with cow's milk allergy: effect of milk challenge and sodium cromoglycate as assessed with polyethyleneglycols (PEG 400 and PEG 1000). *Clin Allergy.* 1986 Nov;16(6):543-51.

Fan AY, Lao L, Zhang RX, Zhou AN, Wang LB, Moudgil KD, Lee DY, Ma ZZ, Zhang WY, Berman BM. Effects of an acetone extract of Boswellia carterii Birdw. (Burseraceae) gum resin on adjuvant-induced arthritis in lewis rats. *J Ethnopharmacol.* 2005 Oct 3;101(1-3):104-9.

Fanaro S, Marten B, Bagna R, Vigi V, Fabris C, Peña-Quintana L, Argüelles F, Scholz-Ahrens KE, Sawatzki G, Zelenka R, Schrezenmeir J, de Vrese M and Bertino E. Galacto-oligosaccharides are bifidogenic and safe at weaning: A double-blind Randomized Multicenter study. *J Pediatr Gastroent Nutr.* 2009 48; 82-88

REFERENCES

Fang SP, Tanaka T, Tago F, Okamoto T, Kojima S. Immunomodulatory effects of gyokuheifusan on INF-gamma/IL-4 (Th1/Th2) balance in ovalbumin (OVA)-induced asthma model mice. *Biol Pharm Bull.* 2005;28:829-33.

FAO/WHO Expert Committee. *Fats and Oils in Human Nutrition.* Food and Nutrition Paper. 1994;(57).

Fawell J, Nieuwenhuijsen MJ. Contaminants in drinking water. *Br Med Bull.* 2003;68:199-208.

Fecka I. Qualitative and quantitative determination of hydrolysable tannins and other polyphenols in herbal products from meadowsweet and dog rose. *Phytochem Anal.* 2009 May;20(3):177-90.

Felley CP, Corthésy-Theulaz I, Rivero JL, Sipponen P, Kaufmann M, Bauerfeind P, Wiesel PH, Brassart D, Pfeifer A, Blum AL, Michetti P. Favourable effect of an acidified milk (LC-1) on Helicobacter pylori gastritis in man. *Eur J Gastroenterol Hepatol.* 2001 Jan;13(1):25-9.

Ferguson BJ. Categorization of eosinophilic chronic rhinosinusitis. *Curr Opin Otolaryngol Head Neck Surg.* 2004 Jun;12(3):237-42.

Fernández-Rivas M, Garrido Fernández S, Nadal JA, Díaz de Durana MD, García BE, González-Mancebo E, Martín S, Barber D, Rico P, Tabar AI. Randomized double-blind, placebo-controlled trial of sublingual immunotherapy with a Pru p 3 quantified peach extract. *Allergy.* 2009 Jun;64(6):876-83.

Fernández-Rivas M, González-Mancebo E, Rodríguez-Pérez R, Benito C, Sánchez-Monge R, Salcedo G, Alonso MD, Rosado A, Tejedor MA, Vila C, Casas ML. Clinically relevant peach allergy is related to peach lipid transfer protein, Pru p 3, in the Spanish population. *J Allergy Clin Immunol.* 2003 Oct;112(4):789-95.

Ferrari M, Benini L, Brotto E, Locatelli F, De Iorio F, Bonella F, Tacchella N, Corradini G, Lo Cascio V, Vantini I. Omeprazole reduces the response to capsaicin but not to methacholine in asthmatic patients with proximal reflux. *Scand J Gastroenterol.* 2007 Mar;42(3):299-307.

Ferrier L, Berard F, Debrauwer L, Chabo C, Langella P, Bueno L, Fioramonti J. Impairment of the intestinal barrier by ethanol involves enteric microflora and mast cell activation in rodents. *Am J Pathol.* 2006 Apr;168(4):1148-54.

Field RW, Krewski D, Lubin JH, Zielinski JM, Alavanja M, Catalan VS, Klotz JB, Létourneau EG, Lynch CF, Lyon JL, Sandler DP, Schoenberg JB, Steck DJ, Stolwijk JA, Weinberg C, Wilcox HB. An overview of the North American residential radon and lung cancer case-control studies. *J Toxicol Environ Health A.* 2006 Apr;69(7):599-631.

Field T, Henteleff T, Hernandez-Reif M, Martinez E, Mavunda K, Kuhn C, Schanberg S. Children with asthma have improved pulmonary functions after massage therapy. *J Pediatr.* 1998 May;132(5):854-8.

Finkelman FD, Boyce JA, Vercelli D, Rothenberg ME. Key advances in mechanisms of asthma, allergy, and immunology in 2009. *J Allergy Clin Immunol.* 2010 Feb;125(2):312-8.

Fiocchi A, Restani P, Bernardo L, Martelli A, Ballabio C, D'Auria E, Riva E. Tolerance of heat-treated kiwi by children with kiwifruit allergy. *Pediatr Allergy Immunol.* 2004 Oct;15(5):454-8.

Fiocchi A, Travaini M, D'Auria E, Banderali G, Bernardo L, Riva E. Tolerance to a rice hydrolysate formula in children allergic to cow's milk and soy. *Clin Exp Allergy.* 2003 Nov;33(11):1576-80.

Fiocchi, A; Restani, P; Riva, E; Qualizza, R; Bruni, P; Restelli, AR; Galli, CL. Meat allergy: I. Specific IgE to BSA and OSA in atopic, beef sensitive children. *J Am Coll Nutr.* 1995 14: 239-244.

Fjeld T, Veiersted B, Sandvik L, Riise G, Levy F. The Effect of Indoor Foliage Plants on Health and Discomfort Symptoms among Office Workers. *Ind Built Environ.* 1998 July;7(4): 204-209.

Flandrin, J, Montanari M. (eds.). *Food: A Culinary History from Antiquity to the Present.* New York: Penguin Books, 1999.

Fleischer DM, Conover-Walker MK, Christie L, Burks AW, Wood RA. Peanut allergy: recurrence and its management. *J Allergy Clin Immunol.* 2004 Nov;114(5):1195-201.

Flinterman AE, van Hoffen E, den Hartog Jager CF, Koppelman S, Pasmans SG, Hoekstra MO, Bruijnzeel-Koomen CA, Knulst AC, Knol EF. Children with peanut allergy recognize predominantly Ara h2 and Ara h6, which remains stable over time. *Clin Exp Allergy.* 2007 Aug;37(8):1221-8.

Foliaki S, Annesi-Maesano I, Tuuau-Potoi N, Waqatakirewa L, Cheng S, Douwes J, Pearce N. Risk factors for symptoms of childhood asthma, allergic rhinoconjunctivitis and eczema in the Pacific: an ISAAC Phase III study. *Int J Tuberc Lung Dis.* 2008 Jul;12(7):799-806.

Forbes EE, Groschwitz K, Abonia JP, Brandt EB, Cohen E, Blanchard C, Ahrens R, Seidu L, McKenzie A, Strait R, Finkelman FD, Foster PS, Matthaei KI, Rothenberg ME, Hogan SP. IL-9- and mast cell-mediated intestinal permeability predisposes to oral antigen hypersensitivity. *J Exp Med.* 2008 Apr 14;205(4):897-913.

Forestier C, Guelon D, Cluytens V, Gillart T, Sirot J, De Champs C. Oral probiotic and prevention of Pseudomonas aeruginosa infections: a randomized, double-blind, placebo-controlled pilot study in intensive care unit patients. *Crit Care.* 2008;12(3):R69.

Forget-Dubois N, Boivin M, Dionne G, Pierce T, Tremblay RE, Pérusse D. A longitudinal twin study of the genetic and environmental etiology of maternal hostile-reactive behavior during infancy and toddlerhood. *Infant Behav Dev.* 2007

Foster S, Hobbs C. *Medicinal Plants and Herbs.* Boston: Houghton Mifflin, 2002.

Fox RD, *Algoculture*. Doctorate Disseration, 1983 Jul.

Francavilla R, Lionetti E, Castellaneta SP, Magistà AM, Maurogiovanni G, Bucci N, De Canio A, Indrio F, Cavallo L, Ierardi E, Miniello VL. Inhibition of Helicobacter pylori infection in humans by Lactobacillus reuteri ATCC 55730 and effect on eradication therapy: a pilot study. *Helicobacter.* 2008 Apr;13(2):127-34.

Francis H, Fletcher G, Anthony C, Pickering C, Oldham L, Hadley E, Custovic A, Niven R. Clinical effects of air filters in homes of asthmatic adults sensitized and exposed to pet allergens. *Clin Exp Allergy.* 2003 Jan;33(1):101-5.

Frank PI, Morris JA, Hazell ML, Linehan MF, Frank TL. Long term prognosis in preschool children with wheeze: longitudinal postal questionnaire study 1993-2004. *BMJ.* 2008 Jun 21;336(7658):1423-6. 2008 Jun 16.

Frawley D, Lad V. *The Yoga of Herbs.* Sante Fe: Lotus Press, 1986.

Freedman BJ. A dietary free from additives in the management of allergic disease. *Clin Allergy.* 1977 Sep;7(5):417-21.

Fremont S, Moneret-Vautrin DA, Franck P, Morisset M, Croizier A, Codreanu F, Kanny G. Prospective study of sensitization and food allergy to flaxseed in 1317 subjects. *Eur Ann Allergy Clin Immunol.* 2010 Jun;42(3):103-11.

Frias J, Song YS, Martínez-Villaluenga C, González de Mejia E, Vidal-Valverde C. Immunoreactivity and amino acid content of fermented soybean products. *J Agric Food Chem.* 2008 Jan 9;56(1):99-105.

Friedman LS, Harvard Health Publ. Ed. *Controlling GERD and Chronic Heartburn.* Boston: Harvard Health, 2008.

Frumkin H. Beyond toxicity: human health and the natural environment. *Am J Prev Med.* 2001;20(3):234-40.

Fu G, Zhong Y, Li C, Li Y, Lin X, Liao B, Tsang EW, Wu K, Huang S. Epigenetic regulation of peanut allergen gene Ara h 3 in developing embryos. *Planta.* 2010 Apr;231(5):1049-60.

Fu JX. Measurement of MEFV in 66 cases of asthma in the convalescent stage and after treatment with Chinese herbs. *Zhong Xi Yi Jie He Za Zhi.* 1989 Nov;9(11):658-9, 644.

Fuiano N, Fusilli S, Passalacqua G, Incorvaia C. Allergen-specific immunoglobulin E in the skin and nasal mucosa of symptomatic and asymptomatic children sensitized to aeroallergens. *J Investig Allergol Clin Immunol.* 2010;20(5):425-30.

Fujii T, Ohtsuka Y, Lee T, Kudo T, Shoji H, Sato H, Nagata S, Shimizu T, Yamashiro Y. Bifidobacterium breve enhances transforming growth factor beta1 signaling by regulating Smad7 expression in preterm in-fants. *J Pediatr Gastroenterol Nutr.* 2006 Jul;43(1):83-8.

Fulgoni VL 3rd. Current protein intake in America: analysis of the National Health and Nutrition Examination Survey, 2003-2004. *Am J Clin Nutr.* 2008 May;87(5):1554S-1557S.

Furrie E. Probiotics and allergy. *Proc Nutr Soc.* 2005 Nov;64(4):465-9.

Furuhjelm C, Warstedt K, Larsson J, Fredriksson M, Böttcher MF, Fälth-Magnusson K, Duchén K. Fish oil supplementation in pregnancy and lactation may decrease the risk of infant allergy. *Acta Paediatr.* 2009 Sep;98(9):1461-7.

Gabory A, Attig L, Junien C. Sexual dimorphism in environmental epigenetic programming. *Mol Cell Endocrinol.* 2009 May 25;304(1-2):8-18. 2009 Mar 9.

Gamboa PM, Cáceres O, Antepara I, Sánchez-Monge R, Ahrazem O, Salcedo G, Barber D, Lombardero M, Sanz ML. Two different profiles of peach allergy in the north of Spain. *Allergy.* 2007 Apr;62(4):408-14.

Gao X, Wang W, Wei S, Li W. Review of pharmacological effects of Glycyrrhiza radix and its bioactive compounds. *Zhongguo Zhong Yao Za Zhi.* 2009 Nov;34(21):2695-700.

Garaczi E, Boros-Gyevi M, Bella Z, Csoma Z, Kemény L, Koreck A. Intranasal phototherapy is more effective than fexofenadine hydrochloride in the treatment of seasonal allergic rhinitis: results of a pilot study. *Photochem Photobiol.* 2011 Mar-Apr;87(2):474-7.

Garavello W, Somigliana E, Acaia B, Gaini I, Pignataro L, Gaini RM. Nasal lavage in pregnant women with seasonal allergic rhinitis: a randomized study. *Int Arch Allergy Immunol.* 2010;151(2):137-41. 2009 Sep 15. 19752567.

Garcia Gomez LJ, Sanchez-Muniz FJ. Review: cardiovascular effect of garlic (Allium sativum). *Arch Latinoam Nutr.* 2000 Sep;50(3):219-29.

García-Compeán D, González MV, Galindo G, Mar DA, Treviño JL, Martínez R, Bosques F, Maldonado H. Prevalence of gastroesophageal reflux disease in patients with extraesophageal symptoms referred from otolaryngology, allergy, and cardiology practices: a prospective study. *Dig Dis.* 2000;18(3):178-82.

Garcia-Marcos L, Canflanca IM, Garrido JB, Varela AL, Garcia-Hernandez G, Guillen Grima F, Gonzalez-Diaz C, Carvajal-Urueña I, Arnedo-Pena A, Busquets-Monge RM, Morales Suarez-Varela M, Blanco-Quiros A. Relationship of asthma and rhinoconjunctivitis with obesity, exercise and Mediterranean diet in Spanish schoolchildren. *Thorax.* 2007 Jun;62(6):503-8.

Gardner ML. Gastrointestinal absorption of intact proteins. Annu Rev Nutr. 1988;8:329-50.

Gary WK, Fanny WS, David SC. Factors associated with difference in prevalence of asthma in children from three cities in China: multicentre epidemiological survey. *BMJ.* 2004;329:1-4.

REFERENCES

Garzi A, Messina M, Frati F, Carfagna L, Zagordo L, Belcastro M, Parmiani S, Sensi L, Marcucci F. An extensively hydrolysed cow's milk formula improves clinical symptoms of gastroesophageal reflux and reduces the gastric emptying time in infants. *Allergol Immunopathol (Madr)*. 2002 Jan-Feb;30(1):36-41.

Gazdik F, Horvathova M, Gazdikova K, Jahnova E. The influence of selenium supplementation on the immunity of corticoid-dependent asthmatics. *Bratisl Lek Listy*. 2002;103(1):17-21.

Gazdik F, Kadrabova J, Gazdikova K. Decreased consumption of corticosteroids after selenium supplementation in corticoid-dependent asthmatics. *Bratisl Lek Listy*. 2002;103(1):22-5.

Geha RS, Beiser A, Ren C, Patterson R, Greenberger PA, Grammer LC, Ditto AM, Harris KE, Shaughnessy MA, Yarnold PR, Corren J, Saxon A. Multicenter, double-blind, placebo-controlled, multiple-challenge evaluation of reported reactions to monosodium glutamate. *J Allergy Clin Immunol*. 2000 Nov;106(5):973-80.

Gerez IF, Shek LP, Chng HH, Lee BW. Diagnostic tests for food allergy. *Singapore Med J*. 2010 Jan;51(1):4-9.

Gergen PJ, Arbes SJ Jr, Calatroni A, Mitchell HE, Zeldin DC. Total IgE levels and asthma prevalence in the US population: results from the National Health and Nutrition Examination Survey 2005-2006. *J Allergy Clin Immunol*. 2009 Sep;124(3):447-53. 2009 Aug 3.

Ghadioungui P. (transl.) *The Ebers Papyrus*. Academy of Scientific Research. Cairo, 1987.

Giampietro PG, Kjellman NI, Oldaeus G, Wouters-Wesseling W, Businco L. Hypoallergenicity of an extensively hydrolyzed whey formula. *Pediatr Allergy Immunol*. 2001 Apr;12(2):83-6.

Gibbons E. *Stalking the Healthful Herbs*. New York: David McKay, 1966.

Gibson RA. Docosa-hexaenoic acid (DHA) accumulation is regulated by the polyunsaturated fat content of the diet: Is it synthesis or is it incorporation? *Asia Pac J Clin Nutr*. 2004;13(Suppl):S78.

Gilbert CR, Arum SM, Smith CM. Vitamin D deficiency and chronic lung disease. *Can Respir J*. 2009 May-Jun;16(3):75-80.

Gill HS, Rutherfurd KJ, Cross ML, Gopal PK. Enhancement of immunity in the elderly by dietary supplementation with the probiotic Bifidobacterium lactis HN019. *Am J Clin Nutr*. 2001 Dec;74(6):833-9.

Gillman A, Douglass JA. What do asthmatics have to fear from food and additive allergy? *Clin Exp Allergy*. 2010 Sep;40(9):1295-302.

Ginde AA, Mansbach JM, Camargo CA Jr. Association between serum 25-hydroxyvitamin D level and upper respiratory tract infection in the Third National Health and Nutrition Examination Survey. *Arch Intern Med*. 2009 Feb 23;169(4):384-90.

Glück U, Gebbers J. Ingested probiotics reduce nasal colonization with pathogenic bacteria (Staphylococcus aureus, Streptococcus pneumoniae, and b-hemolytic streptococci. *Am J. Clin. Nutr*. 2003;77:517-520.

Goedsche K, Förster M, Kroegel C, Uhlemann C. Repeated cold water stimulations (hydrotherapy according to Kneipp) in patients with COPD. *Forsch Komplementmed*. 2007 Jun;14(3):158-66.

Goel V, Dolan RJ. The functional anatomy of humor: segregating cognitive and affective components. *Nat Neurosci*. 2001;4:237-8.

Gohil K, Packer L. Bioflavonoid-Rich Botanical Extracts Show Antioxidant and Gene Regulatory Activity. *Ann N Y Acad Sci*. 2002;957:70-7.

Goldin BR, Adlercreutz H, Dwyer JT, Swenson L, Warram JH, Gorbach SL. Effect of diet on excretion of estrogens in pre- and postmenopausal women. *Cancer Res*. 1981 Sep;41(9 Pt 2):3771-3.

Goldin BR, Adlercreutz H, Gorbach SL, Warram JH, Dwyer JT, Swenson L, Woods MN. Estrogen excretion patterns and plasma levels in vegetarian and omnivorous women. *N Engl J Med*. 1982 Dec 16;307(25):1542-7.

Goldin BR, Swenson L, Dwyer J, Sexton M, Gorbach SL. Effect of diet and Lactobacillus acidophilus supplements on human fecal bacterial enzymes. *J Natl Cancer Inst*. 1980 Feb;64(2):255-61.

Goldstein JL, Aisenberg J, Zakko SF, Berger MF, Dodge WE. Endoscopic ulcer rates in healthy subjects associated with use of aspirin (81 mg q.d.) alone or coadministered with celecoxib or naproxen: a randomized, 1-week trial. *Dig Dis Sci*. 2008 Mar;53(3):647-56.

Golub E. *The Limits of Medicine*. New York: Times Books, 1994.

Gonzales M, Malcoe LH, Myers OB, Espinoza J. Risk factors for asthma and cough among Hispanic children in the southwestern United States of America, 2003-2004. *Rev Panam Salud Publica*. 2007 May;21(5):274-81.

González Alvarez R, Arruzazabala ML. Current views of the mechanism of action of prophylactic antiallergic drugs. *Allergol Immunopathol (Madr)*. 1981 Nov-Dec;9(6):501-8.

González J, Fernández M, García Fragoso L. Exclusive breastfeeding reduces asthma in a group of children from the Caguas municipality of Puerto Rico. *Bol Asoc Med P R*. 2010 Jan-Mar;102(1):10-2.

González Morales JE, Leal de Hernández L, González Spencer D. Asthma associated with gastroesophageal reflux. *Rev Alerg Mex*. 1998 Jan-Feb;45(1):16-21.

González-Pérez A, Aponte Z, Vidaurre CF, Rodríguez LA. Anaphylaxis epidemiology in patients with and patients without asthma: a United Kingdom database review. *J Allergy Clin Immunol*. 2010 May;125(5):1098-1104.e1.

371

González-Sánchez R, Trujillo X, Trujillo-Hernández B, Vásquez C, Huerta M, Elizalde A. Forskolin versus sodium cromoglycate for prevention of asthma attacks: a single-blinded clinical trial. *J Int Med Res.* 2006 Mar-Apr;34(2):200-7.

Gordon BR. Patch testing for allergies. *Curr Opin Otolaryngol Head Neck Surg.* 2010 Jun;18(3):191-4.

Gore KV, Rao AK, Guruswamy MN. Physiological studies with Tylophora asthmatica in bronchial asthma. *Indian J Med Res.* 1980 Jan;71:144-8.

Goren AI, Hellmann S. Changes prevalence of asthma among schoolchildren in Israel. *Eur Respir J.* 1997;10:2279-2284.

Gotteland M, Poliak L, Cruchet S, Brunser O. Effect of regular ingestion of Saccharomyces boulardii plus inulin or Lactobacillus acidophilus LB in children colonized by Helicobacter pylori. *Acta Paediatr.* 2005 Dec;94(12):1747-51.

Govindan S, Viswanathan S, Vijayasekaran V, Alagappan R. A pilot study on the clinical efficacy of Solanum xanthocarpum and Solanum trilobatum in bronchial asthma. *J Ethnopharmacol.* 1999 Aug;66(2):205-10.

Govindan S, Viswanathan S, Vijayasekaran V, Alagappan R. Further studies on the clinical efficacy of Solanum xanthocarpum and Solanum trilobatum in bronchial asthma. *Phytother Res.* 2004 Oct;18(10):805-9.

Grant WB, Holick MF. Benefits and requirements of vitamin D for optimal health: a review. *Altern Med Rev.* 2005 Jun;10(2):94-111.

Grant WB. Hypothesis—ultraviolet-B irradiance and vitamin D reduce the risk of viral infections and thus their sequelae, including autoimmune diseases and some cancers. *Photochem Photobiol.* 2008 Mar-Apr;84(2):356-65. 2008 Jan 7.

Gray H. *Anatomy, Descriptive and Surgical.* 15th Edition. New York: Random House, 1977.

Gray-Davison F. *Ayurvedic Healing.* New York: Keats, 2002.

Greskevitch M, Kullman G, Bang KM, Mazurek JM. Respiratory disease in agricultural workers: mortality and morbidity statistics. *J Agromedicine.* 2007;12(3):5-10.

Griffith HW. *Healing Herbs: The Essential Guide.* Tucson: Fisher Books, 2000.

Grimm T, Chovanová Z, Muchová J, Sumegová K, Liptáková A, Duracková Z, Högger P. Inhibition of NF-kappaB activation and MMP-9 secretion by plasma of human volunteers after ingestion of maritime pine bark extract (Pycnogenol). *J Inflamm (Lond).* 2006 Jan 27;3:1.

Grimm T, Schäfer A, Högger P. Antioxidant activity and inhibition of matrix metalloproteinases by metabolites of maritime pine bark extract (pycnogenol). *Free Radic Biol Med.* 2004 Mar 15;36(6):811-22.

Grimm T, Skrabala R, Chovanová Z, Muchová J, Sumegová K, Liptáková A, Duracková Z, Högger P. Single and multiple dose pharmacokinetics of maritime pine bark extract (pycnogenol) after oral administration to healthy volunteers. *BMC Clin Pharmacol.* 2006 Aug 3;6:4.

Gropper SS, Smith JL, Groff JL. *Advanced nutrition and human metabolism.* Belmonth, CA: Wadsworth Publ, 2008.

Groschwitz KR, Ahrens R, Osterfeld H, Gurish MF, Han X, Abrink M, Finkelman FD, Pejler G, Hogan SP. Mast cells regulate homeostatic intestinal epithelial migration and barrier function by a chymase/Mcpt4-dependent mechanism. *Proc Natl Acad Sci U S A.* 2009 Dec 29;106(52):22381-6.

Grosser BI, Monti-Bloch L, Jennings-White C, Berliner DL. Behavioral and electrophysiological effects of androstadienone, a human pheromone. *Psychoneuroendocrinology.* 2000 Apr;25(3):289-99.

Grzanna R, Lindmark L, Frondoza CG. Ginger—an herbal medicinal product with broad anti-inflammatory actions. *J Med Food.* 2005 Summer;8(2):125-32.

Guandalini S. The influence of gluten: weaning recommendations for healthy children and children at risk for celiac disease. *Nestle Nutr Workshop Ser Pediatr Program.* 2007;60:139-51; discussion 151-5.

Guerin M, Huntley ME, Olaizola M. Haematococcus astaxanthin: applications for human health and nutrition. *Trends Biotechnol.* 2003 May;21(5):210-6.

Guinot P, Brambilla C, Duchier J, Braquet P, Bonvoisin B, Cournot A. Effect of BN 52063, a specific PAF-acether antagonist, on bronchial provocation test to allergens in asthmatic patients. A preliminary study. *Prostaglandins.* 1987 Nov;34(5):723-31.

Gundermann KJ, Müller J. Phytodolor—effects and efficacy of a herbal medicine. *Wien Med Wochenschr.* 2007;157(13-14):343-7.

Gupta I, Gupta V, Parihar A, Gupta S, Lüdtke R, Safayhi H, Ammon HP. Effects of Boswellia serrata gum resin in patients with bronchial asthma: results of a double-blind, placebo-controlled, 6-week clinical study. *Eur J Med Res.* 1998 Nov 17;3(11):511-4.

Gupta R, Sheikh A, Strachan DP, Anderson HR (2006) Time trends in allergic disorders in the UK. *Thorax;* published online. doi: 10.1136/thx.2004.038844.

Gupta S, George P, Gupta V, Tandon VR, Sundaram KR. Tylophora indica in bronchial asthma—a double blind study. *Indian J Med Res.* 1979 Jun;69:981-9.

Gutmanis J. *Hawaiian Herbal Medicine.* Waipahu, HI: Island Heritage, 2001.

Haggag EG, Abou-Moustafa MA, Boucher W, Theoharides TC. The effect of a herbal water-extract on histamine release from mast cells and on allergic asthma. *J Herb Pharmacother.* 2003;3(4):41-54.

REFERENCES

Haines JL, Ter-Minassian M, Bazyk A, Gusella JF, Kim DJ, Terwedow H, Pericak-Vance MA, Rimmler JB, Haynes CS, Roses AD, Lee A, Shaner B, Menold M, Seboun E, Fitoussi RP, Gartioux C, Reyes C, Ribierre F, Gyapay G, Weissenbach J, Hauser SL, Goodkin DE, Lincoln R, Usuku K, Oksenberg JR, et al. A complete genomic screen for multiple sclerosis underscores a role for the major histocompatability complex. The Multiple Sclerosis Genetics Group. *Nat Genet.* 1996 Aug;13(4):469-71..

Halász A, Cserháti E. The prognosis of bronchial asthma in childhood in Hungary: a long-term follow-up. *J Asthma.* 2002 Dec;39(8):693-9.

Halken S, Hansen KS, Jacobsen HP, Estmann A, Faelling AE, Hansen LG, Kier SR, Lassen K, Lintrup M, Mortensen S, Ibsen KK, Osterballe O, Host A. Comparison of a partially hydrolyzed infant formula with two extensively hydrolyzed formulas for allergy prevention: a prospective, randomized study. *Pediatr Allergy Immunol.* 2000 Aug;11(3):149-61.

Halpern GM, Miller AH. *Medicinal Mushrooms: Ancient Remedies for Modern Ailments.* New York: M. Evans, 2002.

Hamasaki Y, Kobayashi I, Hayasaki R, Zaitu M, Muro E, Yamamoto S, Ichimaru T, Miyazaki S. The Chinese herbal medicine, shinpi-to, inhibits IgE-mediated leukotriene synthesis in rat basophilic leukemia-2H3 cells. *J Ethnopharmacol.* 1997 Apr;56(2):123-31.

Hamelmann E, Beyer K, Gruber C, Lau S, Matricardi PM, Nickel R, Niggemann B, Wahn U. Primary prevention of allergy: avoiding risk or providing protection? *Clin Exp Allergy.* 2008 Feb;38(2):233-45.

Hamilton RG. Clinical laboratory assessment of immediate-type hypersensitivity. *J Allergy Clin Immunol.* 2010 Feb;125(2 Suppl 2):S284-96.

Hammond BG, Mayhew DA, Kier LD, Mast RW, Sander WJ. Safety assessment of DHA-rich microalgae from Schizochytrium sp. *Regul Toxicol Pharmacol.* 2002 Apr;35(2 Pt 1):255-65.

Han ER, Choi IS, Kim HK, Kang YW, Park JG, Lim JR, Seo JH, Choi JH. Inhaled corticosteroid-related tooth problems in asthmatics. *J Asthma.* 2009 Mar;46(2):160-4.

Han SN, Leka LS, Lichtenstein AH, Ausman LM, Meydani SN. Effect of a therapeutic lifestyle change diet on immune functions of moderately hypercholesterolemic humans. *J Lipid Res.* 2003 Dec;44(12):2304-10.

Hansen KS, Ballmer-Weber BK, Lüttkopf D, Skov PS, Wüthrich B, Bindslev-Jensen C, Vieths S, Poulsen LK. Roasted hazelnuts—allergenic activity evaluated by double-blind, placebo-controlled food challenge. *Allergy.* 2003 Feb;58(2):132-8.

Hansen KS, Ballmer-Weber BK, Sastre J, Lidholm J, Andersson K, Oberhofer H, Lluch-Bernal M, Ostling J, Mattsson L, Schocker F, Vieths S, Poulsen LK. Component-resolved in vitro diagnosis of hazelnut allergy in Europe. *J Allergy Clin Immunol.* 2009 May;123(5):1134-41, 1141.e1-3.

Hansen KS, Khinchi MS, Skov PS, Bindslev-Jensen C, Poulsen LK, Malling HJ. Food allergy to apple and specific immunotherapy with birch pollen. *Mol Nutr Food Res.* 2004 Nov;48(6):441-8.

Haranath PS, Shyamalakumari S. Experimental study on mode of action of Tylophora asthmatica in bronchial asthma. *Indian J Med Res.* 1975 May;63(5):661-70.

Harrington JJ, Lee-Chiong T Jr. Sleep and older patients. *Clin Chest Med.* 2007 Dec;28(4):673-84, v.

Hartz C, Lauer I, Del Mar San Miguel Moncin M, Cistero-Bahima A, Foetisch K, Lidholm J, Vieths S, Scheurer S. Comparison of IgE-Binding Capacity, Cross-Reactivity and Biological Potency of Allergenic Non-Specific Lipid Transfer Proteins from Peach, Cherry and Hazelnut. *Int Arch Allergy Immunol.* 2010 Jun 17;153(4):335-346.

Harvald B, Hauge M: Hereditary factors elucidated by twin studies. In *Genetics and the Epidemiology of Chronic Disease.* Edited by Neel JV, Shaw MV, Schull WJ. Washington, DC: Dept Health, Education and Welfare, 1965:64-76.

Hassan AM. Selenium status in patients with aspirin-induced asthma. *Ann Clin Biochem.* 2008 Sep;45(Pt 5):508-12.

Hasselmark L, Malmgren R, Zetterström O, Unge G. Selenium supplementation in intrinsic asthma. *Allergy.* 1993 Jan;48(1):30-6.

Hata K, Ishikawa K, Hori K, Konishi T. Differentiation-inducing activity of lupeol, a lupane-type triterpene from Chinese dandelion root (Hokouei-kon), on a mouse melanoma cell line. *Biol Pharm Bull.* 2000 Aug;23(8):962-7.

Hattori K, Sasai M, Yamamoto A, Taniuchi S, Kojima T, Kobayashi Y, Iwamoto H, Yaeshima T, Hayasawa H. Intestinal flora of infants with cow milk hypersensitivity fed on casein-hydrolyzed formula supplemented raffinose. *Arerugi.* 2000 Dec;49(12):1146-55.

Heaney LG, Brightling CE, Menzies-Gow A, Stevenson M, Niven RM; British Thoracic Society Difficult Asthma Network. Refractory asthma in the UK: cross-sectional findings from a UK multicentre registry. *Thorax.* 2010 Sep;65(9):787-94.

Heaney RP, Dowell MS. Absorbability of the calcium in a high-calcium mineral water. *Osteoporos Int.* 1994 Nov;4(6):323-4.

Heap GA, van Heel DA. Genetics and pathogenesis of coeliac disease. *Semin Immunol.* May 13 2009.

Heine RG, Nethercote M, Rosenbaum J, Allen KJ. Emerging management concepts for eosinophilic esophagitis in children. *J Gastroenterol Hepatol.* 2011 May 4.

Hemmer W, Focke M, Marzban G, Swoboda I, Jarisch R, Laimer M. Identification of Bet v 1-related allergens in fig and other Moraceae fruits. *Clin Exp Allergy.* 2010 Apr;40(4):679-87.

Hendel B, Ferreira P. *Water & Salt: The Essence of Life.* Gaithersburg: Natural Resources, 2003.

Herbert V. Vitamin B12: Plant sources, requirements, and assay. *Am J Clin Nutr.* 1988;48:852-858.

Herman PM, Drost LM. Evaluating the clinical relevance of food sensitivity tests: a single subject experiment. *Altern Med Rev.* 2004 Jun;9(2):198-207.

Herzog AM, Black KA, Fountaine DJ, Knotts TR. Reflection and attentional recovery as two distinctive benefits of restorative environments. *J Environ Psychol.* 1997;17:165-70.

Hess-Kosa K. *Indoor Air Quality: Sampling Methodologies.* Boca Raton: CRC Press, 2002.

Heyman M, Grasset E, Ducroc R, Desjeux JF. Antigen absorption by the jejunal epithelium of children with cow's milk allergy. *Pediatr Res.* 1988 Aug;24(2):197-202.

Hide DW, Matthews S, Tariq S, Arshad SH. Allergen avoidance in infancy and allergy at 4 years of age. *Allergy.* 1996 Feb;51(2):89-93.

Hijazi Z, Molla AM, Al-Habashi H, Muawad WM, Molla AM, Sharma PN. Intestinal permeability is increased in bronchial asthma. *Arch Dis Child.* 2004 Mar;89(3):227-9.

Hill J, Micklewright A, Lewis S, Britton J. Investigation of the effect of short-term change in dietary magnesium intake in asthma. *Eur Respir J.* 1997 Oct;10(10):2225-9.

Hirose Y, Murosaki S, Yamamoto Y, Yoshikai Y, Tsuru T. Daily intake of heat-killed Lactobacillus plantarum L-137 augments acquired immunity in healthy adults. *J Nutr.* 2006 Dec;136(12):3069-73.

Hobbs C. *Medicinal Mushrooms.* Summertown, TN: Botanica Press, 2003.

Hobbs C. *Stress & Natural Healing.* Loveland, CO: Interweave Press, 1997.

Hoff S, Seiler H, Heinrich J, Kompauer I, Nieters A, Becker N, Nagel G, Gedrich K, Karg G, Wolfram G, Linseisen J. Allergic sensitisation and allergic rhinitis are associated with n-3 polyunsaturated fatty acids in the diet and in red blood cell membranes. *Eur J Clin Nutr.* 2005 Sep;59(9):1071-80.

Hoffmann D. *Holistic Herbal.* London: Thorsons, 2002.

Hofmann D, Hecker M, Völp A. Efficacy of dry extract of ivy leaves in children with bronchial asthma-a review of randomized controlled trials. *Phytomedicine.* 2003 Mar;10(2-3):213-20.

Höiby AS, Strand V, Robinson DS, Sager A, Rak S. Efficacy, safety, and immunological effects of a 2-year immunotherapy with Depigoid birch pollen extract: a randomized, double-blind, placebo-controlled study. *Clin Exp Allergy.* 2010 Jul;40(7):1062-70.

Holick MF. Sunlight and vitamin D for bone health and prevention of autoimmune diseases, cancers, and cardiovascular disease. *Am J Clin Nutr.* 2004 Dec;80(6 Suppl):1678S-88S.

Holick MF. The vitamin D deficiency pandemic and consequences for nonskeletal health: mechanisms of action. *Mol Aspects Med.* 2008 Dec;29(6):361-8

Holick MF. Vitamin D status: measurement, interpretation, and clinical application. *Ann Epidemiol.* 2009 Feb;19(2):73-8.

Holladay, S.D. Prenatal Immunotoxicant Exposure and Postnatal Autoimmune Disease. *Environ Health Perspect.* 1999; 107(suppl 5):687-691.

Holt GA. *Food & Drug Interactions.* Chicago: Precept Press, 1998, 83.

Homma M, Oka K, Niitsuma T, Itoh H. A novel 11 beta-hydroxysteroid dehydrogenase inhibitor contained in saiboku-to, a herbal remedy for steroid-dependent bronchial asthma. *J Pharm Pharmacol.* 1994 Apr;46(4):305-9.

Hönscheid A, Rink L, Haase H. T-lymphocytes: a target for stimulatory and inhibitory effects of zinc ions. *Endocr Metab Immune Disord Drug Targets.* 2009 Jun;9(2):132-44.

Hooper R, Calvert J, Thompson RL, Deetlefs ME, Burney P. Urban/rural differences in diet and atopy in South Africa. *Allergy.* 2008 Apr;63(4):425-31.

Hope BE, Massey DG, Fournier-Massey G. Hawaiian materia medica for asthma. *Hawaii Med J.* 1993 Jun;52(6):160-6.

Horak E, Morass B, Ulmer H. Association between environmental tobacco smoke exposure and wheezing disorders in Austrian preschool children. *Swiss Med Wkly.* 2007 Nov 3;137(43-44):608-13.

Horrobin DF. Effects of evening primrose oil in rheumatoid arthritis. *Ann Rheum Dis.* 1989 Nov;48(11):965-6.

Hospers IC, de Vries-Vrolijk K, Brand PL. Double-blind, placebo-controlled cow's milk challenge in children with alleged cow's milk allergies, performed in a general hospital: diagnosis rejected in two-thirds of the children. *Ned Tijdschr Geneeskd.* 2006 Jun 10;150(23):1292-7.

Hosseini S, Pishnamazi S, Sadrzadeh SM, Farid F, Farid R, Watson RR. Pycnogenol((R)) in the Management of Asthma. *J Med Food.* 2001 Winter;4(4):201-209.

Hougee S, Vriesema AJ, Wijering SC, Knippels LM, Folkerts G, Nijkamp FP, Knol J, Garssen J. Oral treatment with probiotics reduces allergic symptoms in ovalbumin-sensitized mice: a bacterial strain comparative study. *Int Arch Allergy Immunol.* 2010;151(2):107-17. 2009 Sep 15.

374

REFERENCES

Houle CR, Leo HL, Clark NM. A developmental, community, and psychosocial approach to food allergies in children. *Curr Allergy Asthma Rep.* 2010 Sep;10(5):381-6.

Houssen ME, Ragab A, Mesbah A, El-Samanoudy AZ, Othman G, Moustafa AF, Badria FA. Natural anti-inflammatory products and leukotriene inhibitors as complementary therapy for bronchial asthma. *Clin Biochem.* 2010 Jul;43(10-11):887-90.

Hsieh KH. Evaluation of efficacy of traditional Chinese medicines in the treatment of childhood bronchial asthma: clinical trial, immunological tests and animal study. Taiwan Asthma Study Group. *Pediatr Allergy Immunol.* 1996 Aug;7(3):130-40.

Hsu CH, Lu CM, Chang TT. Efficacy and safety of modified Mai-Men-Dong-Tang for treatment of allergic asthma. *Pediatr Allergy Immunol.* 2005;16:76-81.

Hu C, Kitts DD. Antioxidant, prooxidant, and cytotoxic activities of solvent-fractionated dandelion (Taraxacum officinale) flower extracts in vitro. *J Agric Food Chem.* 2003 Jan 1;51(1):301-10.

Hu C, Kitts DD. Dandelion (Taraxacum officinale) flower extract suppresses both reactive oxygen species and nitric oxide and prevents lipid oxidation in vitro. *Phytomedicine.* 2005 Aug;12(8):588-97.

Hu C, Kitts DD. Luteolin and luteolin-7-O-glucoside from dandelion flower suppress iNOS and COX-2 in RAW264.7 cells. *Mol Cell Biochem.* 2004 Oct;265(1-2):107-13.

Huang D, Ou B, Prior RL. The chemistry behind antioxidant capacity assays. *J Agric Food Chem.* 2005 Mar 23;53(6):1841-56.

Huang M, Wang W, Wei S. Investigation on medicinal plant resources of Glycyrrhiza uralensis in China and chemical assessment of its underground part. *Zhongguo Zhong Yao Za Zhi.* 2010 Apr;35(8):947-52.

Huntley A, Ernst E. Herbal medicines for asthma: a systematic review. *Thorax.* 2000, 55:925-929.

Hur YM, Rushton JP. Genetic and environmental contributions to prosocial behaviour in 2- to 9-year-old South Korean twins. *Biol Lett.* 2007 Dec 22;3(6):664-6.

Husby S. Dietary antigens: uptake and humoral immunity in man. *APMIS Suppl.* 1988;1:1-40.

Hyndman SJ, Vickers LM, Htut T, Maunder JW, Peock A, Higenbottam TW. A randomized trial of dehumidification in the control of house dust mite. *Clin Exp Allergy.* 2000 Aug;30(8):1172-80.

Ibero M, Boné J, Martín B, Martínez J. Evaluation of an extensively hydrolysed casein formula (Damira 2000) in children with allergy to cow's milk proteins. *Allergol Immunopathol (Madr).* 2010 Mar-Apr;38(2):60-8.

Ibrahim AR, Kawamoto S, Nishimura M, Pak S, Aki T, Diaz-Perales A, Salcedo G, Asturias JA, Hayashi T, Ono K. A new lipid transfer protein homolog identified as an IgE-binding antigen from Japanese cedar pollen. *Biosci Biotechnol Biochem.* 2010;74(3):504-9.

Inbar O, Dotan R, Dlin RA, Neuman I, Bar-Or O. Breathing dry or humid air and exercise-induced asthma during swimming. *Eur J Appl Physiol Occup Physiol.* 1980;44(1):43-50.

Indrio F, Ladisa G, Mautone A, Montagna O. Effect of a fermented formula on thymus size and stool pH in healthy term infants. *Pediatr Res.* 2007 Jul;62(1):98-100.

Innis SM, Hansen JW. Plasma fatty acid responses, metabolic effects, and safety of microalgal and fungal oils rich in arachidonic and docosahexaenoic acids in adults. *Am J Clin Nutr.* 1996 Aug;64(2):159-67.

Ionescu JG. New insights in the pathogenesis of atopic disease. *J Med Life.* 2009 Apr-Jun;2(2):146-54.

Iribarren C, Tolstykh IV, Miller MK, Eisner MD. Asthma and the prospective risk of anaphylactic shock and other allergy diagnoses in a large integrated health care delivery system. *Ann Allergy Asthma Immunol.* 2010 May;104(5):371-7.

ISAAC. The International Study of Asthma and Allergies in Childhood (ISAAC) Steering Committee. Worldwide variation in prevalence of symptoms of asthma, allergic rhinoconjunctivitis, and atopic eczema: ISAAC. *Lancet.* 1998;351:1225-1232.

Ishida Y, Nakamura F, Kanzato H, Sawada D, Hirata H, Nishimura A, Kajimoto O, Fujiwara S. Clinical effects of Lactobacillus acidophilus strain L-92 on perennial allergic rhinitis: a double-blind, placebo-controlled study. *J Dairy Sci.* 2005 Feb;88(2):527-33.

Ishtiaq M, Hanif W, Khan MA, Ashraf M, Butt AM. An ethnomedicinal survey and documentation of important medicinal folklore food phytonims of flora of Samahni valley, (Azad Kashmir) Pakistan. *Pak J Biol Sci.* 2007 Jul 1;10(13):2241-56.

Ivory K, Chambers SJ, Pin C, Prieto E, Arqués JL, Nicoletti C. Oral delivery of Lactobacillus casei Shirota modifies allergen-induced immune responses in allergic rhinitis. *Clin Exp Allergy.* 2008 Aug;38(8):1282-9.

Izbicki G, Chavko R, Banauch GI, Weiden MD, Berger KI, Aldrich TK, Hall C, Kelly KJ, Prezant DJ. World trade center "sarcoid-like" granulomatous pulmonary disease in New York City fire department rescue workers. *Chest.* 2007 May;131(5):1414-23.

Izquierdo JL, Martín A, de Lucas P, Rodríguez-González-Moro JM, Almonacid C, Paravisini A. Misdiagnosis of patients receiving inhaled therapies in primary care. *Int J Chron Obstruct Pulmon Dis.* 2010 Aug 9;5:241-9.

Izumi K, Aihara M, Ikezawa Z. Effects of non steroidal antiinflammatory drugs (NSAIDs) on immediate-type food allergy analysis of Japanese cases from 1998 to 2009. *Arerugi.* 2009 Dec;58(12):1629-39.

Jaber R. Respiratory and allergic diseases: from upper respiratory tract infections to asthma. *Prim Care*. 2002 Jun;29(2):231-61.

Jackson DJ, Lemanske RF Jr. The role of respiratory virus infections in childhood asthma inception. *Immunol Allergy Clin North Am*. 2010 Nov;30(4):513-22, vi.

Jacobs DE, Wilson J, Dixon SL, Smith J, Evens A. The relationship of housing and population health: a 30-year retrospective analysis. *Environ Health Perspect*. 2009 Apr;117(4):597-604. 2008 Dec 16.

Jagetia GC, Aggarwal BB. "Spicing up" of the immune system by curcumin. *J Clin Immunol*. 2007 Jan;27(1):19-35.

Jagetia GC, Nayak V, Vidyasagar MS. Evaluation of the antineoplastic activity of guduchi (Tinospora cordifolia) in cultured HeLa cells. *Cancer Lett*. 1998 May 15;127(1-2):71-82.

Jagetia GC, Rao SK. Evaluation of Cytotoxic Effects of Dichloromethane Extract of Guduchi (Tinospora cordifolia Miers ex Hook F & THOMS) on Cultured HeLa Cells. *Evid Based Complement Alternat Med*. 2006 Jun;3(2):267-72.

Jahnova E, Horvathova M, Gazdik F, Weissova S. Effects of selenium supplementation on expression of adhesion molecules in corticoid-dependent asthmatics. *Bratisl Lek Listy*. 2002;103(1):12-6.

Jaiswal M, Prajapati PK, Patgiri BJ Ravishankar B. A Comparative Pharmaco - Clinical Study on Anti-Asthmatic Effect of Shirisharishta Prepared by Bark, Sapwood and Heartwood of Albizia Lebbeck. *J Res Ayurv*. 2006;27(3):67-74.

Jaiswal M, Prajapati PK, Patgiri BJ, Ravishankar B. Clinical Study on Anti-Asthmatic Effect of Shirisharishta Prepared by Bark, Sapwood and Heartwood of Albizia Lebbeck. *Pharmaco*. 2006 27(3): 67-74

Janson C, Anto J, Burney P, Chinn S, de Marco R, Heinrich J, Jarvis D, Kuenzli N, Leynaert B, Luczynska C, Neukirch F, Svanes C, Sunyer J, Wjst M; European Community Respiratory Health Survey II. The European Community Respiratory Health Survey: what are the main results so far? European Community Respiratory Health Survey II. *Eur Respir J*. 2001 Sep;18(3):598-611.

Jarocka-Cyrta E, Baniukiewicz A, Wasilewska J, Pawlak J, Kaczmarski M. Focal villous atrophy of the duodenum in children who have outgrown cow's milk allergy. Chromoendoscopy and magnification endoscopy evaluation. *Med Wieku Rozwoj*. 2007 Apr-Jun;11(2 Pt 1):123-7.

Jayaprakasam B, Doddaga S, Wang R, Holmes D, Goldfarb J, Li XM. Licorice flavonoids inhibit eotaxin-1 secretion by human fetal lung fibroblasts in vitro. *J Agric Food Chem*. 2009 Feb 11;57(3):820-5.

Jennings S, Prescott SL. Early dietary exposures and feeding practices: role in pathogenesis and prevention of allergic disease? *Postgrad Med J*. 2010 Feb;86(1012):94-9.

Jensen B. *Foods that Heal*. Garden City Park, NY: Avery Publ, 1988, 1993.

Jensen B. *Nature Has a Remedy*. Los Angeles: Keats, 2001.

Jeon HJ, Kang HJ, Jung HJ, Kang YS, Lim CJ, Kim YM, Park EH. Anti-inflammatory activity of Taraxacum officinale. *J Ethnopharmacol*. 2008 Jan 4;115(1):82-8.

Jernelöv S, Höglund CO, Axelsson J, Axén J, Grönneberg R, Grunewald J, Stierna P, Lekander M. Effects of examination stress on psychological responses, sleep and allergic symptoms in atopic and non-atopic students. *Int J Behav Med*. 2009;16(4):305-10.

Johansson G, Holmén A, Persson L, Högstedt B, Wassén C, Ottova L, Gustafsson JA. Long-term effects of a change from a mixed diet to a lacto-vegetarian diet on human urinary and faecal mutagenic activity. *Mutagenesis*. 1998 Mar;13(2):167-71.

Johansson G, Holmén A, Persson L, Högstedt B, Wassén C, Ottova L, Gustafsson JA. Dietary influence on some proposed risk factors for colon cancer: fecal and urinary mutagenic activity and the activity of some intestinal bacterial enzymes. *Cancer Detect Prev*. 1997;21(3):258-66.

Johansson G, Holmén A, Persson L, Högstedt B, Wassén C, Ottova L, Gustafsson JA. The effect of a shift from a mixed diet to a lacto-vegetarian diet on human urinary and fecal mutagenic activity. *Carcinogenesis*. 1992 Feb;13(2):153-7.

Johansson G, Ravald N. Comparison of some salivary variables between vegetarians and omnivores. *Eur J Oral Sci*. 1995 Apr;103(2 (Pt 1)):95-8.

Johari H. *Ayurvedic Massage: Traditional Indian Techniques for Balancing Body and Mind*. Rochester, VT: Healing Arts, 1996.

Johnson LM. Gitksan medicinal plants—cultural choice and efficacy. *J Ethnobiol Ethnomed*. 2006 Jun 21;2:29.

Jones MA, Silman AJ, Whiting S, *et al*. Occurrence of rheumatoid arthritis is not increased in the first degree relatives of a population based inception cohort of inflammatory polyarthritis. *Ann Rheum Dis*. 1996;55(2): 89-93.

José RJ, Roberts J, Bakerly ND. The effectiveness of a social marketing model on case-finding for COPD in a deprived inner city population. *Prim Care Respir J*. 2010 Jun;19(2):104-8.

Joseph SP, Borrell LN, Shapiro A. Self-reported lifetime asthma and nativity status in U.S. children and adolescents: results from the National Health and Nutrition Examination Survey 1999-2004. *J Health Care Poor Underserved*. 2010 May;21(2 Suppl):125-39.

REFERENCES

Juergens UR, Dethlefsen U, Steinkamp G, Gillissen A, Repges R, Vetter H. Anti-inflammatory activity of 1.8-cineol (eucalyptol) in bronchial asthma: a double-blind placebo-controlled trial. *Respir Med.* 2003 Mar;97(3):250-6.

Julkunen-Tiitto R. A chemotaxonomic survey of phenolics in leaves of northern Salicaceae species. Phytochemistry. 1986;25(3):663-667.

Jung HA, Yokozawa T, Kim BW, Jung JH, Choi JS. Selective inhibition of prenylated flavonoids from Sophora flavescens against BACE1 and cholinesterases. *Am J Chin Med.* 2010;38(2):415-29.

Jurenka JS. Anti-inflammatory properties of curcumin, a major constituent of Curcuma longa: a review of preclinical and clinical research. *Altern Med Rev.* 2009 Feb;14(2):141-153.

Juvonen R, Bloigu A, Peitso A, Silvennoinen-Kassinen S, Saikku P, Leinonen M, Hassi J, Harju T. Training improves physical fitness and decreases CRP also in asthmatic conscripts. *J Asthma.* 2008 Apr;45(3):237-42.

Kähkönen MP, Hopia AI, Vuorela HJ, Rauha JP, Pihlaja K, Kujala TS, Heinonen M. Antioxidant activity of plant extracts containing phenolic compounds. *J Agric Food Chem.* 1999 Oct;47(10):3954-62.

Kaila M, Vanto T, Valovirta E, Koivikko A, Juntunen-Backman K. Diagnosis of food allergy in Finland: survey of pediatric practices. *Pediatr Allergy Immunol.* 2000 Nov;11(4):246-9.

Kalach N, Benhamou PH, Campeotto F, Dupont Ch. Anemia impairs small intestinal absorption measured by intestinal permeability in children. *Eur Ann Allergy Clin Immunol.* 2007 Jan;39(1):20-2.

Kaliner M, Shelhamer JH, Borson B, Nadel J, Patow C, Marom Z. Human respiratory mucus. *Am Rev Respir Dis.* 1986 Sep;134(3):612-21.

Kalliomäki M, Salminen S, Arvilommi H, Kero P, Koskinen P, Isolauri E. Probiotics in primary prevention of atopic disease: a randomised placebo-controlled trial. *Lancet.* 2001 Apr 7;357(9262):1076-9.

Kamdar T, Bryce PJ. Immunotherapy in food allergy. Immunotherapy. 2010 May;2(3):329-38.

Kang SK, Kim JK, Ahn SH, Oh JE, Kim JH, Lim DH, Son BK. Relationship between silent gastroesophageal reflux and food sensitization in infants and young children with recurrent wheezing. *J Korean Med Sci.* 2010 Mar;25(3):425-8.

Kanny G, Grignon G, Dauca M, Guedenet JC, Moneret-Vautrin DA. Ultrastructural changes in the duodenal mucosa induced by ingested histamine in patients with chronic urticaria. *Allergy.* 1996 Dec;51(12):935-9.

Kapil A, Sharma S. Immunopotentiating compounds from Tinospora cordifolia. *J Ethnopharmacol.* 1997 Oct;58(2):89-95.

Kaplan C. Indoor air pollution from unprocessed solid fuels in developing countries. *Rev Environ Health.* 2010 Jul-Sep;25(3):221-42.

Kaplan M, Mutlu EA, Benson M, Fields JZ, Banan A, Keshavarzian A. Use of herbal preparations in the treatment of oxidant-mediated inflammatory disorders. *Complement Ther Med.* 2007 Sep;15(3):207-16. 2006 Aug 21.

Kaplan R. The nature of the view from home: psychological benefits. *Environ Behav.* 2001;33(4):507-42.

Kaplan R. Wilderness perception and psychological benefits: an analysis of a continuing program. *Leisure Sci.* 1984;6(3):271-90.

Karkoulias K, Patouchas D, Alahiotis S, Tsiamita M, Vrodakis K, Spiropoulos K. Specific sensitization in wheat flour and contributing factors in traditional bakers. *Eur Rev Med Pharmacol Sci.* 2007 May-Jun;11(3):141-8.

Karpińska J, Mikolué B, Motkowski R, Piotrowska-Jastrzebska J. HPLC method for simultaneous determination of retinol, alpha-tocopherol and coenzyme Q10 in human plasma. *J Pharm Biomed Anal.* 2006 Sep 18;42(2):232-6.

Kashiwada Y, Takanaka K, Tsukada H, Miwa Y, Taga T, Tanaka S, Ikeshiro Y. Sesquiterpene glucosides from anti-leukotriene B4 release fraction of Taraxacum officinale. *J Asian Nat Prod Res.* 2001;3(3):191-7.

Katial RK, Strand M, Prasertsuntarasai T, Leung R, Zheng W, Alam R. The effect of aspirin desensitization on novel biomarkers in aspirin-exacerbated respiratory diseases. *J Allergy Clin Immunol.* 2010 Oct;126(4):738-44. 2010 Aug 21.

Kattan JD, Srivastava KD, Sampson HA, Li XM. Pharmacologic and Immunologic Effects of Individual Herbs of Food Allergy Herbal Formula 2 in a Murine Model of Peanut Allergy. *J Allergy Clin Immunol.* 2006;117(2):S34.

Kattan JD, Srivastava KD, Zou ZM, Goldfarb J, Sampson HA, Li XM. Pharmacological and immunological effects of individual herbs in the Food Allergy Herbal Formula-2 (FAHF-2) on peanut allergy. *Phytother Res.* 2008 May;22(5):651-9.

Katz DL, Cushman D, Reynolds J, Njike V, Treu JA, Walker J, Smith E, Katz C. Putting physical activity where it fits in the school day: preliminary results of the ABC (Activity Bursts in the Classroom) for fitness program. *Prev Chronic Dis.* 2010 Jul;7(4):A82. 2010 Jun 15.

Katz Y, Rajuan N, Goldberg MR, Eisenberg E, Heyman E, Cohen A, Leshno M. Early exposure to cow's milk protein is protective against IgE-mediated cow's milk protein allergy. *J Allergy Clin Immunol.* 2010 Jul;126(1):77-82.e1.

Kazaks AG, Uriu-Adams JY, Albertson TE, Shenoy SF, Stern JS. Effect of oral magnesium supplementation on measures of airway resistance and subjective assessment of asthma control and quality of life in men and women with mild to moderate asthma: a randomized placebo controlled trial. *J Asthma.* 2010 Feb;47(1):83-92.

Kazansky DB. MHC restriction and allogeneic immune responses. *J Immunotoxicol.* 2008 Oct;5(4):369-84.

Kazlowska K, Hsu T, Hou CC, Yang WC, Tsai GJ. Anti-inflammatory properties of phenolic compounds and crude extract from Porphyra dentata. *J Ethnopharmacol.* 2010 Mar 2;128(1):123-30.

Ke X, Qian D, Zhu L, Hong S. [Analysis on quality of life and personality characteristics of allergic rhinitis]. *Lin Chung Er Bi Yan Hou Tou Jing Wai Ke Za Zhi.* 2010 Mar;24(5):200-2.

Keita AV, Söderholm JD. The intestinal barrier and its regulation by neuroimmune factors. *Neurogastroenterol Motil.* 2010 Jul;22(7):718-33.

Kekkonen RA, Lummela N, Karjalainen H, Latvala S, Tynkkynen S, Jarvenpaa S, Kautiainen H, Julkunen I, Vapaatalo H, Korpela R. Probiotic intervention has strain-specific anti-inflammatory effects in healthy adults. *World J Gastroenterol.* 2008 Apr 7;14(13):2029-36.

Kekkonen RA, Sysi-Aho M, Seppanen-Laakso T, Julkunen I, Vapaatalo H, Oresic M, Korpela R. Effect of probiotic *Lactobacillus rhamnosus* GG intervention on global serum lipidomic profiles in healthy adults. *World J Gastroenterol.* 2008 May 28;14(20):3188-94.

Kekkonen RA, Vasankari TJ, Vuorimaa T, Haahtela T, Julkunen I, Korpela R. The effect of probiotics on respiratory infections and gastrointestinal symptoms during training in marathon runners. *Int J Sport Nutr Exerc Metab.* 2007 Aug;17(4):352-63.

Kelder P. *Ancient Secret of the Fountain of Youth.* New York: Doubleday, 1998.

Kelly HW, Van Natta ML, Covar RA, Tonascia J, Green RP, Strunk RC; CAMP Research Group. Effect of long-term corticosteroid use on bone mineral density in children: a prospective longitudinal assessment in the childhood Asthma Management Program (CAMP) study. *Pediatrics.* 2008 Jul;122(1):e53-61.

Kelly-Pieper K, Patil SP, Busse P, Yang N, Sampson H, Li XM, Wisnivesky JP, Kattan M. Safety and tolerability of an antiasthma herbal Formula (ASHMI) in adult subjects with asthma: a randomized, double-blinded, placebo-controlled, dose-escalation phase I study. *J Altern Complement Med.* 2009 Jul;15(7):735-43.

Kenia P, Houghton T, Beardsmore C. Does inhaling menthol affect nasal patency or cough? *Pediatr Pulmonol.* 2008 Jun;43(6):532-7.

Keogh JB, Grieger JA, Noakes M, Clifton PM. Flow-Mediated Dilatation Is Impaired by a High-Saturated Fat Diet but Not by a High-Carbohydrate Diet. *Arterioscler Thromb Vasc Biol.* 2005 Mar 17

Kerckhoffs DA, Brouns F, Hornstra G, Mensink RP. Effects on the human serum lipoprotein profile of beta-glucan, soy protein and isoflavones, plant sterols and stanols, garlic and tocotrienols. *J Nutr.* 2002 Sep;132(9):2494-505.

Kerkhof M, Postma DS, Brunekreef B, Reijmerink NE, Wijga AH, de Jongste JC, Gehring U, Koppelman GH. Toll-like receptor 2 and 4 genes influence susceptibility to adverse effects of traffic-related air pollution on childhood asthma. *Thorax.* 2010 Aug;65(8):690-7.

Key T, Appleby P, Davey G, Allen N, Spencer E, Travis R. Mortality in British vegetarians: review and preliminary results from EPIC-Oxford. *Amer. Jour. Clin. Nutr. Suppl.* 2003;78(3): 533S-538S.

Kiecolt-Glaser JK, Heffner KL, Glaser R, Malarkey WB, Porter K, Atkinson C, Laskowski B, Lemeshow S, Marshall GD. How stress and anxiety can alter immediate and late phase skin test responses in allergic rhinitis. *Psychoneuroendocrinology.* 2009 Jun;34(5):670-80.

Kiefte-de Jong JC, Escher JC, Arends LR, Jaddoe VW, Hofman A, Raat H, Moll HA. Infant nutritional factors and functional constipation in childhood: the Generation R study. *Am J Gastroenterol.* 2010 Apr;105(4):940-5.

Kim HM, Shin HY, Lim KH, Ryu ST, Shin TY, Chae HJ, Kim HR, Lyu YS, An NH, Lim KS. Taraxacum officinale inhibits tumor necrosis factor-alpha production from rat astrocytes. *Immunopharmacol Immunotoxicol.* 2000 Aug;22(3):519-30.

Kim JH, An S, Kim JE, Choi GS, Ye YM, Park HS. Beef-induced anaphylaxis confirmed by the basophil activation test. *Allergy Asthma Immunol Res.* 2010 Jul;2(3):206-8.

Kim JH, Ellwood PE, Asher MI. Diet and asthma: looking back, moving forward. *Respir Res.* 2009 Jun 12;10:49.

Kim JH, Kim JE, Choi GS, Hwang EK, An S, Ye YM, Park HS. A case of occupational rhinitis caused by rice powder in the grain industry. *Allergy Asthma Immunol Res.* 2010 Apr;2(2):141-3.

Kim JH, Lee SY, Kim HB, Jin HS, Yu JH, Kim BJ, Kim BS, Kang MJ, Jang SO, Hong SJ. TBXA2R gene polymorphism and responsiveness to leukotriene receptor antagonist in children with asthma. *Clin Exp Allergy.* 2008 Jan;38(1):51-9.

378

REFERENCES

Kim JI, Lee MS, Jung SY, Choi JY, Lee S, Ko JM, Zhao H, Zhao J, Kim AR, Shin MS, Kang KW, Jung HJ, Kim TH, Liu B, Choi SM. Acupuncture for persistent allergic rhinitis: a multi-centre, randomised, controlled trial protocol. *Trials.* 2009 Jul 14;10:54.

Kim JY, Kim DY, Lee YS, Lee BK, Lee KH, Ro JY. DA-9601, Artemisia asiatica herbal extract, ameliorates airway inflammation of allergic asthma in mice. *Mol Cells.* 2006;22:104-12.

Kim NI, Jo Y, Ahn SB, Son BK, Kim SH, Park YS, Kim SH, Ju JE. A case of eosinophilic esophagitis with food hypersensitivity. *J Neurogastroenterol Motil.* 2010 Jul;16(3):315-8.

Kim SJ, Jung JY, Kim HW, Park T. Anti-obesity effects of Juniperus chinensis extract are associated with increased AMP-activated protein kinase expression and phosphorylation in the visceral adipose tissue of rats. *Biol Pharm Bull.* 2008 Jul;31(7):1415-21.

Kim TE, Park SW, Noh G, Lee S. Comparison of skin prick test results between crude allergen extracts from foods and commercial allergen extracts in atopic dermatitis by double-blind placebo-controlled food challenge for milk, egg, and soybean. *Yonsei Med J.* 2002 Oct;43(5):613-20.

Kim YH, Kim KS, Han CS, Yang HC, Park SH, Ko KI, Lee SH, Kim KH, Lee NH, Kim JM, Son K. Inhibitory effects of natural plants of Jeju Island on elastase and MMP-1 expression. *Int J Cosmet Sci.* 2007 Dec;29(6):487-8.

Kimata H. Differential effects of laughter on allergen-specific immunoglobulin and neurotrophin levels in tears. *Percept Mot Skills.* 2004 Jun;98(3 Pt 1):901-8.

Kimata H. Effect of viewing a humorous vs. nonhumorous film on bronchial responsiveness in patients with bronchial asthma. *Physiol Behav.* 2004 Jun;81(4):681-4.

Kimata H. Emotion with tears decreases allergic responses to latex in atopic eczema patients with latex allergy. *J Psychosom Res.* 2006 Jul;61(1):67-9.

Kimata H. Increase in dermcidin-derived peptides in sweat of patients with atopic eczema caused by a humorous video. *J Psychosom Res.* 2007 Jan;62(1):57-9.

Kimata H. Laughter counteracts enhancement of plasma neurotrophin levels and allergic skin wheal responses by mobile phone-mediated stress. *Behav Med.* 2004 Winter;29(4):149-52.

Kimata H. Modulation of fecal polyamines by viewing humorous films in patients with atopic dermatitis. *Eur J Gastroenterol Hepatol.* 2010 Jun;22(6):724-8.

Kimata H. Reduction of allergic responses in atopic infants by mother's laughter. *Eur J Clin Invest.* 2004 Sep;34(9):645-6.

Kimata H. Viewing a humorous film decreases IgE production by seminal B cells from patients with atopic eczema. *J Psychosom Res.* 2009 Feb;66(2):173-5.

Kimata H. Viewing humorous film improves nighttime wakening in children with atopic dermatitis. *Indian Pediatr.* 2007 Apr;44(4):281-5.

Kimata M, Inagaki N, Nagai H. Effects of luteolin and other flavonoids on IgE-mediated allergic reactions. *Planta Med.* 2000 Feb;66(1):25-9.

Kimata M, Shichijo M, Miura T, Serizawa I, Inagaki N, Nagai H. Effects of luteolin, quercetin and baicalein on immunoglobulin E-mediated mediator release from human cultured mast cells. *Clin Exp Allergy.* 2000 Apr;30(4):501-8.

Kimmatkar N, Thawani V, Hingorani L, Khiyani R. Efficacy and tolerability of Boswellia serrata extract in treatment of osteoarthritis of knee—a randomized double blind placebo controlled trial. *Phytomedicine.* 2003 Jan;10(1):3-7.

Kinaciyan T, Jahn-Schmid B, Radakovics A, Zwölfer B, Schreiber C, Francis JN, Ebner C, Bohle B. Successful sublingual immunotherapy with birch pollen has limited effects on concomitant food allergy to apple and the immune response to the Bet v 1 homolog Mal d 1. *J Allergy Clin Immunol.* 2007 Apr;119(4):937-43.

Kinross JM, von Roon AC, Holmes E, Darzi A, Nicholson JK. The human gut microbiome: implications for future health care. *Curr Gastroenterol Rep.* 2008 Aug;10(4):396-403.

Kippelen P, Larsson J, Anderson SD, Brannan JD, Dahlén B, Dahlén SE. Effect of sodium cromoglycate on mast cell mediators during hyperpnea in athletes. *Med Sci Sports Exerc.* 2010 Oct;42(10):1853-60.

Kirjavainen PV, Salminen SJ, Isolauri E. Probiotic bacteria in the management of atopic disease: underscoring the importance of viability. *J Pediatr Gastroenterol Nutr.* 2003 Feb;36(2):223-7.

Kisiel W, Barszcz B. Further sesquiterpenoids and phenolics from Taraxacum officinale. *Fitoterapia.* 2000 Jun;71(3):269-73.

Kisiel W, Michalska K. Sesquiterpenoids and phenolics from Taraxacum hondoense. *Fitoterapia.* 2005 Sep;76(6):520-4.

Klein R, Landau MG. *Healing: The Body Betrayed.* Minneapolis: DCI:Chronimed, 1992.

Klein-Galczinsky C. Pharmacological and clinical effectiveness of a fixed phytogenic combination trembling poplar (Populus tremula), true goldenrod (Solidago virgaurea) and ash (Fraxinus excelsior) in mild to moderate rheumatic complaints. *Wien Med Wochenschr.* 1999;149(8-10):248-53.

Klemola T, Vanto T, Juntunen-Backman K, Kalimo K, Korpela R, Varjonen E. Allergy to soy formula and to extensively hydrolyzed whey formula in infants with cow's milk allergy: a prospective, randomized study with a follow-up to the age of 2 years. *J Pediatr.* 2002 Feb;140(2):219-24.

Kloss J. *Back to Eden.* Twin Oaks, WI: Lotus Press, 1939-1999.

Knutson TW, Bengtsson U, Dannaeus A, Ahlstedt S, Knutson L. Effects of luminal antigen on intestinal albumin and hyaluronan permeability and ion transport in atopic patients. *J Allergy Clin Immunol.* 1996 Jun;97(6):1225-32.

Ko J, Busse PJ, Shek L, Noone SA, Sampson HA, Li XM. Effect of Chinese Herbal Formulas on T Cell Responses in Patients with Peanut Allergy or Asthma. *J Allergy Clin Immunol* .2005;115:S34.

Ko J, Lee JI, Munoz-Furlong A, Li XM, Sicherer SH. Use of complementary and alternative medicine by food-allergic patients. *Ann Allergy Asthma Immunol.* 2006;97:365-9.

Kobayashi I, Hamasaki Y, Sato R, Zaitu M, Muro E, Yamamoto S, Ichimaru T, Miyazaki S. Saiboku-To, a herbal extract mixture, selectively inhibits 5-lipoxygenase activity in leukotriene synthesis in rat basophilic leukemia-1 cells. *J Ethnopharmacol.* 1995 Aug 11;48(1):33-41.

Kohlhammer Y, Döring A, Schäfer T, Wichmann HE, Heinrich J; KORA Study Group. Swimming pool attendance and hay fever rates later in life. *Allergy.* 2006 Nov;61(11):1305-9. PubMed PMID: 17002706.

Kohlhammer Y, Zutavern A, Rzehak P, Woelke G, Heinrich J. Influence of physical inactivity on the prevalence of hay fever. *Allergy.* 2006 Nov;61(11):1310-5.

Kokwaro JO. *Medicinal Plants of East Africa.* Nairobi: Univ of Neirobi Press, 2009.

Kong LF, Guo LH, Zheng XY. Effect of yiqi bushen huoxue herbs in treating children asthma and on levels of nitric oxide, endothelin-1 and serum endothelial cells. *Zhongguo Zhong Xi Yi Jie He Za Zhi.* 2001 Sep;21(9):667-9.

Koo HN, Hong SH, Song BK, Kim CH, Yoo YH, Kim HM. Taraxacum officinale induces cytotoxicity through TNF-alpha and IL-1alpha secretion in Hep G2 cells. *Life Sci.* 2004 Jan 16;74(9):1149-57.

Kootstra HS, Vlieg-Boerstra BJ, Dubois AE. Assessment of the reduced allergenic properties of the Santana apple. *Ann Allergy Asthma Immunol.* 2007 Dec;99(6):522-5.

Kositz C, Schroecksnadel K, Grander G, Schennach H, Kofler H, Fuchs D. High serum tryptophan concentration in pollinosis patients is associated with unresponsiveness to pollen extract therapy. *Int Arch Allergy Immunol.* 2008;147(1):35-40.

Kotzampassi K, Giamarellos-Bourboulis EJ, Voudouris A, Kazamias P, Eleftheriadis E. Benefits of a synbiotic formula (Synbiotic 2000Forte) in critically Ill trauma patients: early results of a randomized controlled trial. *World J Surg.* 2006 Oct;30(10):1848-55.

Kovács T, Mette H, Per B, Kun L, Schmelczer M, Barta J, Jean-Claude D, Nagy J. Relationship between intestinal permeability and antibodies against food antigens in IgA nephropathy. *Orv Hetil.* 1996 Jan 14;137(2):65-9.

Kowalchik C, Hylton W (eds). *Rodale's Illustrated Encyclopedia of Herbs.* Emmaus, PA: 1987.

Kowalczyk E, Krzesiński P, Kura M, Niedworok J, Kowalski J, Blaszczyk J. Pharmacological effects of flavonoids from Scutellaria baicalensis. *Przegl Lek.* 2006;63(2):95-6.

Kozlowski LT, Mehta NY, Sweeney CT, Schwartz SS, Vogler GP, Jarvis MJ, West RJ. Filter ventilation and nicotine content of tobacco in cigarettes from Canada, the United Kingdom, and the United States. *Tob Control.* 1998 Winter;7(4):369-75.

Kreig M. *Black Market Medicine.* New York: Bantam, 1968.

Kremmyda LS, Vlachava M, Noakes PS, Diaper ND, Miles EA, Calder PC. Atopy Risk in Infants and Children in Relation to Early Exposure to Fish, Oily Fish, or Long-Chain Omega-3 Fatty Acids: A Systematic Review. *Clin Rev Allergy Immunol.* 2009 Dec 9.

Krogulska A, Dynowski J, Wasowska-Królikowska K. Bronchial reactivity in schoolchildren allergic to food. *Ann Allergy Asthma Immunol.* 2010 Jul;105(1):31-8.

Krogulska A, Wasowska-Królikowska K, Dynowski J. Evaluation of bronchial hyperreactivity in children with asthma undergoing food challenges. *Pol Merkur Lekarski.* 2007 Jul;23(133):30-5.

Krogulska A, Wasowska-Królikowska K, Polakowska E, Chrul S. Cytokine profile in children with asthma undergoing food challenges. *J Investig Allergol Clin Immunol.* 2009;19(1):43-8.

Krogulska A, Wasowska-Królikowska K, Polakowska E, Chrul S. Evaluation of receptor expression on immune system cells in the peripheral blood of asthmatic children undergoing food challenges. Int Arch Allergy Immunol. 2009;150(4):377-88. 2009 Jul 1.

Krogulska A, Wasowska-Królikowska K, Trzeźwińska B. Food challenges in children with asthma. *Pol Merkur Lekarski.* 2007 Jul;23(133):22-9.

Kroidl RF, Schwichtenberg U, Frank E. Bronchial asthma due to storage mite allergy. Pneumologie. 2007 Aug;61(8):525-30.

Krueger AP, Reed EJ. Biological impact of small air ions. Science. 1976 Sep 24;193(4259):1209-13.

REFERENCES

Krüger P, Kanzer J, Hummel J, Fricker G, Schubert-Zsilavecz M, Abdel-Tawab M. Permeation of Boswellia extract in the Caco-2 model and possible interactions of its constituents KBA and AKBA with OATP1B3 and MRP2. *Eur J Pharm Sci.* 2009 Feb 15;36(2-3):275-84.

Kubota A, He F, Kawase M, Harata G, Hiramatsu M, Iino H. Diversity of intestinal bifidobacteria in patients with Japanese cedar pollinosis and possible influence of probiotic intervention. *Curr Microbiol.* 2011 Jan;62(1):71-7.

Kubota A, He F, Kawase M, Harata G, Hiramatsu M, Salminen S, Iino H. Lactobacillus strains stabilize intestinal microbiota in Japanese cedar pollinosis patients. *Microbiol Immunol.* 2009 Apr;53(4):198-205.

Kuitunen M, Kukkonen K, Juntunen-Backman K, Korpela R, Poussa T, Tuure T, Haahtela T, Savilahti E. Probiotics prevent IgE-associated allergy until age 5 years in Cesarean-delivered children but not in the total cohort. *J Allergy Clin Immunol.* 2009 Feb;123(2):335-41.

Kuitunen M, Savilahti E, Sarnesto A. Human alpha-lactalbumin and bovine beta-lactoglobulin absorption in infants. *Allergy.* 1994 May;49(5):354-60.

Kuitunen M, Savilahti E. Mucosal IgA, mucosal cow's milk antibodies, serum cow's milk antibodies and gastrointestinal permeability in infants. *Pediatr Allergy Immunol.* 1995 Feb;6(1):30-5.

Kukkonen K, Kuitunen M, Haahtela T, Korpela R, Poussa T, Savilahti E. High intestinal IgA associates with reduced risk of IgE-associated allergic diseases. *Pediatr Allergy Immunol.* 2010 Feb;21(1 Pt 1):67-73.

Kukkonen K, Savilahti E, Haahtela T, Juntunen-Backman K, Korpela R, Poussa T, Tuure T, Kuitunen M. Probiotics and prebiotic galacto-oligosaccharides in the prevention of allergic diseases: a randomized, double-blind, placebo-controlled trial. *J Allergy Clin Immunol.* 2007 Jan;119(1):192-8.

Kulka M. The potential of natural products as effective treatments for allergic inflammation: implications for allergic rhinitis. *Curr Top Med Chem.* 2009;9(17):1611-24.

Kull I, Bergström A, Lilja G, Pershagen G, Wickman M. Fish consumption during the first year of life and development of allergic diseases during childhood. *Allergy.* 2006 Aug;61(8):1009-15.

Kull I, Melen E, Alm J, Hallberg J, Svartengren M, van Hage M, Pershagen G, Wickman M, Bergström A. Breast-feeding in relation to asthma, lung function, and sensitization in young schoolchildren. *J Allergy Clin Immunol.* 2010 May;125(5):1013-9.

Kumar A, Panghal S, Mallapur SS, Kumar M, Ram V, Singh BK. Antiinflammatory Activity of Piper longum Fruit Oil. *Indian J Pharm Sci.* 2009 Jul;71(4):454-6.

Kumar A, Saluja AK, Shah UD, Mayavanshi AV. Pharmacological potential of Albizzia lebbeck: A Review. *Pharmacog.* 2007 Jan-May; 1(1) 171-174.

Kumar R, Singh BP, Srivastava P, Sridhara S, Arora N, Gaur SN. Relevance of serum IgE estimation in allergic bronchial asthma with special reference to food allergy. *Asian Pac J Allergy Immunol.* 2006 Dec;24(4):191-9.

Kummeling I, Mills EN, Clausen M, Dubakiene R, Pérez CF, Fernández-Rivas M, Knulst AC, Kowalski ML, Lidholm J, Le TM, Metzler C, Mustakov T, Popov T, Potts J, van Ree R, Sakellariou A, Töndury B, Tzannis K, Burney P. The EuroPrevall surveys on the prevalence of food allergies in children and adults: background and study methodology. *Allergy.* 2009 Oct;64(10):1493-7.

Kung HC, Hoyert DL, Xu J, Murphy SL. Deaths: Final Data for 2005. *National Vital Statistics Reports.* 2008;56(10). http://www.cdc.gov/nchs/data/ nvsr/nvsr56/nvsr56_10.pdf. Accessed: 2008 Jun.

Kunisawa J, Kiyono H. Aberrant interaction of the gut immune system with environmental factors in the development of food allergies. *Curr Allergy Asthma Rep.* 2010 May;10(3):215-21.

Kurth T, Barr RG, Gaziano JM, Buring JE. Randomised aspirin assignment and risk of adult-onset asthma in the Women's Health Study. *Thorax.* 2008 Jun;63(6):514-8. 2008 Mar 13.

Kusunoki T, Morimoto T, Nishikomori R, Yasumi T, Heike T, Mukaida K, Fujii T, Nakahata T. Breastfeeding and the prevalence of allergic diseases in schoolchildren: Does reverse causation matter? *Pediatr Allergy Immunol.* 2010 Feb;21(1 Pt 1):60-6.

Kuvaeva IB. Permeability of the gastronintestinal tract for macromolecules in health and disease. *Hum Physiol.* 1979 Mar-Apr;4(2):272-83.

Kuz'mina IaS, Vavilova NN. Kinesitherapy of patients with bronchial asthma and excessive body weight at the early stage of rehabilitation treatment. *Vopr Kurortol Fizioter Lech Fiz Kult.* 2009 Sep-Oct;(5):17-20.

Kuznetsova TA, Shevchenko NM, Zviagintseva TN, Besednova NN. Biological activity of fucoidans from brown algae and the prospects of their use in medicine]. *Antibiot Khimioter.* 2004;49(5):24-30.

Kvamme JM, Wilsgaard T, Florholmen J, Jacobsen BK. Body mass index and disease burden in elderly men and women: the Tromso Study. *Eur J Epidemiol.* 2010 Mar;25(3):183-93. 2010 Jan 20.

Lad V. *Ayurreda: The Science of Self-Healing.* Twin Lakes, WI: Lotus Press.

Lamaison JL, Carnat A, Petitjean-Freytet C. Tannin content and inhibiting activity of elastase in Rosaceae. *Ann Pharm Fr.* 1990;48(6):335-40.

Laney AS, Cragin LA, Blevins LZ, Sumner AD, Cox-Ganser JM, Kreiss K, Moffatt SG, Lohff CJ. Sarcoidosis, asthma, and asthma-like symptoms among occupants of a historically water-damaged office building. *Indoor Air.* 2009 Feb;19(1):83-90.

Lang CJ, Hansen M, Roscioli E, Jones J, Murgia C, Leigh Ackland M, Zalewski P, Anderson G, Ruffin R. Dietary zinc mediates inflammation and protects against wasting and metabolic derangement caused by sustained cigarette smoke exposure in mice. *Biometals.* 2011 Feb;24(1):23-39. 2010 Aug 29.

Lange NE, Rifas-Shiman SL, Camargo CA Jr, Gold DR, Gillman MW, Litonjua AA. Maternal dietary pattern during pregnancy is not associated with recurrent wheeze in children. *J Allergy Clin Immunol.* 2010 Aug;126(2):250-5, 255.e1-4.

Lappe FM. *Diet for a Small Planet.* New York: Ballantine, 1971.

Larenas-Linnemann D, Matta JJ, Shah-Hosseini K, Michels A, Mösges R. Skin prick test evaluation of Dermatophagoides pteronyssinus diagnostic extracts from Europe, Mexico, and the United States. *Ann Allergy Asthma Immunol.* 2010 May;104(5):420-5.

Lau BH, Riesen SK, Truong KP, Lau EW, Rohdewald P, Barreta RA. Pycnogenol as an adjunct in the management of childhood asthma. *J Asthma.* 2004;41(8):825-32.

Laubereau B, Filipiak-Pittroff B, von Berg A, Grübl A, Reinhardt D, Wichmann HE, Koletzko S; GINI Study Group. Caesarean section and gastrointestinal symptoms, atopic dermatitis, and sensitisation during the first year of life. *Arch Dis Child.* 2004 Nov;89(11):993-7.

Laurière M, Pecquet C, Bouchez-Mahiout I, Snégaroff J, Bayrou O, Raison-Peyron N, Vigan M. Hydrolysed wheat proteins present in cosmetics can induce immediate hypersensitivities. *Contact Dermatitis.* 2006 May;54(5):283-9.

LaValle JB. *The Cox-2 Connection.* Rochester, VT: Healing Arts, 2001.

Lazarou J, Pomeranz BH, Corey PN. Incidence of adverse drug reactions in hospitalized patients: a meta-analysis of prospective studies. *JAMA.* 1998 Apr.

Lean G. US study links more than 200 diseases to pollution. *London Independent.* 2004 Nov 14.

Leander M, Cronqvist A, Janson C, Uddenfeldt M, Rask-Andersen A. Health-related quality of life predicts onset of asthma in a longitudinal population study. *Respir Med.* 2009 Feb;103(2):194-200.

Lecheler J, Pfannebecker B, Nguyen DT, Petzold U, Munzel U, Kremer HJ, Maus J. Prevention of exercise-induced asthma by a fixed combination of disodium cromoglycate plus reproterol compared with montelukast in young patients. *Arzneimittelforschung.* 2008;58(6):303-9.

Lee E, Haa K, Yook JM, Jin MH, Seo CS, Son KH, Kim HP, Bae KH, Kang SS, Son JK, Chang HW. Anti-asthmatic activity of an ethanol extract from Saururus chinensis. *Biol Pharm Bull.* 2006 Feb;29(2):211-5.

Lee JH, Noh J, Noh G, Kim HS, Mun SH, Choi WS, Cho S, Lee S. Allergen-specific B cell subset responses in cow's milk allergy of late eczematous reactions in atopic dermatitis. *Cell Immunol.* 2010;262(1):44-51.

Lee JY, Kim CJ. Determination of allergenic egg proteins in food by protein-, mass spectrometry-, and DNA-based methods. *J AOAC Int.* 2010 Mar-Apr;93(2):462-77.

Lee KH, Yeh MH, Kao ST, Hung CM, Chen BC, Liu CJ, Yeh CC. Xia-bai-san inhibits lipopolysaccharide-induced activation of intercellular adhesion molecule-1 and nuclear factor-kappa B in human lung cells. *J Ethnopharmacol.* 2009 Jul 30;124(3):530-8.

Lee YS, Kim SH, Jung SH, Kim JK, Pan CH, Lim SS. Aldose reductase inhibitory compounds from Glycyrrhiza uralensis. *Biol Pharm Bull.* 2010;33(5):917-21.

Léger D, Annesi-Maesano I, Carat F, Rugina M, Chanal I, Pribil C, El Hasnaoui A, Bousquet J. Allergic rhinitis and its consequences on quality of sleep: An unexplored area. *Arch Intern Med.* 2006 Sep 18;166(16):1744-8.

Lehmann B. The vitamin D3 pathway in human skin and its role for regulation of biological processes. *Photochem Photobiol.* 2005 Nov-Dec;81(6):1246-51.

Lehto M, Airaksinen L, Puustinen A, Tillander S, Hannula S, Nyman T, Toskala E, Alenius H, Lauerma A. Thaumatin-like protein and baker's respiratory allergy. *Ann Allergy Asthma Immunol.* 2010 Feb;104(2):139-46.

Leitzmann C. Vegetarian diets: what are the advantages? *Forum Nutr.* 2005;(57):147-56.

Léonard R, Wopfner N, Pabst M, Stadlmann J, Petersen BO, Duus JØ, Himly M, Radauer C, Gadermaier G, Razzazi-Fazeli E, Ferreira F, Altmann F. A new allergen from ragweed (Ambrosia artemisiifolia) with homology to art v 1 from mugwort. *J Biol Chem.* 2010 Aug 27;285(35):27192-200.

Leu YL, Shi LS, Damu AG. Chemical constituents of Taraxacum formosanum. *Chem Pharm Bull.* 2003 May;51(5):599-601.

Leu YL, Wang YL, Huang SC, Shi LS. Chemical constituents from roots of Taraxacum formosanum. *Chem Pharm Bull.* 2005 Jul;53(7):853-5.

Leung DY, Sampson HA, Yunginger JW, Burks AW Jr, Schneider LC, Wortel CH, Davis FM, Hyun JD, Shanahan WR Jr; Avon Longitudinal Study of Parents and Children Study Team. Effect of anti-IgE therapy in patients with peanut allergy. *N Engl J Med.* 2003 Mar 13;348(11):986-93.

Leung DY, Shanahan WR Jr, Li XM, Sampson HA. New approaches for the treatment of anaphylaxis. *Novartis Found Symp.* 2004;257:248-60; discussion 260-4, 276-85.

Lewerin C, Jacobsson S, Lindstedt G, Nilsson-Ehle H. Serum biomarkers for atrophic gastritis and antibodies against Helicobacter pylori in the elderly: Implications for vitamin B12, folic acid and iron status and response to oral vitamin therapy. *Scand J Gastroenterol.* 2008;43(9):1050-6.

REFERENCES

Lewis SA, Grimshaw KE, Warner JO, Hourihane JO. The promiscuity of immunoglobulin E binding to peanut allergens, as determined by Western blotting, correlates with the severity of clinical symptoms. *Clin Exp Allergy*. 2005 Jun;35(6):767-73.

Lewis WH, Elvin-Lewis MPF. *Medical Botany: Plants Affecting Man's Health*. New York: Wiley, 1977.

Lewontin R. *The Genetic Basis of Evolutionary Change*. New York: Columbia Univ Press, 1974.

Leyel CF. *Culpeper's English Physician & Complete Herbal*. Hollywood, CA: Wilshire, 1971.

Leynadier F. Mast cells and basophils in asthma. Ann Biol Clin (Paris). 1989;47(6):351-6.

Li J, Sun B, Huang Y, Lin X, Zhao D, Tan G, Wu J, Zhao H, Cao L, Zhong N. A multicentre study assessing the prevalence of sensitizations in patients with asthma and/or rhinitis in China. *Allergy*. 2009;64:1083-1092.

Li MH, Zhang HL, Yang BY. Effects of ginkgo leaf concentrated oral liquor in treating asthma. *Zhongguo Zhong Xi Yi Jie He Za Zhi*. 1997 Apr;17(4):216-8. 5.

Li Q, Li XL, Yang X, Bao JM, Shen XH. Effects of antiallergic herbal agents on cystic fibrosis transmembrane conductance regulator in nasal mucosal epithelia of allergic rhinitis rabbits. *Chin Med J (Engl)*. 2009 Dec 20;122(24):3020-4.

Li S, Li W, Wang Y, Asada Y, Koike K. Prenylflavonoids from Glycyrrhiza uralensis and their protein tyrosine phosphatase-1B inhibitory activities. *Bioorg Med Chem Lett*. 2010 Sep 15;20(18):5398-401.

Li XM, Huang CK, Zhang TF, Teper AA, Srivastava K, Schofield BH, Sampson HA. The chinese herbal medicine formula MSSM-002 suppresses allergic airway hyperreactivity and modulates TH1/TH2 responses in a murine model of allergic asthma. *J Allergy Clin Immunol*. 2000;106:660-8.

Li XM, Srivastava K. Traditional Chinese medicine for the therapy of allergic disorders. *Curr Opin Otolaryngol Head Neck Surg*. 2006 Jun;14(3):191-6.

Li XM, Zhang TF, Huang CK, Srivastava K, Teper AA, Zhang L, Schofield BH, Sampson HA. Food Allergy Herbal Formula-1 (FAHF-1) blocks peanut-induced anaphylaxis in a murine model. *J Allergy Clin Immunol*. 2001;108:639-46.

Li XM, Zhang TF, Sampson H, Zou ZM, Beyer K, Wen MC, Schofield B. The potential use of Chinese herbal medicines in treating allergic asthma. *Ann Allergy Asthma Immunol*. 2004;93:S35-S44.

Li XM. Beyond allergen avoidance: update on developing therapies for peanut allergy. *Curr Opin Allergy Clin Immunol*. 2005;5:287-92.

Li YQ, Yuan W, Zhang SL. Clinical and experimental study of xiao er ke cuan ling oral liquid in the treatment of infantile bronchopneumonia. *Zhongguo Zhong Xi Yi Jie He Za Zhi*. 1992 Dec;12(12):719-21, 737, 708.

Lied GA, Lillestol K, Valeur J, Berstad A. Intestinal B cell-activating factor: an indicator of non-IgE-mediated hypersensitivity reactions to food? *Aliment Pharmacol Ther*. 2010 Jul;32(1):66-73.

Lillestol K, Berstad A, Lind R, Florvaag E, Arslan Lied G, Tangen T. Anxiety and depression in patients with self-reported food hypersensitivity. *Gen Hosp Psychiatry*. 2010 Jan-Feb;32(1):42-8.

Lima JA, Fischer GB, Sarria EE, Mattiello R, Solé D. Prevalence of and risk factors for wheezing in the first year of life. *J Bras Pneumol*. 2010 Oct;36(5):525-31. English, Portuguese.

Limb SL, Brown KC, Wood RA, Wise RA, Eggleston PA, Tonascia J, Hamilton RG, Adkinson NF Jr. Adult asthma severity in individuals with a history of childhood asthma. *J Allergy Clin Immunol*. 2005 Jan;115(1):61-6.

Lindahl O, Lindwall L, Spångberg A, Stenram A, Ockerman PA. Vegan regimen with reduced medication in the treatment of bronchial asthma. *J Asthma*. 1985;22(1):45-55.

Ling WH, Hänninen O. Shifting from a conventional diet to an uncooked vegan diet reversibly alters fecal hydrolytic activities in humans. J Nutr. 1992 Apr;122(4):924-30.

Lininger S, Gaby A, Austin S, Brown D, Wright J, Duncan A. *The Natural Pharmacy*. New York: Three Rivers, 1999.

Linsalata M, Russo F, Berloco P, Caruso ML, Matteo GD, Cifone MG, Simone CD, Ierardi E, Di Leo A. The influence of Lactobacillus brevis on ornithine decarboxylase activity and polyamine profiles in Helicobacter pylori-infected gastric mucosa. Helicobacter. 2004 Apr;9(2):165-72.

Lipski E. *Digestive Wellness*. Los Angeles, CA: Keats, 2000.

Liu AH, Jaramillo R, Sicherer SH, Wood RA, Bock SA, Burks AW, Massing M, Cohn RD, Zeldin DC. National prevalence and risk factors for food allergy and relationship to asthma: results from the National Health and Nutrition Examination Survey 2005-2006. *J Allergy Clin Immunol*. 2010 Oct;126(4):798-806.e13.

Liu F, Zhang J, Liu Y, Zhang N, Holtappels G, Lin P, Liu S, Bachert C. Inflammatory profiles in nasal mucosa of patients with persistent vs intermittent allergic rhinitis. *Allergy*. 2010 Sep;65(9):1149-57.

Liu GM, Cao MJ, Huang YY, Cai QF, Weng WY, Su WJ. Comparative study of in vitro digestibility of major allergen tropomyosin and other food proteins of Chinese mitten crab (Eriocheir sinensis). *J Sci Food Agric*. 2010 Aug 15;90(10):1614-20.

Liu HY, Giday Z, Moore BF. Possible pathogenetic mechanisms producing bovine milk protein inducible malabsorption: a hypothesis. *Ann Allergy*. 1977 Jul;39(1):1-7.

Liu JY, Hu JH, Zhu QG, Li FQ, Wang J, Sun HJ. Effect of matrine on the expression of substance P receptor and inflammatory cytokines production in human skin keratinocytes and fibroblasts. *Int Immunopharmacol.* 2007 Jun;7(6):816-23.

Liu T, Valdez R, Yoon PW, Crocker D, Moonesinghe R, Khoury MJ. The association between family history of asthma and the prevalence of asthma among US adults: National Health and Nutrition Examination Survey, 1999-2004. *Genet Med.* 2009 May;11(5):323-8.

Liu X, Beaty TH, Deindl P, Huang SK, Lau S, Sommerfeld C, Fallin MD, Kao WH, Wahn U, Nickel R. Associations between specific serum IgE response and 6 variants within the genes IL4, IL13, and IL4RA in German children: the German Multicenter Atopy Study. *J Allergy Clin Immunol.* 2004 Mar;113(3):489-95.

Liu XJ, Cao MA, Li WH, Shen CS, Yan SQ, Yuan CS. Alkaloids from Sophora flavescens Aition. *Fitoterapia.* 2010 Sep;81(6):524-7.

Liu Z, Bhattacharyya S, Ning B, Midoro-Horiuti T, Czerwinski EW, Goldblum RM, Mort A, Kearney CM. Plant-expressed recombinant mountain cedar allergen Jun a 1 is allergenic and has limited pectate lyase activity. *Int Arch Allergy Immunol.* 2010;153(4):347-58.

Lloyd JU. *American Materia Medica, Therapeutics and Pharmacognosy.* Portland, OR: Eclectic Medical Publications, 1989-1983.

Lloyd Spencer J. Immunization via the anal mucosa and adjacent skin to protect against respiratory virus infections and allergic rhinitis: a hypothesis. *Med Hypotheses.* 2010 Mar;74(3):542-6.

Lloyd-Still JD, Powers CA, Hoffman DR, Boyd-Trull K, Lester LA, Benisek DC, Arterburn LM. Bioavailability and safety of a high dose of docosahexaenoic acid triacylglycerol of algal origin in cystic fibrosis patients: a randomized, controlled study. *Nutrition.* 2006 Jan;22(1):36-46.

Locke GR 3rd, Talley NJ, Fett SL, Zinsmeister AR, Melton LJ 3rd. Prevalence and clinical spectrum of gastroesophageal reflux: a population-based study in Olmsted County, Minnesota. *Gastroenterology.* 1997 May;112(5):1448-56.

Loizzo MR, Saab AM, Tundis R, Statti GA, Menichini F, Lampronti I, Gambari R, Cinatl J, Doerr HW. Phytochemical analysis and in vitro antiviral activities of the essential oils of seven Lebanon species. *Chem Biodivers.* 2008 Mar;5(3):461-70.

Lomax AR, Calder PC. Probiotics, immune function, infection and inflammation: a review of the evidence from studies conducted in humans. *Curr Pharm Des.* 2009;15(13):1428-518.

Longo G, Barbi E, Berti I, Meneghetti R, Pittalis A, Ronfani L, Ventura A. Specific oral tolerance induction in children with very severe cow's milk-induced reactions. *J Allergy Clin Immunol.* 2008 Feb;121(2):343-7.

Lopes EA, Fanelli-Galvani A, Prisco CC, Gonçalves RC, Jacob CM, Cabral AL, Martins MA, Carvalho CR. Assessment of muscle shortening and static posture in children with persistent asthma. *Eur J Pediatr.* 2007 Jul;166(7):715-21.

López N, de Barros-Mazón S, Vilela MM, Silva CM, Ribeiro JD. Genetic and environmental influences on atopic immune response in early life. *J Investig Allergol Clin Immunol.* 1999 Nov-Dec;9(6):392-8.

Lopez-Garcia E, Schulze MB, Meigs JB, Manson JE, Rifai N, Stampfer MJ, Willett WC, Hu FB. Consumption of trans fatty acids is related to plasma biomarkers of inflammation and endothelial dysfunction. *J Nutr.* 2005 Mar;135(3):562-6.

Lu MK, Shih YW, Chang Chien TT, Fang LH, Huang HC, Chen PS. α-Solanine inhibits human melanoma cell migration and invasion by reducing matrix metalloproteinase-2/9 activities. *Biol Pharm Bull.* 2010;33(10):1685-91.

Lucas A, Brooke OG, Cole TJ, Morley R, Bamford MF. Food and drug reactions, wheezing, and eczema in preterm infants. *Arch Dis Child.* 1990 Apr;65(4):411-5. 8; .

Lucendo AJ, Lucendo B. An update on the immunopathogenesis of eosinophilic esophagitis. *Expert Rev Gastroenterol Hepatol.* 2010 Apr;4(2):141-8.

Lunardi AC, Marques da Silva CC, Rodrigues Mendes FA, Marques AP, Stelmach R, Fernandes Carvalho CR. Musculoskeletal dysfunction and pain in adults with asthma. *J Asthma.* 2011 Feb;48(1):105-10.

Lv X, Xi L, Han D, Zhang L. Evaluation of the psychological status in seasonal allergic rhinitis patients. *ORL J Otorhinolaryngol Relat Spec.* 2010;72(2):84-90.

Lykken DT, Tellegen A, DeRubeis R: Volunteer bias in twin research: the rule of two-thirds. *Soc Biol* 1978, 25(1): 1-9. Phillips DI: Twin studies in medical research: can they tell us whether diseases are genetically determined? *Lancet* 1993;341(8851): 1008-1009.

Ma J, Xiao L, Knowles SB. Obesity, insulin resistance and the prevalence of atopy and asthma in US adults. *Allergy.* 2010 Nov;65(11):1455-63.

Ma XP, Muzhapaer D. Efficacy of sublingual immunotherapy in children with dust mite allergic asthma. *Zhongguo Dang Dai Er Ke Za Zhi.* 2010 May;12(5):344-7.

Mabey R, ed. *The New Age Herbalist.* New York: Simon & Schuster, 1941.

Macdonald TT, Monteleone G. Immunity, inflammation, and allergy in the gut. *Science.* 2005 Mar 25;307(5717):1920-5.

REFERENCES

Maciorkowska E, Kaczmarski M, Andrzej K. Endoscopic evaluation of upper gastrointestinal tract mucosa in children with food hypersensitivity. *Med Wieku Rozwoj.* 2000 Jan-Mar;4(1):37-48.

Mackerras D, Cunningham J, Hunt A, Brent P. Re: "effect of supplemental folic acid in pregnancy on childhood asthma: a prospective birth cohort study". *Am J Epidemiol.* 2010 Mar 15;171(6):746-7; author reply 747. 2010 Feb 9.

MacRedmond R, Singhera G, Attridge S, Bahzad M, Fava C, Lai Y, Hallstrand TS, Dorscheid DR. Conjugated linoleic acid improves airway hyper-reactivity in overweight mild asthmatics. *Clin Exp Allergy.* 2010 Jul;40(7):1071-8.

Macsali F, Real FG, Omenaas ER, Bjorge L, Janson C, Franklin K, Svanes C. Oral contraception, body mass index, and asthma: a cross-sectional Nordic-Baltic population survey. *J Allergy Clin Immunol.* 2009 Feb;123(2):391-7.

Madden JA, Plummer SF, Tang J, Garaiova I, Plummer NT, Herbison M, Hunter JO, Shimada T, Cheng L, Shirakawa T. Effect of probiotics on preventing disruption of the intestinal microflora following antibiotic therapy: a double-blind, placebo-controlled pilot study. *Int Immunopharmacol.* 2005 Jun;5(6):1091-7.

Maeda N, Inomata N, Morita A, Kirino M, Ikezawa Z. Correlation of oral allergy syndrome due to plant-derived foods with pollen sensitization in Japan. *Ann Allergy Asthma Immunol.* 2010 Mar;104(3):205-10.

Maes HH, Silberg JL, Neale MC, Eaves LJ. Genetic and cultural transmission of antisocial behavior: an extended twin parent model. *Twin Res Hum Genet.* 2007 Feb;10(1):136-50.

Mai XM, Kull I, Wickman M, Bergström A. Antibiotic use in early life and development of allergic diseases: respiratory infection as the explanation. *Clin Exp Allergy.* 2010 Aug;40(8):1230-7.

Mainardi T, Kapoor S, Bielory L. Complementary and alternative medicine: herbs, phytochemicals and vitamins and their immunologic effects. *J Allergy Clin Immunol.* 2009 Feb;123(2):283-94; quiz 295-6.

Majamaa H, Isolauri E. Probiotics: a novel approach in the management of food allergy. *J Allergy Clin Immunol.* 1997 Feb;99(2):179-85.

Makrides M, Neumann M, Gibson R. Effect of maternal docosahexaenoic acid (DHA) supplementation on breast milk composition. *Europ Jrnl of Clin Nutr.* 1996;50:352-357.

Maliakal PP, Wanwimolruk S. Effect of herbal teas on hepatic drug metabolizing enzymes in rats. *J Pharm Pharmacol.* 2001 Oct;53(10):1323-9.

Mälkönen T, Alanko K, Jolanki R, Luukkonen R, Aalto-Korte K, Lauerma A, Susitaival P. Long-term follow-up study of occupational hand eczema. Br J Dermatol. 2010 Aug 13.

Mallol J, Solé D, Baeza-Bacab M, Aguirre-Camposano V, Soto-Quiros M, Baena-Cagnani C; Latin American ISAAC Group. Regional variation in asthma symptom prevalence in Latin American children. *J Asthma.* 2010 Aug;47(6):644-50.

Maneechotesuwan K, Supawita S, Kasetsinsombat K, Wongkajornsilp A, Barnes PJ. Sputum indoleamine-2, 3-dioxygenase activity is increased in asthmatic airways by using inhaled corticosteroids. *J Allergy Clin Immunol.* 2008 Jan;121(1):43-50.

Mansfield LE, Posey CR. Daytime sleepiness and cognitive performance improve in seasonal allergic rhinitis treated with intranasal fluticasone propionate. *Allergy Asthma Proc.* 2007 Mar-Apr;28(2):226-9.

Mansson HL. Fatty acids in bovine milk fat. *Food Nutr Res.* 2008;52. doi: 10.3402/fnr.v52i0.1821.

Manz F. Hydration and disease. *J Am Coll Nutr.* 2007 Oct;26(5 Suppl):535S-541S.

Marcucci F, Duse M, Frati F, Incorvaia C, Marseglia GL, La Rosa M. The future of sublingual immunotherapy. *Int J Immunopathol Pharmacol.* 2009 Oct-Dec;22(4 Suppl):31-3.

Margioris AN. Fatty acids and postprandial inflammation. *Curr Opin Clin Nutr Metab Care.* 2009 Mar;12(2):129-37.

Maria KW, Behrens T, Brasky TM. Are asthma and allergies in children and adolescents increasing? Results from ISAAC Phase I and Phase II surveys in Munster, Germany. Allergy. 2003;58:572-579.

Marth K, Novatchkova M, Focke-Tejkl M, Jenisch S, Jäger S, Kabelitz D, Valenta R. Tracing antigen signatures in the human IgE repertoire. *Mol Immunol.* 2010 Aug;47(14):2323-9.

Martin IR, Wickens K, Patchett K, Kent R, Fitzharris P, Siebers R, Lewis S, Crane J, Holbrook N, Town GI, Smith S. Cat allergen levels in public places in New Zealand. *N Z Med J.* 1998 Sep 25;111(1074):356-8.

Martinez M. Docosahexaenoic acid therapy in docosahexaenoic acid-deficient patients with disorders of peroxisomal biogenesis. *Versicherungsmedizin.* 1996;31 Suppl:145-152

Martínez-Augustin O, Boza JJ, Del Pino JI, Lucena J, Martínez-Valverde A, Gil A. Dietary nucleotides might influence the humoral immune response against cow's milk proteins in preterm neonates. *Biol Neonate.* 1997;71(4):215-23.

Martin-Venegas R, Roig-Perez S, Ferrer R, Moreno JJ. Arachidonic acid cascade and epithelial barrier function during Caco-2 cell differentiation. J Lipid Res. 2006 Apr;3.

Maslowski KM, Mackay CR. Diet, gut microbiota and immune responses. *Nat Immunol.* 2011 Jan;12(1):5-9.

Masoli M, Fabian D, Holt S, Beasley R. The global burden of asthma: executive summary of the GINA Dissemination Committee Report. *Allergy.* 2004;59:469-478.

Massey DG, Chien YK, Fournier-Massey G. Mamane: scientific therapy for asthma? *Hawaii Med J.* 1994;53:350-1. 363.

Massicot JG, Cohen SG. Epidemiologic and socioeconomic aspects of allergic diseases. *J Allergy Clin Immunol.* 1986 Nov;78(5 Pt 2):954-8.

Matasar MJ, Neugut AI. Epidemiology of anaphylaxis in the United States. *Curr Allergy Asthma Rep.* 2003;3;30-35.

Matheson MC, Haydn Walters E, Burgess JA, Jenkins MA, Giles GG, Hopper JL, Abramson MJ, Dharmage SC. Childhood immunization and atopic disease into middle-age—a prospective cohort study. *Pediatr Allergy Immunol.* 2010 Mar;21(2 Pt 1):301-6.

Matricardi PM, Bockelbrink A, Beyer K, Keil T, Niggemann B, Grüber C, Wahn U, Lau S. Primary versus secondary immunoglobulin E sensitization to soy and wheat in the Multi-Centre Allergy Study cohort. *Clin Exp Allergy.* 2008 Mar;38(3):493-500.

Matsui EC, Matsui W. Higher serum folate levels are associated with a lower risk of atopy and wheeze. *J Allergy Clin Immunol.* 2009 Jun;123(6):1253-9.e2. 2009 May 5.

Matsumoto Y, Noguchi E, Imoto Y, Nanatsue K, Takeshita K, Shibasaki M, Arinami T, Fujieda S. Upregulation of IL17RB during natural allergen exposure in patients with seasonal allergic rhinitis. *Allergol Int.* 2011 Mar;60(1):87-92.

Mattila P, Renkonen J, Toppila-Salmi S, Parviainen V, Joenväärä S, Alff-Tuomala S, Nicorici D, Renkonen R. Time-series nasal epithelial transcriptomics during natural pollen exposure in healthy subjects and allergic patients. *Allergy.* 2010 Feb;65(2):175-83.

Mayes MD. Epidemiologic studies of environmental agents and systemic autoimmune diseases. *Environ Health Perspect.* 1999 Oct;107 Suppl 5:743-8.

McAlindon TE. Nutraceuticals: do they work and when should we use them? *Best Pract Res Clin Rheumatol.* 2006 Feb;20(1):99-115.

McCarney RW, Lasserson TJ, Linde K, Brinkhaus B. An overview of two Cochrane systematic reviews of complementary treatments for chronic asthma: acupuncture and homeopathy. *Respir Med.* 2004 Aug;98(8):687-96.

McCarney RW, Linde K, Lasserson TJ. Homeopathy for chronic asthma. *Cochrane Database Syst Rev.* 2004;(1):CD000353.

McConnaughey E. *Sea Vegetables.* Happy Camp, CA: Naturegraph, 1985.

McDougall J, McDougall M. *The McDougal Plan.* Clinton, NJ: New Win, 1983.

McHugh MK, Symanski E, Pompeii LA, Delclos GL. Prevalence of asthma by industry and occupation in the U.S. working population. *Am J Ind Med.* 2010 May;53(5):463-75.

McHugh MK, Symanski E, Pompeii LA, Delclos GL. Prevalence of asthma among adult females and males in the United States: results from the National Health and Nutrition Examination Survey (NHANES), 2001-2004. *J Asthma.* 2009 Oct;46(8):759-66.

McKeever TM, Lewis SA, Cassano PA, Ocké M, Burney P, Britton J, Smit HA. Patterns of dietary intake and relation to respiratory disease, forced expiratory volume in 1 s, and decline in 5-y forced expiratory volume. *Am J Clin Nutr.* 2010 Aug;92(2):408-15. 2010 Jun 16.

McKenzie H, Main J, Pennington CR, Parratt D. Antibody to selected strains of Saccharomyces cerevisiae (baker's and brewer's yeast) and Candida albicans in Crohn's disease. *Gut.* 1990 May;31(5):536-8.

McLachlan CN. beta-casein A1, ischaemic heart disease mortality, and other illnesses. *Med Hypotheses.* 2001 Feb;56(2):262-72.

McNally ME, Atkinson SA, Cole DE. Contribution of sulfate and sulfoesters to total sulfur intake in infants fed human milk. *J Nutr.* 1991 Aug;121(8):1250-4.

McNaught CE, Woodcock NP, Anderson AD, MacFie J. A prospective randomised trial of probiotics in critically ill patients. *Clin Nutr.* 2005 Apr;24(2):211-9.

Meglio P, Bartone E, Plantamura M, Arabito E, Giampietro PG. A protocol for oral desensitization in children with IgE-mediated cow's milk allergy. *Allergy.* 2004 Sep;59(9):980-7.

Mehra PN, Puri HS. Studies on Gaduchi satwa. *Indian J Pharm.* 1969;31:180-2.

Meier B, Shao Y, Julkunen-Tiitto R, Bettschart A, Sticher O. A chemotaxonomic survey of phenolic compounds in Swiss willow species. Planta Med. 1992;58:A698.

Meier B, Sticher O, Julkunen-Tiitto R. Pharmaceutical aspects of the use of willows in herbal remedies. Planta Med. 1988;54(6):559-560.

Melcion C, Verroust P, Baud L, Ardaillou N, Morel-Maroger L, Ardaillou R. Protective effect of procyanidolic oligomers on the heterologous phase of glomerulonephritis induced by anti-glomerular basement membrane antibodies. *C R Seances Acad Sci III.* 1982 Dec 6;295(12):721-6.

Men, Research, And The History Of Hay Fever. *OldAndSold.com*, 1943; Accessed May 16, 2011

Mendes FA, Gonçalves RC, Nunes MP, Saraiva-Romanholo BM, Cukier A, Stelmach R, Jacob-Filho W, Martins MA, Carvalho CR. Effects of aerobic training on psychosocial morbidity and symptoms in patients with asthma: a randomized clinical trial. *Chest.* 2010 Aug;138(2):331-7. 2010 Apr 2.

REFERENCES

Merchant RE and Andre CA. 2001. A review of recent clinical trials of the nutritional supplement Chlorella pyrenoidosa in the treatment of fibromyalgia, hypertension, and ulcerative colitis. *Altern Ther Health Med.* May-Jun;7(3):79-91.

Messina M. Insights gained from 20 years of soy research. *J Nutr.* 2010 Dec;140(12):2289S-2295S. 2010 Oct 27.

Metsälä J, Lundqvist A, Kaila M, Gissler M, Klaukka T, Virtanen SM. Maternal and perinatal characteristics and the risk of cow's milk allergy in infants up to 2 years of age: a case-control study nested in the Finnish population. *Am J Epidemiol.* 2010 Jun 15;171(12):1310-6.

Meyer A, Kirsch H, Domergue F, Abbadi A, Sperling P, Bauer J, Cirpus P, Zank TK, Moreau H, Roscoe TJ, Zahringer U, Heinz E. Novel fatty acid elongases and their use for the reconstitution of docosahexaenoic acid biosynthesis. *J Lipid Res.* 2004 Oct;45(10):1899-909.

Meyer AL, Elmadfa I, Herbacek I, Micksche M. Probiotic, as well as conventional yogurt, can enhance the stimulated production of proinflammatory cytokines. *J Hum Nutr Diet.* 2007 Dec;20(6):590-8.

Michaelsen KF. Probiotics, breastfeeding and atopic eczema. *Acta Derm Venereol Suppl (Stockh).* 2005 Nov;(215):21-4.

Michail S. The role of probiotics in allergic diseases. *Allergy Asthma Clin Immunol.* 2009 Oct 22;5(1):5.

Michalska K, Kisiel W. Sesquiterpene lactones from Taraxacum obovatum. *Planta Med.* 2003 Feb;69(2):181-3.

Michelson PH, Williams LW, Benjamin DK, Barnato AE. Obesity, inflammation, and asthma severity in childhood: data from the National Health and Nutrition Examination Survey 2001-2004. *Ann Allergy Asthma Immunol.* 2009 Nov;103(5):381-5.

Mickleborough TD, Lindley MR, Ray S. Dietary salt, airway inflammation, and diffusion capacity in exercise-induced asthma. *Med Sci Sports Exerc.* 2005 Jun;37(6):904-14.

Mikoluc B, Motkowski R, Karpinska J, Piotrowska-Jastrzebska J. Plasma levels of vitamins A and E, coenzyme Q10, and anti-ox-LDL antibody titer in children treated with an elimination diet due to food hypersensitivity. *Int J Vitam Nutr Res.* 2009 Sep;79(5-6):328-36.

Miller AL. The etiologies, pathophysiology, and alternative/complementary treatment of asthma. *Altern Med Rev.* 2001 Feb;6(1):20-47.

Miller GT. *Living in the Environment.* Belmont, CA: Wadsworth, 1996.

Mindell E, Hopkins V. *Prescription Alternatives.* New Canaan, CT: Keats, 1998.

Miranda H, Outeiro TF. The sour side of neurodegenerative disorders: the effects of protein glycation. *J Pathol.* 2010 May;221(1):13-25.

Mitchell AE, Hong YJ, Koh E, Barrett DM, Bryant DE, Denison RF, Kaffka S. Ten-year comparison of the influence of organic and conventional crop management practices on the content of flavonoids in tomatoes. *J Agric Food Chem.* 2007 Jul 25;55(15):6154-9.

Mittag D, Akkerdaas J, Ballmer-Weber BK, Vogel L, Wensing M, Becker WM, Koppelman SJ, Knulst AC, Helbling A, Hefle SL, Van Ree R, Vieths S. Ara h 8, a Bet v 1-homologous allergen from peanut, is a major allergen in patients with combined birch pollen and peanut allergy. *J Allergy Clin Immunol.* 2004 Dec;114(6):1410-7.

Mittag D, Vieths S, Vogel L, Becker WM, Rihs HP, Helbling A, Wüthrich B, Ballmer-Weber BK. Soybean allergy in patients allergic to birch pollen: clinical investigation and molecular characterization of allergens. *J Allergy Clin Immunol.* 2004 Jan;113(1):148-54.

Miyake Y, Sasaki S, Tanaka K, Hirota Y. Dairy food, calcium and vitamin D intake in pregnancy, and wheeze and eczema in infants. *Eur Respir J.* 2010 Jun;35(6):1228-34. 2009 Oct 19.

Miyazawa T, Itahashi K, Imai T. Management of neonatal cow's milk allergy in high-risk neonates. *Pediatr Int.* 2009 Aug;51(4):544-7.

Moattari A, Aleyasin S, Arabpour M, Sadeghi S. Prevalence of Human Metapneumovirus (hMPV) in Children with Wheezing in Shiraz-Iran. *Iran J Allergy Asthma Immunol.* 2010 Dec;9(4):250-4.

Mokhtar N, Chan SC. Use of complementary medicine amongst asthmatic patients in primary care. *Med J Malaysia.* 2006 Mar;61(1):125-7.

Monarca S, Zerbini I, Simonati C, Gelatti U. Drinking water hardness and chronic degenerative diseases. Part II. Cardiovascular diseases. *Ann. Ig.* 2003;15:41-56.

Moneret-Vautrin DA, Kanny G, Thévenin F. Asthma caused by food allergy. *Rev Med Interne.* 1996;17(7):551-7.

Moneret-Vautrin DA, Morisset M. Adult food allergy. *Curr Allergy Asthma Rep.* 2005 Jan;5(1):80-5.

Monks H, Gowland MH, Mackenzie H, Erlewyn-Lajeunesse M, King R, Lucas JS, Roberts G. How do teenagers manage their food allergies? *Clin Exp Allergy.* 2010 Aug 2.

Moorhead KJ, Morgan HC. *Spirulina: Nature's Superfood.* Kailua-Kona, HI: Nutrex, 1995.

Moreira A, Delgado L, Haahtela T, Fonseca J, Moreira P, Lopes C, Mota J, Santos P, Rytilä P, Castel-Branco MG. Physical training does not increase allergic inflammation in asthmatic children. *Eur Respir J.* 2008 Dec;32(6):1570-5.

Moreira P, Moreira A, Padrão P, Delgado L. The role of economic and educational factors in asthma: evidence from the Portuguese health survey. *Public Health.* 2008 Apr;122(4):434-9. 2007 Oct 17.

387

Morel AF, Dias GO, Porto C, Simionatto E, Stuker CZ, Dalcol II. Antimicrobial activity of extractives of Solidago microglossa. *Fitoterapia*. 2006 Sep;77(6):453-5.

Morisset M, Moneret-Vautrin DA, Guenard L, Cuny JM, Frentz P, Hatahet R, Hanss Ch, Beaudouin E, Petit N, Kanny G. Oral desensitization in children with milk and egg allergies obtains recovery in a significant proportion of cases. A randomized study in 60 children with cow's milk allergy and 90 children with egg allergy. *Eur Ann Allergy Clin Immunol*. 2007 Jan;39(1):12-9.

Morisset M, Moneret-Vautrin DA, Kanny G, Guénard L, Beaudouin E, Flabbée J, Hatahet R. Thresholds of clinical reactivity to milk, egg, peanut and sesame in immunoglobulin E-dependent allergies: evaluation by double-blind or single-blind placebo-controlled oral challenges. *Clin Exp Allergy*. 2003 Aug;33(8):1046-51.

Moussaieff A, Shein NA, Tsenter J, Grigoriadis S, Simeonidou C, Alexandrovich AG, Trembovler V, Ben-Neriah Y, Schmitz ML, Fiebich BL, Munoz E, Mechoulam R, Shohami E. Incensole acetate: a novel neuroprotective agent isolated from Boswellia carterii. *J Cereb Blood Flow Metab*. 2008 Jul;28(7):1341-52.

Moyle A. *Nature Cure for Asthma and Hay Fever*. Wellingborough, U.K.: Thorsons, 1978.

Mozaffarian D, Aro A, Willett WC. Health effects of trans-fatty acids: experimental and observational evidence. *Eur J Clin Nutr*. 2009 May;63 Suppl 2:S5-21.

Müller S, Pühl S, Vieth M, Stolte M. Analysis of symptoms and endoscopic findings in 117 patients with histological diagnoses of eosinophilic esophagitis. *Endoscopy*. 2007 Apr;39(4):339-44.

Murray M, Pizzorno J. *Encyclopedia of Natural Medicine*. 2nd Edition. Roseville, CA: Prima Publishing, 1998.

Nadkarni AK, Nadkarni KM. *Indian Materia Medica*. (Vols 1 and 2). Bombay, India: Popular Pradashan, 1908, 1976.

Nagai T, Arai Y, Emori M, Nunome SY, Yabe T, Takeda T, Yamada H. Anti-allergic activity of a Kampo (Japanese herbal) medicine "Sho-seiryu-to (Xiao-Qing-Long-Tang)" on airway inflammation in a mouse model. *Int Immunopharmacol*. 2004 Oct;4(10-11):1353-65.

Nagel G, Linseisen J. Dietary intake of fatty acids, antioxidants and selected food groups and asthma in adults. *Eur J Clin Nutr*. 2005 Jan;59(1):8-15.

Nagel G, Weinmayr G, Kleiner A, Garcia-Marcos L, Strachan DP; ISAAC Phase Two Study Group. Effect of diet on asthma and allergic sensitisation in the International Study on Allergies and Asthma in Childhood (ISAAC) Phase Two. *Thorax*. 2010 Jun;65(6):516-22.

Naghii MR, Samman S. The role of boron in nutrition and metabolism. *Prog Food Nutr Sci*. 1993 Oct-Dec;17(4):331-49.

Nair PK, Rodriguez S, Ramachandran R, Alamo A, Melnick SJ, Escalon E, Garcia PI Jr, Wnuk SF, Ramachandran C. Immune stimulating properties of a novel polysaccharide from the medicinal plant Tinospora cordifolia. *Int Immunopharmacol*. 2004 Dec 15;4(13):1645-59.

Nakano T, Shimojo N, Morita Y, Arima T, Tomiita M, Kohno Y. Sensitization to casein and beta-lactoglobulin (BLG) in children with cow's milk allergy (CMA). *Arerugi*. 2010 Feb;59(2):117-22.

Napoli, J.E., Brand-Miller, J.C., Conway, P. (2003) Bifidogenic effects of feeding infant formula containing galactooligosaccharides in healthy formula-fed infants. *Asia Pac J Clin Nutr*. 12(Suppl): S60

Nariya M, Shukla V, Jain S, Ravishankar B. Comparison of enteroprotective efficacy of triphala formulations (Indian Herbal Drug) on methotrexate-induced small intestinal damage in rats. *Phytother Res*. 2009 Aug;23(8):1092-8.

Naruszewicz M, Johansson ML, Zapolska-Downar D, Bukowska H. Effect of Lactobacillus plantarum 299v on cardiovascular disease risk factors in smokers. *Am J Clin Nutr*. 2002 Dec;76(6):1249-55.

National Cooperation Group on Childhood Asthma. A nationwide survey in China on prevalence of asthma in urban children. *Chin J Pediatr*. pp. 123-127.

National Toxicology Program. Final Report on Carcinogens Background Document for Formaldehyde. *Rep Carcinog Backgr Doc*. 2010 Jan;(10-5981):i-512.

NDL, BHNRC, ARS, USDA. *Oxygen Radical Absorbance Capacity (ORAC) of Selected Foods - 2007*. Beltsville, MD: USDA-ARS. 2007.

Nentwich I, Michková E, Nevoral J, Urbanek R, Szépfalusi Z. Cow's milk-specific cellular and humoral immune responses and atopy skin symptoms in infants from atopic families fed a partially (pHF) or extensively (eHF) hydrolyzed infant formula. *Allergy*. 2001 Dec;56(12):1144-56.

Newall CA, Anderson LA, Phillipson JD (eds). *Herbal Medicines: A Guide for Health-Care Professionals*. London: Pharmaceut Press; 1996.

Newmark T, Schulick P. *Beyond Aspirin*. Prescott, AZ: Holm, 2000.

Neyestani TR, Shariatzadeh N, Gharavi A, Kalayi A, Khalaji N. Physiological dose of lycopene suppressed oxidative stress and enhanced serum levels of immunoglobulin M in patients with Type 2 diabetes mellitus: a possible role in the prevention of long-term complications. *J Endocrinol Invest*. 2007 Nov;30(10):833-8.

Ngai SP, Jones AY, Hui-Chan CW, Ko FW, Hui DS. Effect of Acu-TENS on post-exercise expiratory lung volume in subjects with asthma-A randomized controlled trial. *Respir Physiol Neurobiol*. 2009 Jul 31;167(3):348-53. 2009 Jun 18.

Nicholls SJ, Lundman P, Harmer JA, Cutri B, Griffiths KA, Rye KA, Barter PJ, Celermajer DS. Consumption of saturated fat impairs the anti-inflammatory properties of high-density lipoproteins and endothelial function. *J Am Coll Cardiol.* 2006 Aug 15;48(4):715-20.

Nicolaou N, Poorafshar M, Murray C, Simpson A, Winell H, Kerry G, Härlin A, Woodcock A, Ahlstedt S, Custovic A. Allergy or tolerance in children sensitized to peanut: prevalence and differentiation using component-resolved diagnostics. *J Allergy Clin Immunol.* 2010 Jan;125(1):191-7.e1-13.

Niederau C, Göpfert E. The effect of chelidonium- and turmeric root extract on upper abdominal pain due to functional disorders of the biliary system. Results from a placebo-controlled double-blind study. *Med Klin.* 1999 Aug 15;94(8):425-30.

Nielsen RG, Bindslev-Jensen C, Kruse-Andersen S, Husby S. Severe gastroesophageal reflux disease and cow milk hypersensitivity in infants and children: disease association and evaluation of a new challenge procedure. *J Pediatr Gastroenterol Nutr.* 2004 Oct;39(4):383-91.

Niggemann B, von Berg A, Bollrath C, Berdel D, Schauer U, Rieger C, Haschke-Becher E, Wahn U. Safety and efficacy of a new extensively hydrolyzed formula for infants with cow's milk protein allergy. *Pediatr Allergy Immunol.* 2008 Jun;19(4):348-54.

Nightingale JA, Rogers DF, Hart LA, Kharitonov SA, Chung KF, Barnes PJ. Effect of inhaled endotoxin on induced sputum in normal, atopic, and atopic asthmatic subjects. *Thorax.* 1998 Jul;53(7):563-71.

Niimi A, Nguyen LT, Usmani O, Mann B, Chung KF. Reduced pH and chloride levels in exhaled breath condensate of patients with chronic cough. *Thorax.* 2004 Jul;59(7):608-12.

Ninan TK, Russell G. Respiratory symptoms and atopy in Aberdeen schoolchildren: evidence from two surveys 25 years apart. BMJ. 1992;304:873-875.

Njoroge GN, Bussmann RW. Traditional management of ear, nose and throat (ENT) diseases in Central Kenya. *J Ethnobiol Ethnomed.* 2006 Dec 27;2:54.

Nobaek S, Johansson ML, Molin G, Ahrné S, Jeppsson B. Alteration of intestinal microflora is associated with reduction in abdominal bloating and pain in patients with irritable bowel syndrome. *Am J Gastroenterol.* 2000 May;95(5):1231-8.

Nodake Y, Fukumoto S, Fukasawa M, Sakakibara R, Yamasaki N. Reduction of the immunogenicity of beta-lactoglobulin from cow's milk by conjugation with a dextran derivative. *Biosci Biotechnol Biochem.* 2010;74(4):721-6.

Noh J, Lee JH, Noh G, Bang SY, Kim HS, Choi WS, Cho S, Lee SS. Characterisation of allergen-specific responses of IL-10-producing regulatory B cells (Br1) in Cow Milk Allergy. *Cell Immunol.* 2010;264(2):143-9.

Noorbakhsh R, Mortazavi SA, Sankian M, Shahidi F, Assarehzadegan MA, Varasteh A. Cloning, expression, characterization, and computational approach for cross-reactivity prediction of manganese superoxide dismutase allergen from pistachio nut. *Allergol Int.* 2010 Sep;59(3):295-304.

Novembre E, Dini L, Bernardini R, Resti M, Vierucci A. Unusual reactions to food additives. *Pediatr Med Chir.* 1992 Jan-Feb;14(1):39-42.

Nowak-Wegrzyn A, Fiocchi A. Is oral immunotherapy the cure for food allergies? *Curr Opin Allergy Clin Immunol.* 2010 Jun;10(3):214-9.

Nsouli TM. Long-term use of nasal saline irrigation: harmful or helpful? *Amer Acad of Allergy, Asthma and Immunol.* 2009; Abstract O32.

Nurmatov U, Devereux G, Sheikh A. Nutrients and foods for the primary prevention of asthma and allergy: Systematic review and meta-analysis. *J Allergy Clin Immunol.* 2010 Dec 23.

Nusem D, Panasoff J. Beer anaphylaxis. *Isr Med Assoc J.* 2009 Jun;11(6):380-1.

Nwaru BI, Erkkola M, Ahonen S, Kaila M, Haapala AM, Kronberg-Kippilä C, Salmelin R, Veijola R, Ilonen J, Simell O, Knip M, Virtanen SM. Age at the introduction of solid foods during the first year and allergic sensitization at age 5 years. *Pediatrics.* 2010 Jan;125(1):50-9. 2009 Dec 7.

O'Connor J., Bensky D. (ed). *Shanghai College of Traditional Chinese Medicine: Acupuncture: A Comprehensive Text.* Seattle: Eastland Press, 1981.

O'Neil C, Helbling AA, Lehrer SB. Allergic reactions to fish. *Clin Rev Allergy.* 1993 Summer;11(2):183-200.

O'Neil C, Helbling AA, Lehrer SB. Allergic reactions to fish. *Clin Rev Allergy.* 1993;11(2):183-200.

Odamaki T, Xiao JZ, Iwabuchi N, Sakamoto M, Takahashi N, Kondo S, Miyaji K, Iwatsuki K, Togashi H, Enomoto T, Benno Y. Influence of Bifidobacterium longum BB536 intake on faecal microbiota in individuals with Japanese cedar pollinosis during the pollen season. *J Med Microbiol.* 2007 Oct;56(Pt 10):1301-8.

Oehme FW (ed.). *Toxicity of heavy metals in the environment. Part 1.* New York: M.Dekker, 1979.

Ogawa T, Hashikawa S, Asai Y, Sakamoto H, Yasuda K, Makimura Y. A new synbiotic, Lactobacillus casei subsp. casei together with dextran, reduces murine and human allergic reaction. *FEMS Immunol Med Microbiol.* 2006 Apr;46(3):400-9.

Oh CK, Lücker PW, Wetzelsberger N, Kuhlmann F. The determination of magnesium, calcium, sodium and potassium in assorted foods with special attention to the loss of electrolytes after various forms of food preparations. *Mag.-Bull.* 1986;8:297-302.

Oh SY, Chung J, Kim MK, Kwon SO, Cho BH. Antioxidant nutrient intakes and corresponding biomarkers associated with the risk of atopic dermatitis in young children. *Eur J Clin Nutr.* 2010 Mar;64(3):245-52. 2010 Jan 27.

Ok IS, Kim SH, Kim BK, Lee JC, Lee YC. Pinellia ternata, Citrus reticulata, and their combinational prescription inhibit eosinophil infiltration and airway hyperresponsiveness by suppressing CCR3+ and Th2 cytokines production in the ovalbumin-induced asthma model. *Mediators Inflamm.* 2009;2009:413270.

Oldak E, Kurzatkowska B, Stasiak-Barmuta A. Natural course of sensitization in children: follow-up study from birth to 6 years of age, I. Evaluation of total serum IgE and specific IgE antibodies with regard to atopic family history. *Rocz Akad Med Bialymst.* 2000;45:87-95.

Onbasi K, Sin AZ, Doganavsargil B, Onder GF, Bor S, Sebik F. Eosinophil infiltration of the oesophageal mucosa in patients with pollen allergy during the season. *Clin Exp Allergy.* 2005 Nov;35(11):1423-31.

Oreskovic NM, Sawicki GS, Kinane TB, Winickoff JP, Perrin JM. Travel patterns to school among children with asthma. *Clin Pediatr.* 2009 Jul;48(6):632-40. 2009 May 6.

Ortiz-Andrellucchi A, Sánchez-Villegas A, Rodríguez-Gallego C, Lemes A, Molero T, Soria A, Peña-Quintana L, Santana M, Ramírez O, García J, Cabrera F, Cobo J, Serra-Majem L. Immunomodulatory effects of the intake of fermented milk with Lactobacillus casei DN114001 in lactating mothers and their children. *Br J Nutr.* 2008 Oct;100(4):834-45.

Osguthorpe JD. Immunotherapy. *Curr Opin Otolaryngol Head Neck Surg.* 2010 Jun;18(3):206-12.

Otto SJ, van Houwelingen AC, Hornstra G. The effect of supplementation with docosahexaenoic and arachidonic acid derived from single cell oils on plasma and erythrocyte fatty acids of pregnant women in the second trimester. *Prostaglandins Leukot Essent Fatty Acids.* 2000 Nov;63(5):323-8.

Ou CC, Tsao SM, Lin MC, Yin MC. Protective action on human LDL against oxidation and glycation by four organosulfur compounds derived from garlic. *Lipids.* 2003 Mar;38(3):219-24.

Ouwehand AC, Bergsma N, Parhiala R, Lahtinen S, Gueimonde M, Finne-Soveri H, Strandberg T, Pitkälä K, Salminen S. Bifidobacterium microbiota and parameters of immune function in elderly subjects. *FEMS Immunol Med Microbiol.* 2008 Jun;53(1):18-25.

Ouwehand AC, Nermes M, Collado MC, Rautonen N, Salminen S, Isolauri E. Specific probiotics alleviate allergic rhinitis during the birch pollen season. *World J Gastroenterol.* 2009 Jul 14;15(26):3261-8.

Ouwehand AC, Nermes M, Collado MC, Rautonen N, Salminen S, Isolauri E. Specific probiotics alleviate allergic rhinitis during the birch pollen season. *World J Gastroenterol.* 2009 Jul 14;15(26):3261-8.

Ouwehand AC, Tiihonen K, Saarinen M, Putaala H, Rautonen N. Influence of a combination of Lactobacillus acidophilus NCFM and lactitol on healthy elderly: intestinal and immune parameters. *Br J Nutr.* 2009 Feb;101(3):367-75.

Ozdemir O. Any benefits of probiotics in allergic disorders? *Allergy Asthma Proc.* 2010 Mar;31(2):103-11.

Paganelli R, Pallone F, Montano S, Le Moli S, Matricardi PM, Fais S, Paoluzi P, D'Amelio R, Aiuti F. Isotypic analysis of antibody response to a food antigen in inflammatory bowel disease. *Int Arch Allergy Appl Immunol.* 1985;78(1):81-5.

Pahud JJ, Schwarz K. Research and development of infant formulae with reduced allergenic properties. *Ann Allergy.* 1984 Dec;53(6 Pt 2):609-14.

Pakhale S, Doucette S, Vandemheen K, Boulet LP, McIvor RA, Fitzgerald JM, Hernandez P, Lemiere C, Sharma S, Field SK, Alvarez GG, Dales RE, Aaron SD. A comparison of obese and nonobese people with asthma: exploring an asthma-obesity interaction. *Chest.* 2010 Jun;137(6):1316-23. 2010 Feb 12.

Palacin A, Bartra J, Muñoz R, Diaz-Perales A, Valero A, Salcedo G. Anaphylaxis to wheat flour-derived foodstuffs and the lipid transfer protein syndrome: a potential role of wheat lipid transfer protein Tri a 14. *Int Arch Allergy Immunol.* 2010;152(2):178-83.

Palacios R, Sugawara I. Hydrocortisone abrogates proliferation of T cells in autologous mixed lymphocyte reaction by rendering the interleukin-2 Producer T cells unresponsive to interleukin-1 and unable to synthesize the T-cell growth factor. *Scand J Immunol.* 1982 Jan;15(1):25-31. 7.

Palacios R. HLA-DR antigens render interleukin-2-producer T lymphocytes sensitive to interleukin-1. *Scand J Immunol.* 1981 Sep;14(3):321-6.

Palmer DJ, Gold MS, Makrides M. Effect of cooked and raw egg consumption on ovalbumin content of human milk: a randomized, double-blind, cross-over trial. *Clin Exp Allergy.* 2005 Feb;35(2):173-8.

Panghal S, Mallapur SS, Kumar M, Ram V, Singh BK. Antiinflammatory Activity of Piper longum Fruit Oil. *Indian J Pharm Sci.* 2009 Jul;71(4):454-6.

Pant H, Ferguson BJ, Macardle PJ. The role of allergy in rhinosinusitis. *Curr Opin Otolaryngol Head Neck Surg.* 2009 Jun;17(3):232-8.

Pant H, Kette FE, Smith WB, Wormald PJ, Macardle PJ. Fungal-specific humoral response in eosinophilic mucus chronic rhinosinusitis. *Laryngoscope.* 2005 Apr;115(4):601-6.

Panzani R, Ariano R, Mistrello G. Cypress pollen does not cross-react to plant-derived foods. *Eur Ann Allergy Clin Immunol.* 2010 Jun;42(3):125-6.

Parcell S. Sulfur in human nutrition and applications in medicine. *Altern Med Rev.* 2002 Feb;7(1):22-44.

Park BJ, Tsunetsugu Y, Kasetani T, Kagawa T, Miyazaki Y. The physiological effects of Shinrin-yoku (taking in the forest atmosphere or forest bathing): evidence from field experiments in 24 forests across Japan. *Environ Health Prev Med.* 2010 Jan;15(1):18-26.

Parra D, De Morentin BM, Cobo JM, Mateos A, Martinez JA. Monocyte function in healthy middle-aged people receiving fermented milk containing Lactobacillus casei. *J Nutr Health Aging.* 2004;8(4):208-11.

Parra MD, Martínez de Morentin BE, Cobo JM, Mateos A, Martínez JA. Daily ingestion of fermented milk containing Lactobacillus casei DN114001 improves innate-defense capacity in healthy middle-aged people. *J Physiol Biochem.* 2004 Jun;60(2):85-91.

Partridge MR, Dockrell M, Smith NM: The use of complementary medicines by those with asthma. Respir Med 2003, 97:436-438.

Pastorello EA, Farioli L, Conti A, Pravettoni V, Bonomi S, Iametti S, Fortunato D, Scibilia J, Bindslev-Jensen C, Ballmer-Weber B, Robino AM, Ortolani C. Wheat IgE-mediated food allergy in European patients: alpha-amylase inhibitors, lipid transfer proteins and low-molecular-weight glutenins. Allergenic molecules recognized by double-blind, placebo-controlled food challenge. *Int Arch Allergy Immunol.* 2007;144(1):10-22.

Pastorello EA, Pompei C, Pravettoni V, Farioli L, Calamari AM, Scibilia J, Robino AM, Conti A, Iametti S, Fortunato D, Bonomi S, Ortolani C. Lipid-transfer protein is the major maize allergen maintaining IgE-binding activity after cooking at 100 degrees C, as demonstrated in anaphylactic patients and patients with positive double-blind, placebo-controlled food challenge results. *J Allergy Clin Immunol.* 2003 Oct;112(4):775-83.

Patchett K, Lewis S, Crane J, Fitzharris P. Cat allergen (Fel d 1) levels on school children's clothing and in primary school classrooms in Wellington, New Zealand. *J Allergy Clin Immunol.* 1997 Dec;100(6 Pt 1):755-9.

Patel DS, Rafferty GF, Lee S, Hannam S, Greenough A. Work of breathing and volume targeted ventilation in respiratory distress. *Arch Dis Child Fetal Neonatal Ed.* 2010 Nov;95(6):F443-6.

Patriarca G, Nucera E, Pollastrini E, Roncallo C, De Pasquale T, Lombardo C, Pedone C, Gasbarrini G, Buonomo A, Schiavino D. Oral specific desensitization in food-allergic children. *Dig Dis Sci.* 2007 Jul;52(7):1662-72.

Patriarca G, Nucera E, Roncallo C, Pollastrini E, Bartolozzi F, De Pasquale T, Buonomo A, Gasbarrini G, Di Campli C, Schiavino D. Oral desensitizing treatment in food allergy: clinical and immunological results. *Aliment Pharmacol Ther.* 2003 Feb;17(3):459-65.

Patwardhan B, Gautam M. Botanical immunodrugs: scope and opportunities. *Drug Discov Today.* 2005 Apr 1;10(7):495-502.

Payment P, Franco E, Richardson L, Siemiatyck, J. Gastrointestinal health effects associated with the consumption of drinking water produced by point-of-use domestic reverse-osmosis filtration units. *Appl. Environ. Microbiol.* 1991;57:945-948.

Peat JK, van den Berg RH, Green WF, Mellis CM, Leeder SR, Woolcock AJ. Changing prevalence of asthma in Australian children. *BMJ.* 1994;308:1591-1596.

Peat JK. The rising trend in allergic illness: which environmental factors are important? Clin Exp Allergy. 1994 Sep;24(9):797-800.

Pehowich DJ, Gomes AV, Barnes JA. Fatty acid composition and possible health effects of coconut constituents. *West Indian Med J.* 2000 Jun;49(2):128-33.

Perez-Galvez A, Martin HD, Sies H, Stahl W. Incorporation of carotenoids from paprika oleoresin into human chylomicrons. *Br J Nutr.* 2003 Jun;89(6):787-93.

Perez-Pena R. Secrets of the Mummy's Medicine Chest. *NY Times.* 2005 Sept 10.

Pessi T, Sütas Y, Hurme M, Isolauri E. Interleukin-10 generation in atopic children following oral Lactobacillus rhamnosus GG. *Clin Exp Allergy.* 2000 Dec;30(12):1804-8.

Peters JI, McKinney JM, Smith B, Wood P, Forkner E, Galbreath AD. Impact of obesity in asthma: evidence from a large prospective disease management study. *Ann Allergy Asthma Immunol.* 2011 Jan;106(1):30-5.

Peterson CG, Hansson T, Skott A, Bengtsson U, Ahlstedt S, Magnussons J. Detection of local mast-cell activity in patients with food hypersensitivity. *J Investig Allergol Clin Immunol.* 2007;17(5):314-20.

Peterson KA, Samuelson WM, Ryujin DT, Young DC, Thomas KL, Hilden K, Fang JC. The role of gastroesophageal reflux in exercise-triggered asthma: a randomized controlled trial. *Dig Dis Sci.* 2009 Mar;54(3):564-71. 2008 Aug 8.

Petlevski R, Hadzija M, Slijepcević M, Juretić D, Petrik J. Glutathione S-transferases and malondialdehyde in the liver of NOD mice on short-term treatment with plant mixture extract P-9801091. *Phytother Res.* 2003 Apr;17(4):311-4.

Pfefferle PI, Sel S, Ege MJ, Büchele G, Blümer N, Krauss-Etschmann S, Herzum I, Albers CE, Lauener RP, Roponen M, Hirvonen MR, Vuitton DA, Riedler J, Brunekreef B, Dalphin JC, Braun-Fahrländer C, Pekkanen J, von Mutius E, Renz H; PASTURE Study Group. Cord blood allergen-specific IgE is associated with reduced IFN-gamma production by cord blood cells: the Protection against Allergy-Study in Rural Environments (PASTURE) Study. *J Allergy Clin Immunol.* 2008 Oct;122(4):711-6.

Pfundstein B, El Desouky SK, Hull WE, Haubner R, Erben G, Owen RW. Polyphenolic compounds in the fruits of Egyptian medicinal plants (Terminalia bellerica, Terminalia chebula and Terminalia horrida): characterization, quantitation and determination of antioxidant capacities. *Phytochemistry.* 2010 Jul;71(10):1132-48.

Physicians' Desk Reference. Montvale, NJ: Thomson, 2003-2008.

Pierce SK, Klinman NR. Antibody-specific immunoregulation. *J Exp Med.* 1977 Aug 1;146(2):509-19.

Piirainen L, Haahtela S, Helin T, Korpela R, Haahtela T, Vaarala O. Effect of Lactobacillus rhamnosus GG on rBet v1 and rMal d1 specific IgA in the saliva of patients with birch pollen allergy. *Ann Allergy Asthma Immunol.* 2008 Apr;100(4):338-42.

Pike MG, Heddle RJ, Boulton P, Turner MW, Atherton DJ. Increased intestinal permeability in atopic eczema. *J Invest Dermatol.* 1986 Feb;86(2):101-4.

Pines JM, Prabhu A, Hilton JA, Hollander JE, Datner EM. The effect of emergency department crowding on length of stay and medication treatment times in discharged patients with acute asthma. *Acad Emerg Med.* 2010 Aug;17(8):834-9.

Pitten FA, Scholler M, Krüger U, Effendy I, Kramer A. Filamentous fungi and yeasts on mattresses covered with different encasings. *Eur J Dermatol.* 2001 Nov-Dec;11(6):534-7.

Pitt-Rivers R, Trotter WR. *The Thyroid Gland.* London: Butterworth Publ, 1954.

Plaschke P, Janson C, Norrman E, Björnsson E, Ellbjär S, Järvholm B. Association between atopic sensitization and asthma and bronchial hyperresponsiveness in swedish adults: pets, and not mites, are the most important allergens. *J Allergy Clin Immunol.* 1999 Jul;104(1):58-65.

Plaut M, Valentine MD. Clinical practice. Allergic rhinitis. *N Engl J Med.* 2005 Nov 3;353(18):1934-44.

Plaut TE, Jones TB. *Dr. Tom Plaut's Asthma guide for people of all ages.* Amherst, MA: Pedipress, 1999.

Plaza V, Miguel E, Bellido-Casado J, Lozano MP, Ríos L, Bolíbar I. [Usefulness of the Guidelines of the Spanish Society of Pulmonology and Thoracic Surgery (SEPAR) in identifying the causes of chronic cough]. Arch Bronconeumol. 2006 Feb;42(2):68-73.

Plohmann B, Bader G, Hiller K, Franz G. Immunomodulatory and antitumoral effects of triterpenoid saponins. *Pharmazie.* 1997 Dec;52(12):953-7.

Poblocka-Olech L, Krauze-Baranowska M. SPE-HPTLC of procyanidins from the barks of different species and clones of Salix. *J Pharm Biomed Anal.* 2008 Nov 4;48(3):965-8.

Pohjavuori E, Viljanen M, Korpela R, Kuitunen M, Tiittanen M, Vaarala O, Savilahti E. Lactobacillus GG effect in increasing IFN-gamma production in infants with cow's milk allergy. *J Allergy Clin Immunol.* 2004 Jul;114(1):131-6.

Polito A, Aboab J, Annane D. The hypothalamic pituitary adrenal axis in sepsis. *Novartis Found Symp.* 2007;280:182-203.

Polk S, Sunyer J, Muñoz-Ortiz L, Barnes M, Torrent M, Figueroa C, Harris J, Vall O, Antó JM, Cullinan P. A prospective study of Fel d1 and Der p1 exposure in infancy and childhood wheezing. *Am J Respir Crit Care Med.* 2004 Aug 1;170(3):273-8.

Pollini F, Capristo C, Boner AL. Upper respiratory tract infections and atopy. *Int J Immunopathol Pharmacol.* 2010 Jan-Mar;23(1 Suppl):32-7.

Ponsonby AL, McMichael A, van der Mei I. Ultraviolet radiation and autoimmune disease: insights from epidemiological research. *Toxicology.* 2002 Dec 27;181-182:71-8.

Postlethwait EM. Scavenger receptors clear the air. *J Clin Invest.* 2007 Mar;117(3):601-4.

Postma DS. Gender Differences in Asthma Development and Progression. *Gender Medicine.* 2007;4:S133-146.

Postolache TT, Lapidus M, Sander ER, Langenberg P, Hamilton RG, Soriano JJ, McDonald JS, Furst N, Bai J, Scrandis DA, Cabassa JA, Stiller JW, Balis T, Guzman A, Togias A, Tonelli LH. Changes in allergy symptoms and depression scores are positively correlated in patients with recurrent mood disorders exposed to seasonal peaks in aeroallergens. *ScientificWorldJournal.* 2007 Dec 17;7:1968-77.

Potterton D. (Ed.) *Culpeper's Color Herbal.* New York: Sterling, 1983.

Poulos LM, Waters AM, Correll PK, Loblay RH, Marks GB. Trends in hospitalizations for anaphylaxis, angioedema, and urticaria in Australia, 1993-1994 to 2004-2005. *J Allergy Clin Immunol.* 2007 Oct;120(4):878-84.

Powe DG, Groot Kormelink T, Sisson M, Blokhuis BJ, Kramer MF, Jones NS, Redegeld FA. Evidence for the involvement of free light chain immunoglobulins in allergic and nonallergic rhinitis. *J Allergy Clin Immunol.* 2010 Jan;125(1):139-45.e1-3.

Prescott SL, Wickens K, Westcott L, Jung W, Currie H, Black PN, Stanley TV, Mitchell EA, Fitzharris P, Siebers R, Wu L, Crane J; Probiotic Study Group. Supplementation with Lactobacillus rhamnosus or Bifidobacterium lactis probiotics in pregnancy increases cord blood interferon-gamma and breast milk transforming growth factor-beta and immunoglobin A detection. *Clin Exp Allergy.* 2008 Oct;38(10):1606-14.

REFERENCES

Priftis KN, Panagiotakos DB, Anthracopoulos MB, Papadimitriou A, Nicolaidou P. Aims, methods and preliminary findings of the Physical Activity, Nutrition and Allergies in Children Examined in Athens (PANACEA) epidemiological study. *BMC Public Health.* 2007 Jul 4;7:140.

Prioult G, Fliss I, Pecquet S. Effect of probiotic bacteria on induction and maintenance of oral tolerance to beta-lactoglobulin in gnotobiotic mice. *Clin Diagn Lab Immunol.* 2003 Sep;10(5):787-92.

Prucksunand C, Indrasukhsri B, Leethochawalit M, Hungspreugs K. Phase II clinical trial on effect of the long turmeric (Curcuma longa Linn) on healing of peptic ulcer. *Southeast Asian J Trop Med Public Health.* 2001 Mar;32(1):208-15.

Pruthi S, Thapa MM. Infectious and inflammatory disorders. *Magn Reson Imaging Clin N Am.* 2009 Aug;17(3):423-38, v.

Qin HL, Zheng JJ, Tong DN, Chen WX, Fan XB, Hang XM, Jiang YQ. Effect of Lactobacillus plantarum enteral feeding on the gut permeability and septic complications in the patients with acute pancreatitis. *Eur J Clin Nutr.* 2008 Jul;62(7):923-30.

Qu C, Srivastava K, Ko J, Zhang TF, Sampson HA, Li XM. Induction of tolerance after establishment of peanut allergy by the food allergy herbal formula-2 is associated with up-regulation of interferon-gamma. *Clin Exp Allergy.* 2007 Jun;37(6):846-55.

Radon K, Danuser B, Iversen M, Jörres R, Monso E, Opravil U, Weber C, Donham KJ, Nowak D. Respiratory symptoms in European animal farmers. *Eur Respir J.* 2001 Apr;17(4):747-54.

Raherison C, Pénard-Morand C, Moreau D, Caillaud D, Charpin D, Kopferschmitt C, Lavaud F, Taytard A, Maesano IA. Smoking exposure and allergic sensitization in children according to maternal allergies. *Ann Allergy Asthma Immunol.* 2008 Apr;100(4):351-7.

Rahman MM, Bhattacharya A, Fernandes G. Docosahexaenoic acid is more potent inhibitor of osteoclast differentiation in RAW 264.7 cells than eicosapentaenoic acid. *J Cell Physiol.* 2008 Jan;214(1):201-9.

Raithel M, Weidenhiller M, Abel R, Baenkler HW, Hahn EG. Colorectal mucosal histamine release by mucosa oxygenation in comparison with other established clinical tests in patients with gastrointestinally mediated allergy. *World J Gastroenterol.* 2006 Aug 7;12(29):4699-705.

Raloff J. Ill Winds. *Science News.* 2001;160(14):218.

Rampton DS, Murdoch RD, Sladen GE. Rectal mucosal histamine release in ulcerative colitis. *Clin Sci (Lond).* 1980 Nov;59(5):389-91.

Rancé F, Kanny G, Dutau G, Moneret-Vautrin DA. Food allergens in children. *Arch Pediatr.* 1999;6(Suppl 1):61S-66S.

Randal Bollinger R, Barbas AS, Bush EL, Lin SS, Parker W. Biofilms in the large bowel suggest an apparent function of the human vermiform appendix. *J Theor Biol.* 2007 Dec 21;249(4):826-31.

Ranjbaran Z, Keefer L, Stepanski E, Farhadi A, Keshavarzian A. The relevance of sleep abnormalities to chronic inflammatory conditions. *Inflamm Res.* 2007 Feb;56(2):51-7.

Rao SK, Rao PS, Rao BN. Preliminary investigation of the radiosensitizing activity of guduchi (Tinospora cordifolia) in tumor-bearing mice. *Phytother Res.* 2008 Nov;22(11):1482-9.

Rapin JR, Wiernsperger N. Possible links between intestinal permeablity and food processing: A potential therapeutic niche for glutamine. *Clinics (Sao Paulo).* 2010 Jun;65(6):635-43.

Rappoport J. Both sides of the pharmaceutical death coin. *Townsend Letter for Doctors and Patients.* 2006 Oct.

Rauha JP, Remes S, Heinonen M, Hopia A, Kähkönen M, Kujala T, Pihlaja K, Vuorela H, Vuorela P. Antimicrobial effects of Finnish plant extracts containing flavonoids and other phenolic compounds. *Int J Food Microbiol.* 2000 May 25;56(1):3-12.

Rauma A. Antioxidant status in vegetarians versus omnivores. *Nutrition.* 2003;16(2): 111-119.

Rautava S, Isolauri E. Cow's milk allergy in infants with atopic eczema is associated with aberrant production of interleukin-4 during oral cow's milk challenge. *J Pediatr Gastroenterol Nutr.* 2004 Nov;39(5):529-35.

Rebhun J. Coexisting immune complex diseases in atopy. *Ann Allergy.* 1980 Dec;45(6):368-71.

Reger D, Goode S, Mercer E. Chemistry: Principles & Practice. Fort Worth, TX: Harcourt Brace, 1993.

Reha CM, Ebru A. Specific immunotherapy is effective in the prevention of new sensitivities. *Allergol Immunopathol (Madr).* 2007 Mar-Apr;35(2):44-51.

Renkonen R, Renkonen J, Joenväärä S, Mattila P, Parviainen V, Toppila-Salmi S. Allergens are transported through the respiratory epithelium. *Expert Rev Clin Immunol.* 2010 Jan;6(1):55-9.

Reuter A, Lidholm J, Andersson K, Ostling J, Lundberg M, Scheurer S, Enrique E, Cistero-Bahima A, San Miguel-Moncin M, Ballmer-Weber BK, Vieths S. A critical assessment of allergen component-based in vitro diagnosis in cherry allergy across Europe. *Clin Exp Allergy.* 2006 Jun;36(6):815-23.

Reznik M, Sharif I, Ozuah PO. Rubbing ointments and asthma morbidity in adolescents. *J Altern Complement Med.* 2004 Dec;10(6):1097-9. Uu

Riccia DN, Bizzini F, Perilli MG, Polimeni A, Trinchieri V, Amicosante G, Cifone MG. Anti-inflammatory effects of Lactobacillus brevis (CD2) on periodontal disease. *Oral Dis.* 2007 Jul;13(4):376-85.

Riccioni G, Barbara M, Bucciarelli T, di Ilio C, D'Orazio N. Antioxidant vitamin supplementation in asthma. *Ann Clin Lab Sci.* 2007 Winter;37(1):96-101.

Riccioni G, Bucciarelli T, Mancini B, Di Ilio C, Della Vecchia R, D'Orazio N. Plasma lycopene and antioxidant vitamins in asthma: the PLAVA study. *J Asthma*. 2007 Jul-Aug;44(6):429-32.

Riccioni G, D'Orazio N. The role of selenium, zinc and antioxidant vitamin supplementation in the treatment of bronchial asthma: adjuvant therapy or not? *Expert Opin Investig Drugs*. 2005 Sep;14(9):1145-55.

Riccioni G, Di Stefano F, De Benedictis M, Verna N, Cavallucci E, Paolini F, Di Sciascio MB, Della Vecchia R, Schiavone C, Boscolo P, Conti P, Di Gioacchino M. Seasonal variability of non-specific bronchial responsiveness in asthmatic patients with allergy to house dust mites. *Allergy Asthma Proc*. 2001 Jan-Feb;22(1):5-9.

Riedler J, Braun-Fahrländer C, Eder W, Schreuer M, Waser M, Maisch S, Carr D, Schierl R, Nowak D, von Mutius E; ALEX Study Team. Exposure to farming in early life and development of asthma and allergy: a cross-sectional survey. *Lancet*. 2001 Oct 6;358(9288):1129-33.

Rimkiene S, Ragazinskiene O, Savickiene N. The cumulation of Wild pansy (Viola tricolor L.) accessions: the possibility of species preservation and usage in medicine. *Medicina (Kaunas)*. 2003;39(4):411-6.

Rinne M, Kalliomaki M, Arvilommi H, Salminen S, Isolauri E. Effect of probiotics and breastfeeding on the bifidobacterium and lactobacillus/enterococcus microbiota and humoral immune responses. *J Pediatr*. 2005 Aug;147(2):186-91.

Río ME, Zago Beatriz L, Garcia H, Winter L. The nutritional status change the effectiveness of a dietary supplement of lactic bacteria on the emerging of respiratory tract diseases in children. *Arch Latinoam Nutr*. 2002 Mar;52(1):29-34.

Robert AM, Groult N, Six C, Robert L. The effect of procyanidolic oligomers on mesenchymal cells in culture II—Attachment of elastic fibers to the cells. *Pathol Biol*. 1990 Jun;38(6):601-7.

Roberts G, Lack G. Diagnosing peanut allergy with skin prick and specific IgE testing. *J Allergy Clin Immunol*. 2005 Jun;115(6):1291-6.

Robinson L, Cherewatenko VS, Reeves S. *Epicor: The Key to a Balanced Immune System*. Sherman Oaks, CA: Health Point, 2009.

Rodriguez J, Crespo JF, Burks W, Rivas-Plata C, Fernandez-Anaya S, Vives R, Daroca P. Randomized, double-blind, crossover challenge study in 53 subjects reporting adverse reactions to melon (Cucumis melo). *J Allergy Clin Immunol*. 2000 Nov;106(5):968-72.

Rodriguez-Fragoso L, Reyes-Esparza J, Burchiel SW, Herrera-Ruiz D, Torres E. Risks and benefits of commonly used herbal medicines in Mexico. *Toxicol Appl Pharmacol*. 2008 Feb 15;227(1):125-35.

Rodríguez-Ortiz PG, Muñoz-Mendoza D, Arias-Cruz A, González-Díaz SN, Herrera-Castro D, Vidaurri-Ojeda AC. Epidemiological characteristics of patients with food allergy assisted at Regional Center of Allergies and Clinical Immunology of Monterrey. *Rev Alerg Mex*. 2009 Nov-Dec;56(6):185-91.

Roduit C, Scholtens S, de Jongste JC, Wijga AH, Gerritsen J, Postma DS, Brunekreef B, Hoekstra MO, Aalberse R, Smit HA. Asthma at 8 years of age in children born by caesarean section. *Thorax*. 2009 Feb;64(2):107-13.

Roessler A, Friedrich U, Vogelsang H, Bauer A, Kaatz M, Hipler UC, Schmidt I, Jahreis G. The immune system in healthy adults and patients with atopic dermatitis seems to be affected differently by a probiotic intervention. *Clin Exp Allergy*. 2008 Jan;38(1):93-102.

Roger A, Justicia JL, Navarro LÁ, Eseverri JL, Ferrès J, Malet A, Alvà V. Observational study of the safety of an ultra-rush sublingual immunotherapy regimen to treat rhinitis due to house dust mites. *Int Arch Allergy Immunol*. 2011;154(1):69-75. 2010 Jul 27.

Romeo J, Wärnberg J, Nova E, Díaz LE, González-Gross M, Marcos A. Changes in the immune system after moderate beer consumption. *Ann Nutr Metab*. 2007;51(4):359-66.

Romieu I, Barraza-Villarreal A, Escamilla-Núñez C, Texcalac-Sangrador JL, Hernandez-Cadena L, Díaz-Sánchez D, De Batlle J, Del Rio-Navarro BE. Dietary intake, lung function and airway inflammation in Mexico City school children exposed to air pollutants. *Respir Res*. 2009 Dec 10;10:122.

Ronteltap A, van Schaik J, Wensing M, Rynja FJ, Knulst AC, de Vries JH. Sensory testing of recipes masking peanut or hazelnut for double-blind placebo-controlled food challenges. *Allergy*. 2004 Apr;59(4):457-60. Clark S, Bock SA, Gaeta TJ, Brenner BE, Cydulka RK, Camargo CA; Multicenter Airway Research Collaboration-8 Investigators. Multicenter study of emergency department visits for food allergies. *J Allergy Clin Immunol*. 2004 Feb;113(2):347-52.

Rook GA, Hernandez-Pando R. Pathogenetic role, in human and murine tuberculosis, of changes in the peripheral metabolism of glucocorticoids and antiglucocorticoids. *Psychoneuroendocrinology*. 1997;22 Suppl 1:S109-13.

Ros E, Mataix J. Fatty acid composition of nuts—implications for cardiovascular health. *Br J Nutr*. 2006 Nov;96 Suppl 2:S29-35.

Rosenfeldt V, Benfeldt E, Valerius NH, Paerregaard A, Michaelsen KF. Effect of probiotics on gastrointestinal symptoms and small intestinal permeability in children with atopic dermatitis. *J Pediatr*. 2004 Nov;145(5):612-6.

Rosenkranz SK, Swain KE, Rosenkranz RR, Beckman B, Harms CA. Modifiable lifestyle factors impact airway health in non-asthmatic prepubescent boys but not girls. *Pediatr Pulmonol*. 2010 Dec 30.

REFERENCES

Rosenlund H, Bergström A, Alm JS, Swartz J, Scheynius A, van Hage M, Johansen K, Brunekreef B, von Mutius E, Ege MJ, Riedler J, Braun-Fahrländer C, Waser M, Pershagen G; PARSIFAL Study Group. Allergic disease and atopic sensitization in children in relation to measles vaccination and measles infection. *Pediatrics.* 2009 Mar;123(3):771-8.

Rozycki VR, Baigorria CM, Freyre MR, Bernard CM, Zannier MS, Charpentier M. Nutrient content in vegetable species from the Argentine Chaco. *Arch Latinoam Nutr.* 1997 Sep;47(3):265-70.

Rubin E., Farber JL. *Pathology.* 3rd Ed. Philadelphia: Lippincott-Raven, 1999.

Rudders SA, Espinola JA, Camargo CA Jr. North-south differences in US emergency department visits for acute allergic reactions. *Ann Allergy Asthma Immunol.* 2010 May;104(5):413-6.

Rynard PB, Palij B, Galloway CA, Roughley FR. Resperin inhalation treatment for chronic respiratory diseases. *Can Fam Physician.* 1968 Oct;14(10):70-1.

Saarinen KM, Juntunen-Backman K, Järvenpää AL, Klemetti P, Kuitunen P, Lope L, Renlund M, Siivola M, Vaarala O, Savilahti E. Breast-feeding and the development of cows' milk protein allergy. *Adv Exp Med Biol.* 2000;478:121-30.

Sahagún-Flores JE, López-Peña LS, de la Cruz-Ramírez Jaimes J, García-Bravo MS, Peregrina-Gómez R, de Alba-García JE. Eradication of Helicobacter pylori: triple treatment scheme plus Lactobacillus vs. triple treatment alone. *Cir Cir.* 2007 Sep-Oct;75(5):333-6.

Sahakian NM, White SK, Park JH, Cox-Ganser JM, Kreiss K. Identification of mold and dampness-associated respiratory morbidity in 2 schools: comparison of questionnaire survey responses to national data. *J Sch Health.* 2008 Jan;78(1):32-7.

Sahin-Yilmaz A, Nocon CC, Corey JP. Immunoglobulin E-mediated food allergies among adults with allergic rhinitis. *Otolaryngol Head Neck Surg.* 2010 Sep;143(3):379-85.

Salem N, Wegher B, Mena P, Uauy R. Arachidonic and docosahexaenoic acids are biosynthesized from their 18-carbon precursors in human infants. *Proc Natl Acad Sci.* 1996;93:49-54.

Salib RJ, Howarth PH. Remodelling of the upper airways in allergic rhinitis: is it a feature of the disease? *Clin Exp Allergy.* 2003 Dec;33(12):1629-33.

Salim AS. Sulfhydryl-containing agents in the treatment of gastric bleeding induced by nonsteroidal anti-inflammatory drugs. *Can J Surg.* 1993 Feb;36(1):53-8.

Salmi H, Kuitunen M, Viljanen M, Lapatto R. Cow's milk allergy is associated with changes in urinary organic acid concentrations. *Pediatr Allergy Immunol.* 2010 Mar;21(2 Pt 2):e401-6.

Salminen S, Isolauri E, Salminen E. Clinical uses of probiotics for stabilizing the gut mucosal barrier: successful strains and future challenges. *Antonie Van Leeuwenhoek.* 1996 Oct;70(2-4):347-58.

Salom IL, Silvis SE, Doscherholmen A. Effect of cimetidine on the absorption of vitamin B12. *Scand J Gastroenterol.* 1982;17:129-31.

Salome CM, Marks GB. Sex, asthma and obesity: an intimate relationship? *Clin Exp Allergy.* 2011 Jan;41(1):6-8.

Salpietro CD, Gangemi S, Briuglia S, Meo A, Merlino MV, Muscolino G, Bisignano G, Trombetta D, Saija A. The almond milk: a new approach to the management of cow-milk allergy/intolerance in infants. *Minerva Pediatr.* 2005 Aug;57(4):173-80.

Salvi SS, Barnes PJ. Chronic obstructive pulmonary disease in non-smokers. *Lancet.* 2009 Aug 29;374(9691):733-43.

Sancho AI, Hoffmann-Sommergruber K, Alessandri S, Conti A, Giuffrida MG, Shewry P, Jensen BM, Skov P, Vieths S. Authentication of food allergen quality by physicochemical and immunological methods. *Clin Exp Allergy.* 2010 Jul;40(7):973-86.

Santos A, Dias A, Pinheiro JA. Predictive factors for the persistence of cow's milk allergy. *Pediatr Allergy Immunol.* 2010 Apr 27.

Sanz Ortega J, Martorell Aragonés A, Michavila Gómez A, Nieto García A; Grupo de Trabajo para el Estudio de la Alergia Alimentaria. Incidence of IgE-mediated allergy to cow's milk proteins in the first year of life. *An Esp Pediatr.* 2001 Jun;54(6):536-9.

Sato Y, Akiyama H, Matsuoka H, Sakata K, Nakamura R, Ishikawa S, Inakuma T, Totsuka M, Sugita-Konishi Y, Ebisawa M, Teshima R. Dietary carotenoids inhibit oral sensitization and the development of food allergy. *J Agric Food Chem.* 2010 Jun 23;58(12):7180-6.

Satyanarayana S, Sushruta K, Sarma GS, Srinivas N, Subba Raju GV. Antioxidant activity of the aqueous extracts of spicy food additives—evaluation and comparison with ascorbic acid in in-vitro systems. *J Herb Pharmacother.* 2004;4(2):1-10.

Savage JH, Kaeding AJ, Matsui EC, Wood RA. The natural history of soy allergy. *J Allergy Clin Immunol.* 2010 Mar;125(3):683-6.

Savilahti EM, Karinen S, Salo HM, Klemetti P, Saarinen KM, Klemola T, Kuitunen M, Hautaniemi S, Savilahti E, Vaarala O. Combined T regulatory cell and Th2 expression profile identifies children with cow's milk allergy. *Clin Immunol.* 2010 Jul;136(1):16-20.

395

Savilahti EM, Rantanen V, Lin JS, Karinen S, Saarinen KM, Goldis M, Mäkelä MJ, Hautaniemi S, Savilahti E, Sampson HA. Early recovery from cow's milk allergy is associated with decreasing IgE and increasing IgG4 binding to cow's milk epitopes. *J Allergy Clin Immunol.* 2010 Jun;125(6):1315-1321.e9.

Sazanova NE, Varnacheva LN, Novikova AV, Pletneva NB. Immunological aspects of food intolerance in children during first years of life. *Pediatriia.* 1992;(3):14-8.

Scadding G, Bjarnason I, Brostoff J, Levi AJ, Peters TJ. Intestinal permeability to 51Cr-labelled ethylenediaminetetraacetate in food-intolerant subjects. *Digestion.* 1989;42(2):104-9.

Scalabrin DM, Johnston WH, Hoffman DR, P'Pool VL, Harris CL, Mitmesser SH. Growth and tolerance of healthy term infants receiving hydrolyzed infant formulas supplemented with Lactobacillus rhamnosus GG: randomized, double-blind, controlled trial. *Clin Pediatr (Phila).* 2009 Sep;48(7):734-44.

Schauenberg P, Paris F. *Guide to Medicinal Plants.* New Canaan, CT: Keats Publ, 1977.

Schauss AG, Wu X, Prior RL, Ou B, Huang D, Owens J, Agarwal A, Jensen GS, Hart AN, Shanbrom E. Antioxidant capacity and other bioactivities of the freeze-dried Amazonian palm berry, Euterpe oleraceae mart. (acai). *J Agric Food Chem.* 2006 Nov 1;54(22):8604-10.

Schempp H, Weiser D, Elstner EF. Biochemical model reactions indicative of inflammatory processes. Activities of extracts from Fraxinus excelsior and Populus tremula. *Arzneimittelforschung.* 2000 Apr;50(4):362-72.

Schillaci D, Arizza V, Dayton T, Camarda L, Di Stefano V. In vitro anti-biofilm activity of Boswellia spp. oleogum resin essential oils. *Lett Appl Microbiol.* 2008 Nov;47(5):433-8.

Schmid B, Kötter I, Heide L. Pharmacokinetics of salicin after oral administration of a standardised willow bark extract. *Eur J Clin Pharmacol.* 2001 Aug;57(5):387-91.

Schmitt DA, Maleki SJ (2004) Comparing the effects of boiling, frying and roasting on the allergenicity of peanuts. *J Allergy Clin Immunol.* 113: S155.

Schnappinger M, Sausenthaler S, Linseisen J, Hauner H, Heinrich J. Fish consumption, allergic sensitisation and allergic diseases in adults. *Ann Nutr Metab.* 2009;54(1):67-74.

Schnappinger M, Sausenthaler S, Linseisen J, Hauner H, Heinrich J. Fish consumption, allergic sensitisation and allergic diseases in adults. *Ann Nutr Metab.* 2009;54(1):67-74.

Schönfeld P. Phytanic Acid toxicity: implications for the permeability of the inner mitochondrial membrane to ions. *Toxicol Mech Methods.* 2004;14(1-2):47-52.

Schottner M, Gansser D, Spiteller G. Lignans from the roots of Urtica dioica and their metabolites bind to human sex hormone binding globulin (SHBG). *Planta Med.* 1997;65:529-532.

Schouten B, van Esch BC, Hofman GA, Boon L, Knippels LM, Willemsen LE, Garssen J. Oligosaccharide-induced whey-specific CD25(+) regulatory T-cells are involved in the suppression of cow milk allergy in mice. *J Nutr.* 2010 Apr;140(4):835-41.

Schroecksnadel S, Jenny M, Fuchs D. Sensitivity to sulphite additives. *Clin Exp Allergy.* 2010 Apr;40(4):688-9.

Schulick P. *Ginger: Common Spice & Wonder Drug.* Brattleboro, VT: Herbal Free Perss, 1996.

Schulz V, Hansel R, Tyler VE. *Rational Phytotherapy.* Berlin: Springer-Verlag, 1998.

Schumacher P. *Biophysical Therapy Of Allergies.* Stuttgart: Thieme, 2005.

Schütz K, Carle R, Schieber A. Taraxacum—a review on its phytochemical and pharmacological profile. *J Ethnopharmacol.* 2006 Oct 11;107(3):313-23.

Schwab D, Hahn EG, Raithel M. Enhanced histamine metabolism: a comparative analysis of collagenous colitis and food allergy with respect to the role of diet and NSAID use. *Inflamm Res.* 2003 Apr;52(4):142-7.

Schwab D, Müller S, Aigner T, Neureiter D, Kirchner T, Hahn EG, Raithel M. Functional and morphologic characterization of eosinophils in the lower intestinal mucosa of patients with food allergy. *Am J Gastroenterol.* 2003 Jul;98(7):1525-34.

Schwelberger HG. Histamine intolerance: a metabolic disease? *Inflamm Res.* 2010 Mar;59 Suppl 2:S219-21.

Scott-Taylor TH, O'B Hourihane J, Strobel S. Correlation of allergen-specific IgG subclass antibodies and T lymphocyte cytokine responses in children with multiple food allergies. *Pediatr Allergy Immunol.* 2010 Sep;21(6):935-44.

Scurlock AM, Jones SM. An update on immunotherapy for food allergy. *Curr Opin Allergy Clin Immunol.* 2010 Dec;10(6):587-93.

Sealey-Voyksner JA, Khosla C, Voyksner RD, Jorgenson JW. Novel aspects of quantitation of immunogenic wheat gluten peptides by liquid chromatography-mass spectrometry. *J Chromatogr A.* 2010 Jun 18;1217(25):4167-83.

Searing DA, Leung DY. Vitamin D in atopic dermatitis, asthma and allergic diseases. *Immunol Allergy Clin North Am.* 2010 Aug;30(3):397-409.

Senior F. Fallout. *New York Magazine.* Fall: 2003.

Senna G, Gani F, Leo G, Schiappoli M. Alternative tests in the diagnosis of food allergies. *Recenti Prog Med.* 2002 May;93(5):327-34.

Seo K, Jung S, Park M, Song Y, Choung S. Effects of leucocyanidines on activities of metabolizing enzymes and antioxidant enzymes. *Biol Pharm Bull.* 2001 May;24(5):592-3.

REFERENCES

Seo SW, Koo HN, An HJ, Kwon KB, Lim BC, Seo EA, Ryu DG, Moon G, Kim HY, Kim HM, Hong SH. Taraxacum officinale protects against cholecystokinin-induced acute pancreatitis in rats. *World J Gastroenterol.* 2005 Jan 28;11(4):597-9.

Seppo L, Korpela R, Lönnerdal B, Metsäniitty L, Juntunen-Backman K, Klemola T, Paganus A, Vanto T. A follow-up study of nutrient intake, nutritional status, and growth in infants with cow milk allergy fed either a soy formula or an extensively hydrolyzed whey formula. *Am J Clin Nutr.* 2005 Jul;82(1):140-5.

Serra A, Cocuzza S, Poli G, La Mantia I, Messina A, Pavone P. Otologic findings in children with gastroesophageal reflux. *Int J Pediatr Otorhinolaryngol.* 2007 Nov;71(11):1693-7. 2007 Aug 22.

Sevar R. Audit of outcome in 455 consecutive patients treated with homeopathic medicines. *Homeopathy.* 2005 Oct;94(4):215-21.

Shahani KM, Meshbesher BF, Mangalampalli V. *Cultivate Health From Within.* Danbury, CT: Vital Health Publ, 2005.

Shaheen S, Potts J, Gnatiuc L, Makowska J, Kowalski ML, Joos G, van Zele T, van Durme Y, De Rudder I, Wöhrl S, Godnic-Cvar J, Skadhauge L, Thomsen G, Zuberbier T, Bergmann KC, Heinzerling L, Gjomarkaj M, Bruno A, Pace E, Bonini S, Fokkens W, Weersink EJ, Loureiro C, Todo-Bom A, Villanueva CM, Sanjuas C, Zock JP, Janson C, Burney P; Selenium and Asthma Research Integration project; GA2LEN. The relation between paracetamol use and asthma: a GA2LEN European case-control study. *Eur Respir J.* 2008 Nov;32(5):1231-6.

Shaheen SO, Newson RB, Rayman MP, Wong AP, Tumilty MK, Phillips JM, Potts JF, Kelly FJ, White PT, Burney PG. Randomised, double blind, placebo-controlled trial of selenium supplementation in adult asthma. *Thorax.* 2007 Jun;62(6):483-90.

Shakib F, Brown HM, Phelps A, Redhead R. Study of IgG sub-class antibodies in patients with milk intolerance. *Clin Allergy.* 1986 Sep;16(5):451-8.

Sharma P, Sharma BC, Puri V, Sarin SK. An open-label randomized controlled trial of lactulose and probiotics in the treatment of minimal hepatic encephalopathy. *Eur J Gastroent Hepatol.* 2008 Jun;20(6):506-11.

Sharma SC, Sharma S, Gulati OP. Pycnogenol inhibits the release of histamine from mast cells. *Phytother Res.* 2003 Jan;17(1):66-9.

Sharnan J, Kumar L, Singh S. Comparison of results of skin prick tests, enzyme-linked immunosorbent assays and food challenges in children with respiratory allergy. *J Trop Pediatr.* 2001 Dec;47(6):367-8.

Shawcross DL, Wright G, Olde Damink SW, Jalan R. Role of ammonia and inflammation in minimal hepatic encephalopathy. *Metab Brain Dis.* 2007 Mar;22(1):125-38.

Shea KM, Trucker RT, Weber RW, Peden DB. Climate change and allergic disease. *Clin Rev Allergy Immunol.* 2008;6:443-453.

Shea-Donohue T, Stiltz J, Zhao A, Notari L. Mast Cells. *Curr Gastroenterol Rep.* 2010 Aug 14.

Shen FY, Lee MS, Jung SK. Effectiveness of pharmacopuncture for asthma: a systematic review and meta-analysis. *Evid Based Complement Alternat Med.* 2011;2011. pii: 678176.

Sheth SS, Waserman S, Kagan R, Alizadehfar R, Primeau MN, Elliot S, St Pierre Y, Wickett R, Joseph L, Harada L, Dufresne C, Allen M, Allen M, Godefroy SB, Clarke AE. Role of food labels in accidental exposures in food-allergic individuals in Canada. *Ann Allergy Asthma Immunol.* 2010 Jan;104(1):60-5.

Shi S, Zhao Y, Zhou H, Zhang Y, Jiang X, Huang K. Identification of antioxidants from Taraxacum mongolicum by high-performance liquid chromatography-diode array detection-radical-scavenging detection-electrospray ionization mass spectrometry and nuclear magnetic resonance experiments. *J Chromatogr A.* 2008 Oct 31;1209(1-2):145-52

Shi S, Zhou H, Zhang Y, Huang K, Liu S. Chemical constituents from Neo-Taraxacum siphonathum. *Zhongguo Zhong Yao Za Zhi.* 2009 Apr;34(8):1002-4.

Shi SY, Zhou CX, Xu Y, Tao QF, Bai H, Lu FS, Lin WY, Chen HY, Zheng W, Wang LW, Wu YH, Zeng S, Huang KX, Zhao Y, Li XK, Qu J. Studies on chemical constituents from herbs of Taraxacum mongolicum. *Zhongguo Zhong Yao Za Zhi.* 2008 May;33(10):1147-57.

Shibata H, Nabe T, Yamamura H, Kohno S. l-Ephedrine is a major constituent of Mao-Bushi-Saishin-To, one of the formulas of Chinese medicine, which shows immediate inhibition after oral administration of passive cutaneous anaphylaxis in rats. *Inflamm Res.* 2000 Aug;49(8):398-403.

Shichinohe K, Shimizu M, Kurokawa K. Effect of M-711 on experimental asthma in rats. *J Vet Med Sci.* 1996 Jan;58(1):55-9.

Shimauchi H, Mayanagi G, Nakaya S, Minamibuchi M, Ito Y, Yamaki K, Hirata H. Improvement of periodontal condition by probiotics with *Lactobacillus salivarius* WB21: a randomized, double-blind, placebo-controlled study. *J Clin Periodontol.* 2008 Oct;35(10):897-905.

Shimoi T, Ushiyama H, Kan K, Saito K, Kamata K, Hirokado M. Survey of glycoalkaloids content in the various potatoes. *Shokuhin Eiseigaku Zasshi.* 2007 Jun;48(3):77-82.

Shishehbor F, Behroo L, Ghafouriyan Broujerdnia M, Namjoyan F, Latifi SM. Quercetin effectively quells peanut-induced anaphylactic reactions in the peanut sensitized rats. *Iran J Allergy Asthma Immunol.* 2010 Mar;9(1):27-34.

397

Shishodia S, Harikumar KB, Dass S, Ramawat KG, Aggarwal BB. The guggul for chronic diseases: ancient medicine, modern targets. *Anticancer Res.* 2008 Nov-Dec;28(6A):3647-64.

Shivpuri DN, Menon MP, Parkash D. Preliminary studies in Tylophora indica in the treatment of asthma and allergic rhinitis. *J Assoc Physicians India.* 1968 Jan;16(1):9-15.

Shivpuri DN, Menon MP, Prakash D. A crossover double-blind study on Tylophora indica in the treatment of asthma and allergic rhinitis. *J Allergy.* 1969 Mar;43(3):145-50.

Shivpuri DN, Singhal SC, Parkash D. Treatment of asthma with an alcoholic extract of Tylophora indica: a cross-over, double-blind study. *Ann Allergy.* 1972; 30:407-12.

Shoaf, K., Muvey, G.L., Armstrong, G.D., Hutkins, R.W. (2006) Prebiotic galactooligosaccharides reduce adherence of enteropathogenic Escherichia coli to tissue culture cells. *Infect Immun.* Dec;74(12):6920-8.

Sicherer SH, Muñoz-Furlong A, Godbold JH, Sampson HA. US prevalence of self-reported peanut, tree nut, and sesame allergy: 11-year follow-up. *J Allergy Clin Immunol.* 2010 Jun;125(6):1322-6.

Sicherer SH, Noone SA, Koerner CB, Christie L, Burks AW, Sampson HA. Hypoallergenicity and efficacy of an amino acid-based formula in children with cow's milk and multiple food hypersensitivities. *J Pediatr.* 2001 May;138(5):688-93.

Sicherer SH, Sampson HA. Food allergy. *J Allergy Clin Immunol.* 2010 Feb;125(2 Suppl 2):S116-25.

Sidoroff V, Hyvärinen M, Piippo-Savolainen E, Korppi M. Lung function and overweight in school aged children after early childhood wheezing. *Pediatr Pulmonol.* 2010 Dec 30.

Sigstedt SC, Hooten CJ, Callewaert MC, Jenkins AR, Romero AE, Pullin MJ, Kornienko A, Lowrey TK, Slambrouck SV, Steelant WF. Evaluation of aqueous extracts of Taraxacum officinale on growth and invasion of breast and prostate cancer cells. *Int J Oncol.* 2008 May;32(5):1085-90.

Silman AJ, MacGregor AJ, Thomson W, Holligan S, Carthy D, Farhan A, Ollier WE. Twin concordance rates for rheumatoid arthritis: results from a nationwide study. *Br J Rheumatol.* 1993 Oct;32(10):903-7.

Silva MF, Kamphorst AO, Hayashi EA, Bellio M, Carvalho CR, Faria AM, Sabino KC, Coelho MG, Nobrega A, Tavares D, Silva AC. Innate profiles of cytokines implicated on oral tolerance correlate with low- or high-suppression of humoral response. *Immunology.* 2010 Jul;130(3):447-57.

Simeone D, Miele E, Boccia G, Marino A, Troncone R, Staiano A. Prevalence of atopy in children with chronic constipation. *Arch Dis Child.* 2008 Dec;93(12):1044-7.

Simões EA, Carbonell-Estrany X, Rieger CH, Mitchell I, Fredrick L, Groothuis JR; Palivizumab Long-Term Respiratory Outcomes Study Group. The effect of respiratory syncytial virus on subsequent recurrent wheezing in atopic and nonatopic children. *J Allergy Clin Immunol.* 2010 Aug;126(2):256-62. 2010 Jul 10.

Simons FER. What's in a name? The allergic rhinitis-asthma connection. *Clin Exp All Rev.* 2003;3:9-17.

Simonte SJ, Ma S, Mofidi S, Sicherer SH. Relevance of casual contact with peanut butter in children with peanut allergy. *J Allergy Clin Immunol.* 2003 Jul;112(1):180-2.

Simopoulos AP. Essential fatty acids in health and chronic disease. *Am J Clin Nutr.* 1999 Sep;70(3 Suppl):560S-569S.

Simpson A, Tan VY, Winn J, Svensén M, Bishop CM, Heckerman DE, Buchan I, Custovic A. Beyond atopy: multiple patterns of sensitization in relation to asthma in a birth cohort study. *Am J Respir Crit Care Med.* 2010 Jun 1;181(11):1200-6.

Simpson AB, Yousef E, Hossain J. Association between peanut allergy and asthma morbidity. *J Pediatr.* 2010 May;156(5):777-81.

Sin A, Terzioğlu E, Kokuludağ A, Sebik F, Kabakçi T. Serum eosinophil cationic protein (ECP) levels in patients with seasonal allergic rhinitis and allergic asthma. *Allergy Asthma Proc.* 1998 Mar-Apr;19(2):69-73.

Singer P, Shapiro H, Theilla M, Anbar R, Singer J, Cohen J. Anti-inflammatory properties of omega-3 fatty acids in critical illness: novel mechanisms and an integrative perspective. *Intensive Care Med.* 2008 Sep;34(9):1580-92.

Singh BB, Khorsan R, Vinjamury SP, Der-Martirosian C, Kizhakkeveettil A, Anderson TM. Herbal treatments of asthma: a systematic review. *J Asthma.* 2007 Nov;44(9):685-98.

Singh S, Khajuria A, Taneja SC, Johri RK, Singh J, Qazi GN. Boswellic acids: A leukotriene inhibitor also effective through topical application in inflammatory disorders. *Phytomedicine.* 2008 Jun;15(6-7):400-7.

Singh V, Jain NK. Asthma as a cause for, rather than a result of, gastroesophageal reflux. *J Asthma.* 1983;20(4):241-3. 3.

Sirvent S, Palomares O, Vereda A, Villalba M, Cuesta-Herranz J, Rodríguez R. nsLTP and profilin are allergens in mustard seeds: cloning, sequencing and recombinant production of Sin a 3 and Sin a 4. *Clin Exp Allergy.* 2009 Dec;39(12):1929-36.

Skamstrup Hansen K, Vieths S, Vestergaard H, Skov PS, Bindslev-Jensen C, Poulsen LK. Seasonal variation in food allergy to apple. *J Chromatogr B Biomed Sci Appl.* 2001 May 25;756(1-2):19-32.

Skripak JM, Nash SD, Rowley H, Brereton NH, Oh S, Hamilton RG, Matsui EC, Burks AW, Wood RA. A randomized, double-blind, placebo-controlled study of milk oral immunotherapy for cow's milk allergy. *J Allergy Clin Immunol.* 2008 Dec;122(6):1154-60.

REFERENCES

Sletten GB, Halvorsen R, Egaas E, Halstensen TS. Changes in humoral responses to beta-lactoglobulin in tolerant patients suggest a particular role for IgG4 in delayed, non-IgE-mediated cow's milk allergy. *Pediatr Allergy Immunol.* 2006 Sep;17(6):435-43.

Smith J. *Genetic Roulette: The Documented Health Risks of Genetically Engineered Foods.* White River Jct, Vermont: Chelsea Green, 2007.

Smith K, Warholak T, Armstrong E, Leib M, Rehfeld R, Malone D. Evaluation of risk factors and health outcomes among persons with asthma. *J Asthma.* 2009 Apr;46(3):234-7.

Smith LJ, Holbrook JT, Wise R, Blumenthal M, Dozor AJ, Mastronarde J, Williams L; American Lung Association Asthma Clinical Research Centers. Dietary intake of soy genistein is associated with lung function in patients with asthma. *J Asthma.* 2004;41(8):833-43.

Smith S, Sullivan K. Examining the influence of biological and psychological factors on cognitive performance in chronic fatigue syndrome: a randomized, double-blind, placebo-controlled, crossover study. *Int J Behav Med.* 2003;10(2):162-73.

Sofic E, Denisova N, Youdim K, Vatrenjak-Velagic V, De Filippo C, Mehmedagic A, Causevic A, Cao G, Joseph JA, Prior RL. Antioxidant and pro-oxidant capacity of catecholamines and related compounds. Effects of hydrogen peroxide on glutathione and sphingomyelinase activity in pheochromocytoma PC12 cells: potential relevance to age-related diseases. *J Neural Transm.* 2001;108(5):541-57.

Soleo L, Colosio C, Alinovi R, Guarneri D, Russo A, Lovreglio P, Vimercati L, Birindelli S, Cortesi I, Flore C, Carta P, Colombi A, Parrinello G, Ambrosi L. Immunologic effects of exposure to low levels of inorganic mercury. *Med Lav.* 2002 May-Jun;93(3):225-32.

Sompamit K, Kukongviriyapan U, Nakmareong S, Pannangpetch P, Kukongviriyapan V. Curcumin improves vascular function and alleviates oxidative stress in non-lethal lipopolysaccharide-induced endotoxaemia in mice. *Eur J Pharmacol.* 2009 Aug 15;616(1-3):192-9.

Sonibare MA, Gbile ZO. Ethnobotanical survey of anti-asthmatic plants in South Western Nigeria. *Afr J Tradit Complement Altern Med.* 2008 Jun 18;5(4):340-5.

Sontag SJ, O'Connell S, Khandelwal S, Greenlee H, Schnell T, Nemchausky B, Chejfec G, Miller T, Seidel J, Sonnenberg A. Asthmatics with gastroesophageal reflux: long term results of a randomized trial of medical and surgical antireflux therapies. *Am J Gastroenterol.* 2003 May;98(5):987-99.

Sosa M, Saavedra P, Valero C, Guañabens N, Nogués X, del Pino-Montes J, Mosquera J, Alegre J, Gómez-Alonso C, Muñoz-Torres M, Quesada M, Pérez-Cano R, Jódar E, Torrijos A, Lozano-Tonkin C, Díaz-Curiel M; GIUMO Study Group. Inhaled steroids do not decrease bone mineral density but increase risk of fractures: data from the GIUMO Study Group. *J Clin Densitom.* 2006 Apr-Jun;9(2):154-8.

Soyka F, Edmonds A. *The Ion Effect: How Air Electricity Rules your Life and Health.* Bantam, New York: Bantam, 1978.

Spence A. *Basic Human Anatomy.* Menlo Park, CA: Benjamin/Commings, 1986.

Spiller G. *The Super Pyramid.* New York: HRS Press, 1993.

Sporik R, Squillace SP, Ingram JM, Rakes G, Honsinger RW, Platts-Mills TA. Mite, cat, and cockroach exposure, allergen sensitisation, and asthma in children: a case-control study of three schools. *Thorax.* 1999 Aug;54(8):675-80.

Srivastava K, Zou ZM, Sampson HA, Dansky H, Li XM. Direct Modulation of Airway Reactivity by the Chinese Anti-Asthma Herbal Formula ASHMI. *J Allergy Clin Immunol.* 2005;115:S7.

Srivastava KD, Qu C, Zhang T, Goldfarb J, Sampson HA, Li XM. Food Allergy Herbal Formula-2 silences peanut-induced anaphylaxis for a prolonged posttreatment period via IFN-gamma-producing CD8+ T cells. *J Allergy Clin Immunol.* 2009 Feb;123(2):443-51.

Srivastava KD, Zhang TF, Qu C, Sampson HA, Li XM. Silencing Peanut Allergy: A Chinese Herbal Formula, FAHF-2, Completely Blocks Peanut-induced Anaphylaxis for up to 6 Months Following Therapy in a Murine Model Of Peanut Allergy. *J Allergy Clin Immunol.* 2006;117:S328.

Stach A, Emberlin J, Smith M, Adams-Groom B, Myszkowska D. Factors that determine the severity of Betula spp. pollen seasons in Poland (Poznań and Krakow) and the United Kingdom (Worcester and London). *Int J Biometeorol.* 2008 Mar;52(4):311-21.

Staden U, Rolinck-Werninghaus C, Brewe F, Wahn U, Niggemann B, Beyer K. Specific oral tolerance induction in food allergy in children: efficacy and clinical patterns of reaction. *Allergy.* 2007 Nov;62(11):1261-9.

Stahl SM. Selective histamine H1 antagonism: novel hypnotic and pharmacologic actions challenge classical notions of antihistamines. *CNS Spectr.* 2008 Dec;13(12):1027-38.

State Pharmacopoeia Commission of The People's Republic of China. *Pharmacopoeia of the People's Republic of China.* Beijing: Chemical Industry Press; 2005.

Steinman HA, Le Roux M, Potter PC. Sulphur dioxide sensitivity in South African asthmatic children. *S Afr Med J.* 1993 Jun;83(6):387-90.

Stenberg JA, Hambäck PA, Ericson L. Herbivore-induced "rent rise" in the host plant may drive a diet breadth enlargement in the tenant. *Ecology.* 2008 Jan;89(1):126-33.

Stengler M. *The Natural Physician's Healing Therapies.* Stamford, CT: Bottom Line Books, 2008.

Stensrud T, Carlsen KH. Can one single test protocol for provoking exercise-induced bronchoconstriction also be used for assessing aerobic capacity? *Clin Respir J*. 2008 Jan;2(1):47-53.

Steurer-Stey C, Russi EW, Steurer J: Complementary and alternative medicine in asthma: do they work? *Swiss Med Wkly*. 2002, 132:338-344.

Stillerman A, Nachtsheim C, Li W, Albrecht M, Waldman J. Efficacy of a novel air filtration pillow for avoidance of perennial allergens in symptomatic adults. *Ann Allergy Asthma Immunol*. 2010 May;104(5):440-9.

Stirapongsasuti P, Tanglertsampan C, Aunhachoke K, Sangasapaviliya A. Anaphylactic reaction to phuk-waan-ban in a patient with latex allergy. *J Med Assoc Thai*. 2010 May;93(5):616-9.

Stordal K, Johannesdottir GB, Bentsen BS, Knudsen PK, Carlsen KC, Closs O, Handeland M, Holm HK, Sandvik L. Acid suppression does not change respiratory symptoms in children with asthma and gastro-oesophageal reflux disease. *Arch Dis Child*. 2005 Sep;90(9):956-60.

Stratiki Z, Costalos C, Sevastiadou S, Kastanidou O, Skouroliakou M, Giakoumatou A, Petrohilou V. The effect of a bifidobacter supplemented bovine milk on intestinal permeability of preterm infants. *Early Hum Dev*. 2007 Sep;83(9):575-9.

Strinnholm A, Brulin C, Lindh V. Experiences of double-blind, placebo-controlled food challenges (DBPCFC): a qualitative analysis of mothers' experiences. *J Child Health Care*. 2010 Jun;14(2):179-88.

Stuck BA, Czajkowski J, Hagner AE, Klimek L, Verse T, Hörmann K, Maurer JT. Changes in daytime sleepiness, quality of life, and objective sleep patterns in seasonal allergic rhinitis: a controlled clinical trial. *J Allergy Clin Immunol*. 2004 Apr;113(4):663-8.

Stull DE, Schaefer M, Crespi S, Sandor DW. Relative strength of relationships of nasal congestion and ocular symptoms with sleep, mood and productivity. *Curr Med Res Opin*. 2009 Jul;25(7):1785-92.

Stutius LM, Sheehan WJ, Rangsithienchai P, Bharmanee A, Scott JE, Young MC, Dioun AF, Schneider LC, Phipatanakul W. Characterizing the relationship between sesame, coconut, and nut allergy in children. *Pediatr Allergy Immunol*. 2010 Dec;21(8):1114-8.

Sugawara G, Nagino M, Nishio H, Ebata T, Takagi K, Asahara T, Nomoto K, Nimura Y. Perioperative synbiotic treatment to prevent postoperative infectious complications in biliary cancer surgery: a randomized controlled trial. *Ann Surg*. 2006 Nov;244(5):706-14.

Sugnanam KK, Collins JT, Smith PK, Connor F, Lewindon P, Cleghorn G, Withers G. Dichotomy of food and inhalant allergen sensitization in eosinophilic esophagitis. *Allergy*. 2007 Nov;62(11):1257-60.

Sulman FG, Levy D, Lunkan L, Pfeifer Y, Tal E. New methods in the treatment of weather sensitivity. Fortschr Med. 1977 Mar 17;95(11):746-52.

Sulman FG. Migraine and headache due to weather and allied causes and its specific treatment. Ups J Med Sci Suppl. 1980;31:41-4.

Sumantran VN, Kulkarni AA, Harsulkar A, Wele A, Koppikar SJ, Chandwaskar R, Gaire V, Dalvi M, Wagh UV. Hyaluronidase and collagenase inhibitory activities of the herbal formulation Triphala guggulu. *J Biosci*. 2007 Jun;32(4):755-61.

Sumiyoshi M, Sakanaka M, Kimura Y. Effects of Red Ginseng extract on allergic reactions to food in Balb/c mice. *J Ethnopharmacol*. 2010 Aug 14.

Sung JH, Lee JO, Son JK, Park NS, Kim MR, Kim JG, Moon DC. Cytotoxic constituents from Solidago virga-aurea var. gigantea MIQ. *Arch Pharm Res*. 1999 Dec;22(6):633-7.

Suomalainen H, Isolauri E. New concepts of allergy to cow's milk. *Ann Med*. 1994 Aug;26(4):289-96.

Sur S, Camara M, Buchmeier A, Morgan S, Nelson HS. Double-blind trial of pyridoxine (vitamin B6) in the treatment of steroid-dependent asthma. Ann Allergy. 1993 Feb;70(2):147-52.

Sütas Y, Kekki OM, Isolauri E. Late onset reactions to oral food challenge are linked to low serum interleukin-10 concentrations in patients with atopic dermatitis and food allergy. *Clin Exp Allergy*. 2000 Aug;30(8):1121-8.

Svanes C, Heinrich J, Jarvis D, Chinn S, Omenaas E, Gulsvik A, Künzli N, Burney P. Pet-keeping in childhood and adult asthma and hay fever: European community respiratory health survey. *J Allergy Clin Immunol*. 2003 Aug;112(2):289-300.

Svendsen AJ, Holm NV, Kyvik K, et al. Relative importance of genetic effects in rheumatoid arthritis: historical cohort study of Danish nationwide twin population. *BMJ* 2002;324(7332): 264-266.

Sweeney B, Vora M, Ulbricht C, Basch E. Evidence-based systematic review of dandelion (Taraxacum officinale) by natural standard research collaboration. *J Herb Pharmacother*. 2005;5(1):79-93.

Swett. JA. *A Treatise on Disease of the Chest*. New York, 1852.

Swiderska-Kielbik S, Krakowiak A, Wiszniewska M, Dudek W, Walusiak-Skorupa J, Krawczyk-Szulc P, Michowicz A, Palczyński C. Health hazards associated with occupational exposure to birds. *Med Pr*. 2010;61(2):213-22.

Szyf M, McGowan P, Meaney MJ. The social environment and the epigenome. *Environ Mol Mutagen*. 2008 Jan;49(1):46-60.

REFERENCES

Takada Y, Ichikawa H, Badmaev V, Aggarwal BB. Acetyl-11-keto-beta-boswellic acid potentiates apoptosis, inhibits invasion, and abolishes osteoclastogenesis by suppressing NF-kappa B and NF-kappa B-regulated gene expression. *J Immunol.* 2006 Mar 1;176(5):3127-40.

Takahashi N, Eisenhuth G, Lee I, Schachtele C, Laible N, Binion S. Nonspecific antibacterial factors in milk from cows immunized with human oral bacterial pathogens. *J Dairy Sci.* 1992 Jul;75(7):1810-20.

Takasaki M, Konoshima T, Tokuda H, Masuda K, Arai Y, Shiojima K, Ageta H. Anti-carcinogenic activity of Taraxacum plant. I. *Biol Pharm Bull.* 1999 Jun;22(6):602-5.

Takeda K, Suzuki T, Shimada SI, Shida K, Nanno M, Okumura K. Interleukin-12 is involved in the enhancement of human natural killer cell activity by Lactobacillus casei Shirota. *Clin Exp Immunol.* 2006 Oct;146(1):109-15.

Tamaoki J, Chiyotani A, Sakai A, Takemura H, Konno K. Effect of menthol vapour on airway hyperresponsiveness in patients with mild asthma. *Respir Med.* 1995 Aug;89(7):503-4.

Tamura M, Shikina T, Morihana T, Hayama M, Kajimoto O, Sakamoto A, Kajimoto Y, Watanabe O, Nonaka C, Shida K, Nanno M. Effects of probiotics on allergic rhinitis induced by Japanese cedar pollen: randomized double-blind, placebo-controlled clinical trial. *Int Arch Allergy Imml.* 2007;143(1):75-82.

Taniguchi C, Homma M, Takano O, Hirano T, Oka K, Aoyagi Y, Niitsuma T, Hayashi T. Pharmacological effects of urinary products obtained after treatment with saiboku-to, a herbal medicine for bronchial asthma, on type IV allergic reaction. *Planta Med.* 2000 Oct;66(7):607-11.

Tapiero H, Ba GN, Couvreur P, Tew KD. Polyunsaturated fatty acids (PUFA) and eicosanoids in human health and pathologies. *Biomed Pharmacother.* 2002 Jul;56(5):215-22.

Tapsell LC, Hemphill I, Cobiac L, Patch CS, Sullivan DR, Fenech M, Roodenrys S, Keogh JB, Clifton PM, Williams PG, Fazio VA, Inge KE. Health benefits of herbs and spices: the past, the present, the future. *Med J Aust.* 2006 Aug 21;185(4 Suppl):S4-24.

Tasli L, Mat C, De Simone C, Yazici H. Lactobacilli lozenges in the management of oral ulcers of Behçet's syndrome. *Clin Exp Rheumatol.* 2006 Sep-Oct;24(5 Suppl 42):S83-6.

Taussig SJ, Batkin S. Bromelain, the enzyme complex of pineapple (Ananas comosus) and its clinical application. An update. *J Ethnopharmacol.* 1988 Feb-Mar;22(2):191-203.

Taylor AL, Dunstan JA, Prescott SL. Probiotic supplementation for the first 6 months of life fails to reduce the risk of atopic dermatitis and increases the risk of allergen sensitization in high-risk children: a randomized controlled trial. *J Allergy Clin Immunol.* 2007 Jan;119(1):184-91.

Taylor AL, Hale J, Wiltschut J, Lehmann H, Dunstan JA, Prescott SL. Effects of probiotic supplementation for the first 6 months of life on allergen- and vaccine-specific immune responses. *Clin Exp Allergy.* 2006 Oct;36(10):1227-35.

Taylor RB, Lindquist N, Kubanek J, Hay ME. Intraspecific variation in palatability and defensive chemistry of brown seaweeds: effects on herbivore fitness. *Oecologia.* 2003 Aug;136(3):412-23.

Teitelbaum J. *From Fatigue to Fantastic.* New York: Avery, 2001.

Terheggen-Lagro SW, Khouw IM, Schaafsma A, Wauters EA. Safety of a new extensively hydrolysed formula in children with cow's milk protein allergy: a double blind crossover study. *BMC Pediatr.* 2002 Oct 14;2:10.

Terracciano L, Bouygue GR, Sarratud T, Veglia F, Martelli A, Fiocchi A. Impact of dietary regimen on the duration of cow's milk allergy: a random allocation study. *Clin Exp Allergy.* 2010 Apr;40(4):637-42.

Tesse R, Schieck M, Kabesch M. Asthma and endocrine disorders: Shared mechanisms and genetic pleiotropy. *Mol Cell Endocrinol.* 2010 Dec 4. [ahead of print] .

Thakkar K, Boatright RO, Gilger MA, El-Serag HB. Gastroesophageal reflux and asthma in children: a systematic review. *Pediatrics.* 2010 Apr;125(4):e925-30. 2010 Mar 29.

Tham KW, Zuraimi MS, Koh D, Chew FT, Ooi PL. Associations between home dampness and presence of molds with asthma and allergic symptoms among young children in the tropics. *Pediatr Allergy Immunol.* 2007 Aug;18(5):418-24.

Thampithak A, Jaisin Y, Meesarapee B, Chongthammakun S, Piyachaturawat P, Govitrapong P, Supavilai P, Sanvarinda Y. Transcriptional regulation of iNOS and COX-2 by a novel compound from Curcuma comosa in lipopolysaccharide-induced microglial activation. *Neurosci Lett.* 2009 Sep 22;462(2):171-5.

Theler B, Brockow K, Ballmer-Weber BK. Clinical presentation and diagnosis of meat allergy in Switzerland and Southern Germany. *Swiss Med Wkly.* 2009 May 2;139(17-18):264-70.

Theofilopoulos AN, Kono DH. The genes of systemic autoimmunity. *Proc Assoc Am Physicians.* 1999;111(3): 228-240.

Thiruvengadam KV, Haranath K, Sudarsan S, Sekar TS, Rajagopal KR, Zacharian MG, Devarajan TV. Tylophora indica in bronchial asthma (a controlled comparison with a standard anti-asthmatic drug). *J Indian Med Assoc.* 1978 Oct 1;71(7):172-6.

Thomas M. Are breathing exercises an effective strategy for people with asthma? *Nurs Times.* 2009 Mar 17-23;105(10):22-7.

Thomas, R.G., Gebhardt, S.E. 2008. Nutritive value of pomegranate fruit and juice. *Maryland Dietetic Association Annual Meeting, USDA-ARS.* 2008 April 11.

Thompson T, Lee AR, Grace T. Gluten contamination of grains, seeds, and flours in the United States: a pilot study. *J Am Diet Assoc.* 2010 Jun;110(6):937-40.

Tierra L. *The Herbs of Life.* Freedom, CA: Crossing Press, 1992.

Tierra M. *The Way of Herbs.* New York: Pocket Books, 1990.

Tisserand R. *The Art of Aromatherapy.* New York: Inner Traditions, 1979.

Tiwari M. *Ayurveda: A Life of Balance.* Rochester, VT: Healing Arts, 1995.

Tlaskalová-Hogenová H, Stepánková R, Hudcovic T, Tucková L, Cukrowska B, Lodinová-Zádníková R, Kozáková H, Rossmann P, Bártová J, Sokol D, Funda DP, Borovská D, Reháková Z, Sinkora J, Hofman J, Drastich P, Kokesová A. Commensal bacteria (normal microflora), mucosal immunity and chronic inflammatory and autoimmune diseases. *Immunol Lett.* 2004 May 15;93(2-3):97-108.

Todd GR, Acerini CL, Ross-Russell R, Zahra S, Warner JT, McCance D. Survey of adrenal crisis associated with inhaled corticosteroids in the United Kingdom. *Arch Dis Child.* 2002 Dec;87(6):457-61.

Tonkal AM, Morsy TA. An update review on Commiphora molmol and related species. *J Egypt Soc Parasitol.* 2008 Dec;38(3):763-96.

Topçu G, Erenler R, Cakmak O, Johansson CB, Celik C, Chai HB, Pezzuto JM. Diterpenes from the berries of Juniperus excelsa. *Phytochemistry.* 1999 Apr;50(7):1195-9.

Toppila-Salmi S, Renkonen J, Joenväärä S, Mattila P, Renkonen R. Allergen interactions with epithelium. *Curr Opin Allergy Clin Immunol.* 2011 Feb;11(1):29-32.

Tordesillas L, Pacios LF, Palacín A, Cuesta-Herranz J, Madero M, Díaz-Perales A. Characterization of IgE epitopes of Cuc m 2, the major melon allergen, and their role in cross-reactivity with pollen profilins. *Clin Exp Allergy.* 2010 Jan;40(1):174-81.

Torrent M, Sunyer J, Muñoz L, Cullinan P, Iturriaga MV, Figueroa C, Vall O, Taylor AN, Anto JM. Early-life domestic aeroallergen exposure and IgE sensitization at age 4 years. *J Allergy Clin Immunol.* 2006 Sep;118(3):742-8.

Towers GH. FAHF-1 purporting to block peanut-induced anaphylaxis. *J Allergy Clin Immunol.* 2003 May;111(5):1140; author reply 1140-1.

Towle A. *Modern Biology.* Austin: Harcourt Brace, 1993.

Trojanová I, Rada V, Kokoska L, Vlková E. The bifidogenic effect of Taraxacum officinale root. *Fitoterapia.* 2004 Dec;75(7-8):760-3.

Troncone R, Caputo N, Florio G, Finelli E. Increased intestinal sugar permeability after challenge in children with cow's milk allergy or intolerance. *Allergy.* 1994 Mar;49(3):142-6.

Trout L, King M, Feng W, Inglis SK, Ballard ST. Inhibition of airway liquid secretion and its effect on the physical properties of airway mucus. *Am J Physiol.* 1998 Feb;274(2 Pt 1):L258-63.

Tsai JC, Tsai S, Chang WC. Comparison of two Chinese medical herbs, Huangbai and Qianniuzi, on influence of short circuit current across the rat intestinal epithelia. *J Ethnopharmacol.* 2004 Jul;93(1):21-5.

Tsong T. Deciphering the language of cells. *Trends in Biochem Sci.* 1989;14:89-92.

Tucker KL, Olson B, Bakun P, Dallal GE, Selhub J, Rosenberg IH. Breakfast cereal fortified with folic acid, vitamin B-6, and vitamin B-12 increases vitamin concentrations and reduces homocysteine concentrations: a randomized trial. *Am J Clin Nutr.* 2004 May;79(5):805-11.

Tulk HM, Robinson LE. Modifying the n-6/n-3 polyunsaturated fatty acid ratio of a high-saturated fat challenge does not acutely attenuate postprandial changes in inflammatory markers in men with metabolic syndrome. *Metabolism.* 2009 Jul 20.

Tunnicliffe WS, Burge PS, Ayres JG. Effect of domestic concentrations of nitrogen dioxide on airway responses to inhaled allergen in asthmatic patients. *Lancet.* 1994 Dec 24-31;344(8939-8940):1733-6.

Tunnicliffe WS, Fletcher TJ, Hammond K, Roberts K, Custovic A, Simpson A, Woodcock A, Ayres JG. Sensitivity and exposure to indoor allergens in adults with differing asthma severity. *Eur Respir J.* 1999 Mar;13(3):654-9.

Tursi A, Brandimarte G, Giorgetti GM, Elisei W. Mesalazine and/or Lactobacillus casei in maintaining long-term remission of symptomatic uncomplicated diverticular disease of the colon. *Hepatogastroenterology.* 2008 May-Jun;55(84):916-20.

U.S. Food and Drug Administration *Guidance for Industry Botanical Drug Products.* CfDEaR. 2000

Uddenfeldt M, Janson C, Lampa E, Leander M, Norbäck D, Larsson L, Rask-Andersen A. High BMI is related to higher incidence of asthma, while a low fish and fruit diet is related to a lower- Results from a long-term follow-up study of three age groups in Sweden. *Respir Med.* 2010 Jul;104(7):972-80.

Udupa AL, Udupa SL, Guruswamy MN. The possible site of anti-asthmatic action of Tylophora asthmatica on pituitary-adrenal axis in albino rats. *Planta Med.* 1991 Oct;57(5):409-13.

Ueno H, Yoshioka K, Matsumoto T. Usefulness of the skin index in predicting the outcome of oral challenges in children. *J Investig Allergol Clin Immunol.* 2007;17(4):207-10.

Ueno M, Adachi A, Fukumoto T, Nishitani N, Fujiwara N, Matsuo H, Kohno K, Morita E. Analysis of causative allergen of the patient with baker's asthma and wheat-dependent exercise-induced anaphylaxis (WDEIA). *Arerugi.* 2010 May;59(5):552-7.

REFERENCES

Ukabam SO, Mann RJ, Cooper BT. Small intestinal permeability to sugars in patients with atopic eczema. *Br J Dermatol.* 1984 Jun;110(6):649-52.

Ulrich RS, Simons RF, Losito BD, Fiorito E, Miles MA, Zelson M. Stress recovery during exposure to natural and urban environments. J Envir Psychol. 1991;11:201-30.

Unsel M, Sin AZ, Ardeniz O, Erdem N, Ersoy R, Gulbahar O, Mete N, Kokuludağ A. New onset egg allergy in an adult. *J Investig Allergol Clin Immunol.* 2007;17(1):55-8.

Upadhyay AK, Kumar K, Kumar A, Mishra HS. Tinospora cordifolia (Willd.) Hook. f. and Thoms. (Guduchi) - validation of the Ayurvedic pharmacology through experimental and clinical studies. *Int J Ayurveda Res.* 2010 Apr;1(2):112-21.

Urata Y, Yoshida S, Irie Y, Tanigawa T, Amayasu H, Nakabayashi M, Akahori K. Treatment of asthma patients with herbal medicine TJ-96: a randomized controlled trial. *Respir Med.* 2002 Jun;96(6):469-74.

Vally H, Thompson PJ, Misso NL. Changes in bronchial hyperresponsiveness following high- and low-sulphite wine challenges in wine-sensitive asthmatic patients. *Clin Exp Allergy.* 2007 Jul;37(7):1062-6.

van Beelen VA, Roeleveld J, Mooibroek H, Sijtsma L, Bino RJ, Bosch D, Rietjens IM, Alink GM. A comparative study on the effect of algal and fish oil on viability and cell proliferation of Caco-2 cells. *Food Chem Toxicol.* 2007 May;45(5):716-24.

van Elburg RM, Uil JJ, de Monchy JG, Heymans HS. Intestinal permeability in pediatric gastroenterology. *Scand J Gastroenterol Suppl.* 1992;194:19-24.

van Huisstede A, Braunstahl GJ. Obesity and asthma: co-morbidity or causal relationship? *Monaldi Arch Chest Dis.* 2010 Sep;73(3):116-23.

van Kampen V, Merget R, Rabstein S, Sander I, Bruening T, Broding HC, Keller C, Muesken H, Overlack A, Schultze-Werninghaus G, Walusiak J, Raulf-Heimsoth M. Comparison of wheat and rye flour solutions for skin prick testing: a multi-centre study (Stad 1). *Clin Exp Allergy.* 2009 Dec;39(12):1896-902.

van Odijk J, Peterson CG, Ahlstedt S, Bengtsson U, Borres MP, Hulthén L, Magnusson J, Hansson T. Measurements of eosinophil activation before and after food challenges in adults with food hypersensitivity. *Int Arch Allergy Immunol.* 2006;140(4):334-41.

van Zwol A, Moll HA, Fetter WP, van Elburg RM. Glutamine-enriched enteral nutrition in very low birthweight infants and allergic and infectious diseases at 6 years of age. *Paediatr Perinat Epidemiol.* 2011 Jan;25(1):60-6.

Vanderhoof JA. Probiotics in allergy management. *J Pediatr Gastroenterol Nutr.* 2008 Nov;47 Suppl 2:S38-40.

VanHaitsma TA, Mickleborough T, Stager JM, Koceja DM, Lindley MR, Chapman R. Comparative effects of caffeine and albuterol on the bronchoconstrictor response to exercise in asthmatic athletes. *Int J Sports Med.* 2010 Apr;31(4):231-6.

Vanto T, Helppilä S, Juntunen-Backman K, Kalimo K, Klemola T, Korpela R, Koskinen P. Prediction of the development of tolerance to milk in children with cow's milk hypersensitivity. *J Pediatr.* 2004 Feb;144(2):218-22.

Vargas C, Bustos P, Diaz PV, Amigo H, Rona RJ. Childhood environment and atopic conditions, with emphasis on asthma in a Chilean agricultural area. *J Asthma.* 2008 Jan-Feb;45(1):73-8.

Varonier HS, de Haller J, Schopfer C. Prevalence of allergies in children and adolescents. *Helv Paediatr Acta.* 1984;39:129-136.

Varraso R, Fung TT, Barr RG, Hu FB, Willett W, Camargo CA Jr. Prospective study of dietary patterns and chronic obstructive pulmonary disease among US women. *Am J Clin Nutr.* 2007 Aug;86(2):488-95.

Varraso R, Fung TT, Hu FB, Willett W, Camargo CA. Prospective study of dietary patterns and chronic obstructive pulmonary disease among US men. *Thorax.* 2007 Sep;62(9):786-91. 2007 May 15.

Varraso R, Jiang R, Barr RG, Willett WC, Camargo CA Jr. Prospective study of cured meats consumption and risk of chronic obstructive pulmonary disease in men. *Am J Epidemiol.* 2007 Dec 15;166(12):1438-45. 2007 Sep 4. 17785711; .

Vassallo MF, Banerji A, Rudders SA, Clark S, Mullins RJ, Camargo CA Jr. Season of birth and food allergy in children. *Ann Allergy Asthma Immunol.* 2010 Apr;104(4):307-13.

Vempati R, Bijlani RL, Deepak KK. The efficacy of a comprehensive lifestyle modification programme based on yoga in the management of bronchial asthma: a randomized controlled trial. *BMC Pulm Med.* 2009 Jul 30;9:37.

Vendt N, Grünberg H, Tuure T, Malminiemi O, Wuolijoki E, Tillmann V, Sepp E, Korpela R. Growth during the first 6 months of life in infants using formula enriched with Lactobacillus rhamnosus GG: double-blind, randomized trial. *J Hum Nutr Diet.* 2006 Feb;19(1):51-8.

Venkatachalam KV. Human 3'-phosphoadenosine 5'-phosphosulfate (PAPS) synthase: biochemistry, molecular biology and genetic deficiency. *IUBMB Life.* 2003 Jan;55(1):1-11.

Venkatesan N, Punithavathi D, Babu M. Protection from acute and chronic lung diseases by curcumin. *Adv Exp Med Biol.* 2007;595:379-405.

Venter C, Hasan Arshad S, Grundy J, Pereira B, Bernie Clayton C, Voigt K, Higgins B, Dean T. Time trends in the prevalence of peanut allergy: three cohorts of children from the same geographical location in the UK. *Allergy.* 2010 Jan;65(1):103-8.

Venter C, Meyer R. Session 1: Allergic disease: The challenges of managing food hypersensitivity. *Proc Nutr Soc.* 2010 Feb;69(1):11-24.

Venter C, Pereira B, Grundy J, Clayton CB, Arshad SH, Dean T. Prevalence of sensitization reported and objectively assessed food hypersensitivity amongst six-year-old children: A population-based study. *Pediatr Allergy Immunol.* 2006;17: 356-363.

Venter C, Pereira B, Grundy J, Clayton CB, Roberts G, Higgins B, Dean T. Incidence of parentally reported and clinically diagnosed food hypersensitivity in the first year of life. *J Allergy Clin Immunol.* 2006;117: 1118-1124.

Ventura MT, Polimeno L, Amoruso AC, Gatti F, Annoscia E, Marinaro M, Di Leo E, Matino MG, Buquicchio R, Bonini S, Tursi A, Francavilla A. Intestinal permeability in patients with adverse reactions to food. *Dig Liver Dis.* 2006 Oct;38(10):732-6.

Venturi A, Gionchetti P, Rizzello F, Johansson R, Zucconi E, Brigidi P, Matteuzzi D, Campieri M. Impact on the composition of the faecal flora by a new probiotic preparation: preliminary data on maintenance treatment of patients with ulcerative colitis. *Aliment Pharmacol Ther.* 1999 Aug;13(8):1103-8.

Verhasselt V. Oral tolerance in neonates: from basics to potential prevention of allergic disease. *Mucosal Immunol.* 2010 Jul;3(4):326-33.

Verstege A, Mehl A, Rolinck-Werninghaus C, Staden U, Nocon M, Beyer K, Niggemann B. The predictive value of the skin prick test weal size for the outcome of oral food challenges. Clin Exp Allergy. 2005 Sep;35(9):1220-6. Rolinck-Werninghaus C, Staden U, Mehl A, Hamelmann E, Beyer K, Niggemann B. Specific oral tolerance induction with food in children: transient or persistent effect on food allergy? *Allergy.* 2005 Oct;60(10):1320-2.

Vidgren HM, Agren JJ, Schwab U, Rissanen T, Hanninen O, Uusitupa MI. Incorporation of n-3 fatty acids into plasma lipid fractions, and erythrocyte membranes and platelets during dietary supplementation with fish, fish oil, and docosahexaenoic acid-rich oil among healthy young men. *Lipids.* 1997 Jul;32(7):697-705.

Viinanen A, Munhbayarlah S, Zevgee T, Narantsetseg L, Naidansuren Ts, Koskenvuo M, Helenius H, Terho EO. Prevalence of asthma, allergic rhinoconjunctivitis and allergic sensitization in Mongolia. *Allergy.* 2005;60:1370-1377.

Vila R, Mundina M, Tomi F, Furlán R, Zacchino S, Casanova J, Cañigueral S. Composition and antifungal activity of the essential oil of Solidago chilensis. *Planta Med.* 2002 Feb;68(2):164-7.

Viljanen M, Kuitunen M, Haahtela T, Juntunen-Backman K, Korpela R, Savilahti E. Probiotic effects on faecal inflammatory markers and on faecal IgA in food allergic atopic eczema/dermatitis syndrome infants. *Pediatr Allergy Immunol.* 2005 Feb;16(1):65-71.

Viljanen M, Savilahti E, Haahtela T, Juntunen-Backman K, Korpela R, Poussa T, Tuure T, Kuitunen M. Probiotics in the treatment of atopic eczema/dermatitis syndrome in infants: a double-blind placebo-controlled trial. *Allergy.* 2005 Apr;60(4):494-500.

Vinson JA, Proch J, Bose P. MegaNatural((R)) Gold Grapeseed Extract: In Vitro Antioxidant and In Vivo Human Supplementation Studies. *J Med Food.* 2001 Spring;4(1):17-26.

Visitsunthorn N, Pacharn P, Jirapongsananuruk O, Weeravejsukit S, Sripramong C, Sookrung N, Bunnag C. Comparison between Siriraj mite allergen vaccine and standardized commercial mite vaccine by skin prick testing in normal Thai adults. *Asian Pac J Allergy Immunol.* 2010 Mar;28(1):41-5.

Visness CM, London SJ, Daniels JL, Kaufman JS, Yeatts KB, Siega-Riz AM, Liu AH, Calatroni A, Zeldin DC. Association of obesity with IgE levels and allergy symptoms in children and adolescents: results from the National Health and Nutrition Examination Survey 2005-2006. *J Allergy Clin Immunol.* 2009 May;123(5):1163-9, 1169.e1-4.

Visness CM, London SJ, Daniels JL, Kaufman JS, Yeatts KB, Siega-Riz AM, Calatroni A, Zeldin DC. Association of childhood obesity with atopic and nonatopic asthma: results from the National Health and Nutrition Examination Survey 1999-2006. *J Asthma.* 2010 Sep;47(7):822-9.

Vlieg-Boerstra BJ, Dubois AE, van der Heide S, Bijleveld CM, Wolt-Plompen SA, Oude Elberink JN, Kukler J, Jansen DF, Venter C, Duiverman EJ. Ready-to-use introduction schedules for first exposure to allergenic foods in children at home. *Allergy.* 2008 Jul;63(7):903-9.

Vlieg-Boerstra BJ, van der Heide S, Bijleveld CM, Kukler J, Duiverman EJ, Wolt-Plompen SA, Dubois AE. Dietary assessment in children adhering to a food allergen avoidance diet for allergy prevention. *Eur J Clin Nutr.* 2006 Dec;60(12):1384-90.

Voicekovska JG, Orlikov GA, Karpov IuG, Teibe U, Ivanov AD, Baidekalne I, Voicehovskis NV, Maulins E. External respiration function and quality of life in patients with bronchial asthma in correction of selenium deficiency. *Ter Arkh.* 2007;79(8):38-41.

Voĭtsekhovskaia IuG, Skesters A, Orlikov GA, Silova AA, Rusakova NE, Larmane LT, Karpov IuG, Ivanov AD, Maulins E. Assessment of some oxidative stress parameters in bronchial asthma patients beyond add-on selenium supplementation. *Biomed Khim.* 2007 Sep-Oct;53(5):577-84.

Vojdani A. Antibodies as predictors of complex autoimmune diseases. *Int J Immunopathol Pharmacol.* 2008 Apr-Jun;21(2):267-78.

REFERENCES

von Berg A, Filipiak-Pittroff B, Krämer U, Link E, Bollrath C, Brockow I, Koletzko S, Grübl A, Heinrich J, Wichmann HE, Bauer CP, Reinhardt D, Berdel D; GINIplus study group. Preventive effect of hydrolyzed infant formulas persists until age 6 years: long-term results from the German Infant Nutritional Intervention Study (GINI). *J Allergy Clin Immunol.* 2008 Jun;121(6):1442-7.

von Berg A, Koletzko S, Grübl A, Filipiak-Pittroff B, Wichmann HE, Bauer CP, Reinhardt D, Berdel D; German Infant Nutritional Intervention Study Group. The effect of hydrolyzed cow's milk formula for allergy prevention in the first year of life: the German Infant Nutritional Intervention Study, a randomized double-blind trial. *J Allergy Clin Immunol.* 2003 Mar;111(3):533-40.

von Kruedener S, Schneider W, Elstner EF. A combination of Populus tremula, Solidago virgaurea and Fraxinus excelsior as an anti-inflammatory and antirheumatic drug. A short review. *Arzneimittelforschung.* 1995 Feb;45(2):169-71.

von Mutius E, Vercelli D. Farm living: effects on childhood asthma and allergy. *Nat Rev Immunol.* 2010 Dec;10(12):861-8. 2010 Nov 9.

Vulevic J, Drakoularakou A, Yaqoob P, Tzortzis G and Gibson GR; Modulation of the fecal microflora profile and immune function by a novel trans-galactooligosaccharide mixture (B-GOS) in healthy elderly volunteers. *Am J Clin Nutr.* 1988 88;1438-1446.

Waddell L. Food allergies in children: the difference between cow's milk protein allergy and food intolerance. *J Fam Health Care.* 2010;20(3):104.

Wahler D, Gronover CS, Richter C, Foucu F, Twyman RM, Moerschbacher BM, Fischer R, Muth J, Prufer D. Polyphenoloxidase silencing affects latex coagulation in Taraxacum spp. *Plant Physiol.* 2009 Jul 15.

Waite DA, Eyles EF, Tonkin SL, O'Donnell TV. Asthma prevalence in Tokelauan children in two environments. *Clin Allergy.* 1980;10:71-75.

Waked M, Salameh P. Risk factors for asthma and allergic diseases in school children across Lebanon. *J Asthma Allergy.* 2008 Nov 11;2:1-7.

Walders-Abramson N, Wamboldt FS, Curran-Everett D, Zhang L. Encouraging physical activity in pediatric asthma: a case-control study of the wonders of walking (WOW) program. *Pediatr Pulmonol.* 2009 Sep;44(9):909-16.

Walker S, Wing A. Allergies in children. *J Fam Health Care.* 2010;20(1):24-6.

Walker WA. Antigen absorption from the small intestine and gastrointestinal disease. *Pediatr Clin North Am.* 1975 Nov;22(4):731-46.

Walker WA. Antigen handling by the small intestine. *Clin Gastroenterol.* 1986 Jan;15(1):1-20.

Walle UK, Walle T. Transport of the cooked-food mutagen 2-amino-1-methyl-6-phenylimidazo- 4,5-b pyridine (PhIP) across the human intestinal Caco-2 cell monolayer: role of efflux pumps. *Carcinogenesis.* 1999 Nov;20(11):2153-7.

Walsh MG. Toxocara infection and diminished lung function in a nationally representative sample from the United States population. *Int J Parasitol.* 2010 Nov 8.

Walsh SJ, Rau LM: Autoimmune diseases: a leading cause of death among young and middle-aged women in the United States. *Am J Public Health* 2000, 90(9): 1463-1466.

Wang G, Liu CT, Wang ZL, Yan CL, Luo FM, Wang L, Li TQ. Effects of Astragalus membranaceus in promoting T-helper cell type 1 polarization and interferon-gamma production by up-regulating T-bet expression in patients with asthma. *Chin J Integr Med.* 2006 Dec;12(4):262-7.

Wang H, Chang B, Wang B. The effect of herbal medicine including astragalus membranaceus (fisch) bge, codonpsis pilosula and glycyrrhiza uralensis fisch on airway responsiveness. *Zhonghua Jie He He Hu Xi Za Zhi.* 1998 May;21(5):287-8.

Wang J, Lin J, Bardina L, Goldis M, Nowak-Wegrzyn A, Shreffler WG, Sampson HA. Correlation of IgE/IgG4 milk epitopes and affinity of milk-specific IgE antibodies with different phenotypes of clinical milk allergy. *J Allergy Clin Immunol.* 2010 Mar;125(3):695-702, 702.e1-702.e6.

Wang J, Patil SP, Yang N, Ko J, Lee J, Noone S, Sampson HA, Li XM. Safety, tolerability, and immunologic effects of a food allergy herbal formula in food allergic individuals: a randomized, double-blinded, placebo-controlled, dose escalation, phase 1 study. *Ann Allergy Asthma Immunol.* 2010 Jul;105(1):75-84.

Wang J. Management of the patient with multiple food allergies. *Curr Allergy Asthma Rep.* 2010 Jul;10(4):271-7.

Wang JL, Shaw NS, Kao MD. Magnesium deficiency and its lack of association with asthma in Taiwanese elementary school children. *Asia Pac J Clin Nutr.* 2007;16 Suppl 2:579-84.

Wang JS, Hung WP. The effects of a swimming intervention for children with asthma. *Respirology.* 2009 Aug;14(6):838-42.

Wang KY, Li SN, Liu CS, Perng DS, Su YC, Wu DC, Jan CM, Lai CH, Wang TN, Wang WM. Effects of ingesting Lactobacillus- and Bifidobacterium-containing yogurt in subjects with colonized Helicobacter pylori. *Am J Clin Nutr.* 2004 Sep;80(3):737-41.

Wang YH, Yang CP, Ku MS, Sun HL, Lue KH. Efficacy of nasal irrigation in the treatment of acute sinusitis in children. *Int J Pediatr Otorhinolaryngol.* 2009 Dec;73(12):1696-701. 2009 Sep 27.

Wang YM, Huan GX. *Utilization of Classical Formulas.* Beijing, China: Chinese Medicine and Pharmacology Publishing Co, 1998.

Waring G, Levy D. Challenging adverse reactions in children with food allergies. *Paediatr Nurs.* 2010 Jul;22(6):16-22.

Waser M, Michels KB, Bieli C, Flöistrup H, Pershagen G, von Mutius E, Ege M, Riedler J, Schram-Bijkerk D, Brunekreef B, van Hage M, Lauener R, Braun-Fahrländer C; PARSIFAL Study team. Inverse association of farm milk consumption with asthma and allergy in rural and suburban populations across Europe. *Clin Exp Allergy.* 2007 May;37(5):661-70.

Watkins BA, Hannon K, Ferruzzi M, Li Y. Dietary PUFA and flavonoids as deterrents for environmental pollutants. *J Nutr Biochem.* 2007 Mar;18(3):196-205.

Watson R. Preedy VR. Botanical Medicine in Clinical Practice. Oxfordshire: CABI, 2008.

Watzl B, Bub A, Blockhaus M, Herbert BM, Lührmann PM, Neuhäuser-Berthold M, Rechkemmer G. Prolonged tomato juice consumption has no effect on cell-mediated immunity of well-nourished elderly men and women. *J Nutr.* 2000 Jul;130(7):1719-23.

Webber CM, England RW. Oral allergy syndrome: a clinical, diagnostic, and therapeutic challenge. *Ann Allergy Asthma Immunol.* 2010 Feb;104(2):101-8; quiz 109-10, 117.

Webster D, Taschereau P, Belland RJ, Sand C, Rennie RP. Antifungal activity of medicinal plant extracts; preliminary screening studies. *J Ethnopharmacol.* 2008 Jan 4;115(1):140-6.

Wei A, Shibamoto T. Antioxidant activities and volatile constituents of various essential oils. *J Agric Food Chem.* 2007 Mar 7;55(5):1737-42.

Weiler JM, Layton T, Hunt M. Asthma in United States Olympic athletes who participated in the 1996 Summer Games. J Allergy Clin Immunol. 1998 Nov;102(5):722-6. 7.

Weiner MA. *Secrets of Fijian Medicine.* Berkeley, CA: Univ. of Calif., 1969.

Weisgerber M, Webber K, Meurer J, Danduran M, Berger S, Flores G. Moderate and vigorous exercise programs in children with asthma: safety, parental satisfaction, and asthma outcomes. Pediatr Pulmonol. 2008 Dec;43(12):1175-82.

Weiss RF. *Herbal Medicine.* Gothenburg, Sweden: Beaconsfield, 1988.

Wen MC, Huang CK, Srivastava KD, Zhang TF, Schofield B, Sampson HA, Li XM. Ku-Shen (Sophora flavescens Ait), a single Chinese herb, abrogates airway hyperreactivity in a murine model of asthma. *J Allergy Clin Immunol.* 2004;113:218.

Wen MC, Taper A, Srivastava KD, Huang CK, Schofield B, Li XM. Immunology of T cells by the Chinese Herbal Medicine Ling Zhi (Ganoderma lucidum) *J Allergy Clin Immunol.* 2003;111:S320.

Wen MC, Wei CH, Hu ZQ, Srivastava K, Ko J, Xi ST, Mu DZ, Du JB, Li GH, Wallenstein S, Sampson H, Kattan M, Li XM. Efficacy and tolerability of anti-asthma herbal medicine intervention in adult patients with moderate-severe allergic asthma. *J Allergy Clin Immunol.* 2005;116:517-24.

Werbach M. *Nutritional Influences on Illness.* Tarzana, CA: Third Line Press, 1996.

West CE, Hammarström ML, Hernell O. Probiotics during weaning reduce the incidence of eczema. *Pediatr Allergy Immunol.* 2009 Aug;20(5):430-7.

West R. Risk of death in meat and non-meat eaters. *BMJ.* 1994 Oct 8;309(6959):955.

Westerholm-Ormio M, Vaarala O, Tiittanen M, Savilahti E. Infiltration of Foxp3- and Toll-like receptor-4-positive cells in the intestines of children with food allergy. *J Pediatr Gastroenterol Nutr.* 2010 Apr;50(4):367-76.

Wheeler JG, Shema SJ, Bogle ML, Shirrell MA, Burks AW, Pittler A, Helm RM. Immune and clinical impact of Lactobacillus acidophilus on asthma. *Ann Allergy Asthma Immunol.* 1997 Sep;79(3):229-33.

White LB, Foster S. The Herbal Drugstore. Emmaus, PA: Rodale, 2000.

Whitfield KE, Wiggins SA, Belue R, Brandon DT. Genetic and environmental influences on forced expiratory volume in African Americans: the Carolina African-American Twin Study of Aging. *Ethn Dis.* 2004 Spring;14(2):206-11.

WHO. *Guidelines for Drinking-water Quality.* 2nd ed, vol. 2. Geneva: World Health Organization, 1996.

WHO. How trace elements in water contribute to health. *WHO Chronicle.* 1978;32:382-385.

WHO. *INFOSAN Food Allergies. Information Note No. 3.* Geneva, Switzerland: World Health Organization, 2006.

Widdicombe JG, Ernst E. Clinical cough V: complementary and alternative medicine: therapy of cough. *Handb Exp Pharmacol.* 2009;(187):321-42.

Wilkens H, Wilkens JH, Uffmann J, Bövers J, Fröhlich JC, Fabel H. Effect of the platelet-activating factor antagonist BN 52063 on exertional asthma. *Pneumologie.* 1990 Feb;44 Suppl 1:347-8.

Willard T, Jones K. *Reishi Mushroom: Herb of Spiritual Potency and Medical Wonder.* Issaquah, Washington: Sylvan Press, 1990.

Willard T. *Edible and Medicinal Plants of the Rocky Mountains and Neighbouring Territories.* Calgary: 1992.

Willemsen LE, Koetsier MA, Balvers M, Beermann C, Stahl B, van Tol EA. Polyunsaturated fatty acids support epithelial barrier integrity and reduce IL-4 mediated permeability in vitro. *Eur J Nutr.* 2008 Jun;47(4):183-91.

REFERENCES

Williams DM. Considerations in the long-term management of asthma in ambulatory patients. *AM J Health Sits Pham.* 2006;63:S14-21.

Wilson D, Evans M, Guthrie N, Sharma P, Baisley J, Schonlau F, Burki C. A randomized, double-blind, placebo-controlled exploratory study to evaluate the potential of pycnogenol for improving allergic rhinitis symptoms. *Phytother Res.* 2010 Aug;24(8):1115-9.

Wilson K, McDowall L, Hodge D, Chetcuti P, Cartledge P. Cow's milk protein allergy. *Community Pract.* 2010 May;83(5):40-1.

Wilson L. *Nutritional Balancing and Hair Mineral Analysis.* Prescott, AZ: LD Wilson, 1998.

Wilson NM, Charette L, Thomson AH, Silverman M. Gastro-oesophageal reflux and childhood asthma: the acid test. *Thorax.* 1985 Aug;40(8):592-7.

Winchester AM. *Biology and its Relation to Mankind.* New York: Van Nostrand Reinhold, 1969.

Wittenberg JS. *The Rebellious Body.* New York: Insight, 1996.

Woessner KM, Simon RA, Stevenson DD. Monosodium glutamate sensitivity in asthma. *J Allergy Clin Immunol.* 1999 Aug;104(2 Pt 1):305-10.

Wöhrl S, Hemmer W, Focke M, Rappersberger K, Jarisch R. Histamine intolerance-like symptoms in healthy volunteers after oral provocation with liquid histamine. *Allergy Asthma Proc.* 2004 Sep-Oct;25(5):305-11.

Wolvers DA, van Herpen-Broekmans WM, Logman MH, van der Wielen RP, Albers R. Effect of a mixture of micronutrients, but not of bovine colostrum concentrate, on immune function parameters in healthy volunteers: a randomized placebo-controlled study. *Nutr J.* 2006 Nov 21;5:28.

Wolverton BC. *How to grow fresh air: 50 houseplants that purify your home or office.* New York: Penguin, 1997.

Wong GWK, Hui DSC, Chan HH, Fox TF, Leung R, Zhong NS, Chen YZ, Lai CKW. Prevalence of respiratory and atopic disorders in Chinese schoolchildren. *Clinical and Experimental Allergy.* 2001;31:1125-1231.

Wong WM, Lai KC, Lam KF, Hui WM, Hu WH, Lam CL, Xia HH, Huang JQ, Chan CK, Lam SK, Wong BC. Prevalence, clinical spectrum and health care utilization of gastro-oesophageal reflux disease in a Chinese population: a population-based study. *Aliment Pharmacol Ther.* 2003 Sep 15;18(6):595-604.

Wood M. *The Book of Herbal Wisdom.* Berkeley, CA: North Atlantic, 1997.

Wood RA, Kraynak J. *Food Allergies for Dummies.* Hoboken, NJ: Wiley Publ, 2007.

Woods RK, Abramson M, Bailey M, Walters EH. International prevalences of reported food allergies and intolerances. Comparisons arising from the European Community Respiratory Health Survey (ECRHS) 1991-1994. *Eur J Clin Nutr* 2001;55:298-304.

Woods RK, Abramson M, Bailey M, Walters EH. International prevalences of reported food allergies and intolerances. Comparisons arising from the European Community Respiratory Health Survey (ECRHS) 1991-1994. *Eur J Clin Nutr.* 2001 Apr;55(4):298-304.

Woods RK, Abramson M, Raven JM, Bailey M, Weiner JM, Walters EH. Reported food intolerance and respiratory symptoms in young adults. *Eur Respir J.* 1998;11: 151-155.

Wouters EF, Reynaert NL, Dentener MA, Vernooy JH. Systemic and local inflammation in asthma and chronic obstructive pulmonary disease: is there a connection? *Proc Am Thorac Soc.* 2009 Dec;6(8):638-47.

Wright A, Lavoie KL, Jacob A, Rizk A, Bacon SL. Effect of body mass index on self-reported exercise-triggered asthma. *Phys Sportsmed.* 2010 Dec;38(4):61-6.

Wright GR, Howieson S, McSharry C, McMahon AD, Chaudhuri R, Thompson J, Donnelly I, Brooks RG, Lawson A, Jolly L, McAlpine L, King EM, Chapman MD, Wood S, Thomson NC. Effect of improved home ventilation on asthma control and house dust mite allergen levels. *Allergy.* 2009 Nov;64(11):1671-80.

Wright RJ. Epidemiology of stress and asthma: from constricting communities and fragile families to epigenetics. *Immunol Allergy Clin North Am.* 2011 Feb;31(1):19-39.

Wu B, Yu J, Wang Y. Effect of Chinese herbs for tonifying Shen on balance of Th1 /Th2 in children with asthma in remission stage. *Zhongguo Zhong Xi Yi Jie He Za Zhi.* 2007 Feb;27(2):120-2.

Xi L, Han DM, Lü XF, Zhang L. Psychological characteristics in patients with allergic rhinitis and its associated factors analysis.. *Zhonghua Er Bi Yan Hou Tou Jing Wai Ke Za Zhi.* 2009 Dec;44(12):982-5.

Xiao P, Kubo H, Ohsawa M, Higashiyama K, Nagase H, Yan YN, Li JS, Kamei J, Ohmiya S. kappa-Opioid receptor-mediated antinociceptive effects of stereoisomers and derivatives of (+)-matrine in mice. *Planta Med.* 1999 Apr;65(3):230-3.

Xie JY, Dong JC, Gong ZH. Effects on herba epimedii and radix Astragali on tumor necrosis factor-alpha and nuclear factor-kappa B in asthmatic rats. *Zhongguo Zhong Xi Yi Jie He Za Zhi.* 2006 Aug;26(8):723-7.

Xu X, Zhang D, Zhang H, Wolters PJ, Killeen NP, Sullivan BM, Locksley RM, Lowell CA, Caughey GH. Neutrophil histamine contributes to inflammation in mycoplasma pneumonia. *J Exp Med.* 2006 Dec 25;203(13):2907-17.

Yadav RK, Ray RB, Vempati R, Bijlani RL. Effect of a comprehensive yoga-based lifestyle modification program on lipid peroxidation. *Indian J Physiol Pharmacol.* 2005 Jul-Sep;49(3):358-62.

Yadav VS, Mishra KP, Singh DP, Mehrotra S, Singh VK. Immunomodulatory effects of curcumin. *Immunopharmacol Immunotoxicol.* 2005;27(3):485-97.

Yadzir ZH, Misnan R, Abdullah N, Bakhtiar F, Arip M, Murad S. Identification of Ige-binding proteins of raw and cooked extracts of Loligo edulis (white squid). *Southeast Asian J Trop Med Public Health.* 2010 May;41(3):653-9.

Yang Z. Are peanut allergies a concern for using peanut-based formulated foods in developing countries? *Food Nutr Bull.* 2010 Jun;31(2 Suppl):S147-53.

Yeager S. *The Doctor's Book of Food Remedies.* Emmaus, PA: Rodale Press, 1998.

Yeh CC, Lin CC, Wang SD, Chen YS, Su BH, Kao ST. Protective and anti-inflammatory effect of a traditional Chinese medicine, Xia-Bai-San, by modulating lung local cytokine in a murine model of acute lung injury. *Int Immunopharmacol.* 2006 Sep;6(9):1506-14.

Yonekura S, Okamoto Y, Okawa T, Hisamitsu M, Chazono H, Kobayashi K, Sakurai D, Horiguchi S, Hanazawa T. Effects of daily intake of Lactobacillus paracasei strain KW3110 on Japanese cedar pollinosis. *Allergy Asthma Proc.* 2009 Jul-Aug;30(4):397-405.

Yu L, Zhang Y, Chen C, Cui HF, Yan XK. Meta-analysis on randomized controlled clinical trials of acupuncture for asthma. *Zhongguo Zhen Jiu.* 2010 Sep;30(9):787-92.

Yu LC. The epithelial gatekeeper against food allergy. *Pediatr Neonatol.* 2009 Dec;50(6):247-54.

Yusoff NA, Hampton SM, Dickerson JW, Morgan JB. The effects of exclusion of dietary egg and milk in the management of asthmatic children: a pilot study. *J R Soc Promot Health.* 2004 Mar;124(2):74-80.

Zanjanian MH. The intestine in allergic diseases. *Ann Allergy.* 1976 Sep;37(3):208-18.

Zarkadas M, Scott FW, Salminen J, Ham Pong A. Common Allergenic Foods and Their Labelling in Canada. *Can J Allerg Clin Immun.* 1999; 4:118-141.

Zeiger RS, Heller S. The development and prediction of atopy in high-risk children: follow-up at age seven years in a prospective randomized study of combined maternal and infant food allergen avoidance. *J Allergy Clin Immunol.* 1995 Jun;95(6):1179-90.

Zhang CS, Yang AW, Zhang AL, Fu WB, Thien FU, Lewith G, Xue CC. Ear-acupressure for allergic rhinitis: a systematic review. *Clin Otolaryngol.* 2010 Feb;35(1):6-12.

Zhang T, Srivastava K, Wen MC, Yang N, Cao J, Busse P, Birmingham N, Goldfarb J, Li XM. Pharmacology and immunological actions of a herbal medicine ASHMI on allergic asthma. *Phytother Res.* 2010 Jul;24(7):1047-55.

Zhang Z, Lai HJ, Roberg KA, Gangnon RE, Evans MD, Anderson EL, Pappas TE, Dasilva DF, Tisler CJ, Salazar LP, Gern JE, Lemanske RF Jr. Early childhood weight status in relation to asthma development in high-risk children. *J Allergy Clin Immunol.* 2010 Dec;126(6):1157-62. 2010 Nov 4.

Zhao FD, Dong JC, Xie JY. Effects of Chinese herbs for replenishing shen and strengthening qi on some indexes of neuro-endocrino-immune network in asthmatic rats. *Zhongguo Zhong Xi Yi Jie He Za Zhi.* 2007 Aug;27(8):715-9.

Zhao J, Bai J, Shen K, Xiang L, Huang S, Chen A, Huang Y, Wang J, Ye R. Self-reported prevalence of childhood allergic diseases in three cities of China: a multicenter study. *BMC Public Health.* 2010 Sep 13;10:551.

Zheng M. Experimental study of 472 herbs with antiviral action against the herpes simplex virus. *Zhong Xi Yi Jie He Za Zhi.* 1990 Jan;10(1):39-41, 6.

Zhou Q, Zhang B, Verne GN. Intestinal membrane permeability and hypersensitivity in the irritable bowel syndrome. *Pain.* 2009 Nov;146(1-2):41-6.

Zhu DD, Zhu XW, Jiang XD, Dong Z. Thymic stromal lymphopoietin expression is increased in nasal epithelial cells of patients with mugwort pollen sensitive-seasonal allergic rhinitis. *Chin Med J (Engl).* 2009 Oct 5;122(19):2303-7.

Zhu HH, Chen YP, Yu JE, Wu M, Li Z. Therapeutic effect of Xincang Decoction on chronic airway inflammation in children with bronchial asthma in remission stage. *Zhong Xi Yi Jie He Xue Bao.* 2005 Jan;3(1):23-7.

Ziaei Kajbaf T, Asar S, Alipoor MR. Relationship between obesity and asthma symptoms among children in Ahvaz, Iran:A cross sectional study. *Ital J Pediatr.* 2011 Jan;37(1):1.

Zielen S, Kardos P, Madonini E. Steroid-sparing effects with allergen-specific immunotherapy in children with asthma: a randomized controlled trial. *J Allergy Clin Immunol.* 2010 Nov;126(5):942-9. 2010 Jul 10.

Ziment I, Tashkin DP. Alternative medicine for allergy and asthma. *J Allergy Clin Immunol.* 2000 Oct;106(4):603-14.

Ziment I. Alternative therapies for asthma. *Curr Opin Pulm Med.* 1997 Jan;3(1):61-71.

Zizza, C. The nutrient content of the Italian food supply 1961-1992. *Euro J Clin Nutr.* 1997;51: 259-265.

Zoccatelli G, Pokoj S, Foetisch K, Bartra J, Valero A, Del Mar San Miguel-Moncin M, Vieths S, Scheurer S. Identification and characterization of the major allergen of green bean (Phaseolus vulgaris) as a non-specific lipid transfer protein (Pha v 3). *Mol Immunol.* 2010 Apr;47(7-8):1561-8.

Index

(Herbs, foods and other natural solutions are too numerous to index)

CPSIA information can be obtained at www.ICGtesting.com
Printed in the USA
LVOW11s1458141215

466577LV00001B/300/P